SEM Micrograph of the
complex trabeculated
inner side of the apex
in rat right ventricle
from
Endocardial Endothelium:
Functional Morphology
by
Luc J. Andries
© RG Landes Co 1994, 1995

MEDICAL
INTELLIGENCE
UNIT

CYTOKINES AND THE HEART: MOLECULAR MECHANISMS OF SEPTIC CARDIOMYOPATHY

MEDICAL
INTELLIGENCE
UNIT

CYTOKINES AND THE HEART: MOLECULAR MECHANISMS OF SEPTIC CARDIOMYOPATHY

Ursula Müller-Werdan

University of Munich
Klinikum Grosshadern
Munich, Germany

Christopher Reithmann

University of Munich
Klinikum Grosshadern
Munich, Germany

Karl Werdan

University of Munich
Klinikum Grosshadern
Munich, Germany
University of Halle-Wittenberg
Klinikum Kröllwit
Halle, Germany

CHAPMAN & HALL
I(T)P An International Thomson Publishing Company

New York • Albany • Bonn • Boston • Cincinnati • Detroit • London • Madrid • Melbourne •
Mexico City • Pacific Grove • Paris • San Francisco • Singapore • Tokyo • Toronto • Washington

R.G. LANDES COMPANY
AUSTIN

MEDICAL INTELLIGENCE UNIT
CYTOKINES AND THE HEART:
MOLECULAR MECHANISMS OF SEPTIC CARDIOMYOPATHY
R.G. LANDES COMPANY
Austin, Texas, U.S.A.

U.S. and Canada Copyright © 1996 R.G. Landes Company and Chapman & Hall
International Copyright © 1996 Springer-Verlag, Heidelberg, Germany

Please address all inquiries to the Publishers:
R.G. Landes Company, 909 Pine Street, Georgetown, Texas, U.S.A. 78626
Phone: 512/ 863 7762; FAX: 512/ 863 0081

Chapman & Hall, 115 Fifth Avenue, New York, New York, U.S.A. 10003

Springer-Verlag GmbH & Co. KG, Tiergartenstrasse 17, D-69121 Heidelberg, Germany

U.S. and Canada ISBN: 0-412-10111-4
International ISBN: 3-540-60175-9

While the authors, editors and publisher believe that drug selection and dosage and the specifications and usage of equipment and devices, as set forth in this book, are in accord with current recommendations and practice at the time of publication, they make no warranty, expressed or implied, with respect to material described in this book. In view of the ongoing research, equipment development, changes in governmental regulations and the rapid accumulation of information relating to the biomedical sciences, the reader is urged to carefully review and evaluate the information provided herein.

Library of Congress Cataloging-in-Publication Data

Müller-Werdan. Ursula, 1961
    Cytokines and the heart: molecular mechanisms of septic cardiomyopathy /
Ursula Müller-Werdan, C. Reithmann, Karl Werdan.
        p. cm. — (Medical intelligence unit)
    Includes bibliographical references and index.
    ISBN 0-412-10111-4
    1. Myocardium—Diseases—Molecular aspects. 2. Cytokines — Pathophysiology.
    3. Septic shock—Molecular aspects. 4. Heart — Infections—Molecular aspects.
    I. Reithmann, C. (Christopher) II. Werdan, Karl. III. Title. IV. Series.
        [DNLM: 1. Myocardial Diseases—physiopathology. 2. Cytokines —physiology.
    3. Sepsis—physiopathology. 4. Shock, Septic — physiopathology. WG 280 M958c 1995]
RC685.M9M845 1995
616.1'2407—dc20
DNLM/DLC
for Library of Congress   95-32356
                                                              CIP

Publisher's Note

R.G. Landes Company publishes five book series: *Medical Intelligence Unit, Molecular Biology Intelligence Unit, Neuroscience Intelligence Unit, Tissue Engineering Intelligence Unit* and *Biotechnology Intelligence Unit.* The authors of our books are acknowledged leaders in their fields and the topics are unique. Almost without exception, no other similar books exist on these topics.

Our goal is to publish books in important and rapidly changing areas of medicine for sophisticated researchers and clinicians. To achieve this goal, we have accelerated our publishing program to conform to the fast pace in which information grows in biomedical science. Most of our books are published within 90 to 120 days of receipt of the manuscript. We would like to thank our readers for their continuing interest and welcome any comments or suggestions they may have for future books.

Deborah Muir Molsberry
Publications Director
R.G. Landes Company

CONTENTS

AUTHORS

Dr. Ursula Müller-Werdan
University of Munich, Department of Medicine
Klinikum Grosshadern
Munich, Germany

Dr. Christopher Reithmann
University of Munich, Department of Medicine
Klinikum Grosshadern
Munich, Germany

Prof. Dr. Karl Werdan
University of Munich, Department of Medicine
Klinikum Grosshadern
Munich, Germany
University of Halle-Wittenberg, Department of Medicine
Klinikum Kröllwit
Halle, Germany

CHAPTER-COAUTHORS

Dr. Hans-Jörg Berger
University of Munich
Department of Medicine
Klinikum Grosshadern
Munich, Germany
Chapter 3

Dr. Günter Pilz
University of Munich
Department of Medicine
Klinikum Grosshadern
Munich, Germany
Chapter 4

Chang He
University of Munich
Department of Medicine
Klinikum Grosshadern
Munich, Germany
Chapters 4, 7

Dr. Josef Stadler
Technical University of Munich
Department of Surgery
Munich, Germany
Chapter 4

Prof. Dr. Heinz Rupp
University of Marburg
Department of Medicine
Molecular Cardiology
Marburg, Germany
Chapters 4, 7

PREFACE

This book is about the molecular mechanisms underlying septic cardiomyopathy, a main feature of septic shock and multiple organ dysfunction syndrome, which are the leading causes of death in intensive care patients. Cytokines play a very prominent pathogenetic role in this myocardial depression, with septic cardiomyopathy being the cardiac disease entity, where knowledge about cytokine action on the heart has accumulated most.

After briefly introducing the clinical picture and discussing the clinical relevance of septic cardiomyopathy, an effort is taken to unravel separately the effects of toxins and mediators—especially cytokines—in sepsis and shock on the cardiomyocyte. Based on these data, negative inotropic cascades emerge, their significance for septic cardiomyopathy being under investigation. Several specific trigger mechanisms of negative inotropy are operative in septic forms of myocardial depression, which clearly differ—at least in part—from nonseptic heart failure. Elucidating these underlying molecular mechanisms may open up new prospects for a more causal treatment of septic cardiomyopathy in the future. It may also help us build up the just emerging basis of cytokine action on the heart in health and disease in a more general framework.

ACKNOWLEDGMENTS

The backbone of this book is based on our article "Negative Inotropic Cascades in Cardiomyocytes Triggered by Substances Relevant to Sepsis" written for the handbook "Pathophysiology of Shock, Sepsis and Organ Failure", edited in 1993 by G. Schlag, M.D. and H. Redl, Ph.D. We are grateful to the editors as well as to Springer-Verlag, Berlin Heidelberg, for the permission to reproduce figures and part of a revised text of this chapter.

Three of our chapters wer-e written in collaboration with several of our colleagues; we want to express our gratitude to Dr. Hans-Jörg Berger (University of Munich) for helping us write Chapter 3; we thank Drs. Günter Pilz (University of Munich) and Josef Stadler (Technical University of Munich) for helping us with Chapter 4; and we are indebted to Chang He (University of Munich) and Dr. Heinz Rupp (University of Marburg) for their valuable contributions to Chapters 4 and 7.

Susanne Helbig, Petra Ebner, Elisabeth Ronft and Martin Rupff are thanked for their help in preparing the manuscript and drawing the figures.

Our own work presented has been supported by Deutsche Forschungsgemeinschaft (Mu 1010/1-4; Re 714-2/1).

===================== CHAPTER 1 =====================

INTRODUCTION

Despite all the new generations of antibiotics, mortality of sepsis and septic shock could not be substantially lowered during the last decades; it remains as high as 40% (Fig. 1.1), accounting for about 100,000 deaths annually in the United States. This high mortality is of small wonder keeping in mind that the bacterial infection of an organ is only the starting point of a cascade and network (Fig. 1.2), which are primed by the invasion of bacterial toxins into the circulation, followed by an activation of mediator cells (e.g. granulocytes, macrophages) with a consecutive release of mediators, especially cytokines. The final consequence is a multiple organ dysfunction syndrome (MODS), often with fatal outcome.

"Septic acute myocarditis" was defined as a clinical entity already 75 years ago.[1] Nowadays, this impairment of the heart within the scope of MODS is often underscored, because myocardial function in sepsis and septic shock conspicuously is not too bad in comparison to that of healthy individuals. However, the degree of septic cardiomyopathy becomes best evident when cardiac output is considered in relation to the systemic vascular resistance (Fig. 1.3), which is severely lowered due to the sepsis-induced vessel damage and consecutive vasodilatation; a healthy heart could compensate for the pathological fall in afterload by an increase in cardiac output up to 20 l/min, while the observed cardiac outputs in our septic patients are considerably lower, due to the damage of the heart by excess of catecholamines, bacterial toxins, mediators and cardiodepressant factors. Therefore, both clinical as well as experimental findings strongly support the concept of a severely impaired heart function within the scope of septic MODS.[2] When this cardiac dysfunction develops, prognosis is bad.[3] Symptomatic support of myocardial depression is at best of only little benefit,[4] attracting attention to more causal treatment regimens based on the underlying mechanisms of septic cardiomyopathy.

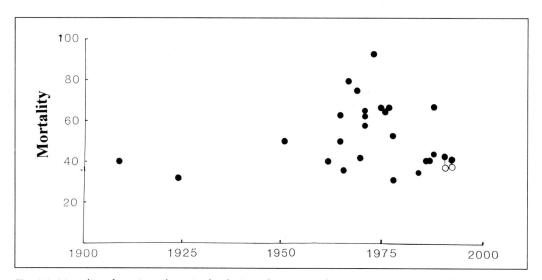

Fig. 1.1. Mortality of sepsis and septic shock. Data from more than 3000 patients are collected from the literature, with every point (●) representing information from a large sepsis study of the according year. In case of double points (●-○), the results of placebo-controlled sepsis treatment trials (○ verum group; ● placebo group) are given.

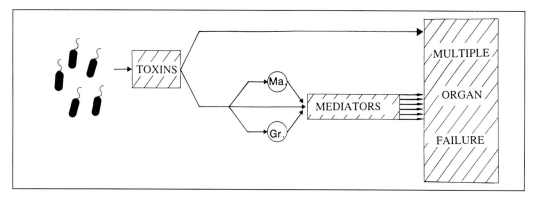

Fig. 1.2. Development of multiple organ dysfunction syndrome in sepsis.

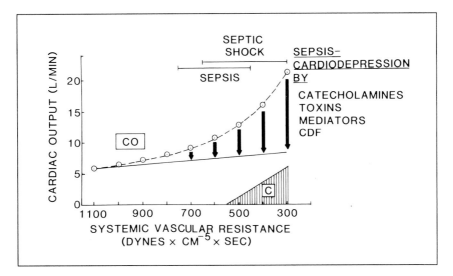

Fig. 1.3. Myocardial depression in sepsis. To compensate for a progressive vasodilatation (decrease in systemic vascular resistance), the calculated rise in cardiac output (- - - - -) should be necessary to maintain a mean arterial pressure of 90 mm Hg (according to: [mean arterial pressure − mean right atrial pressure (10 mm Hg)] = systemic vascular resistance (dynes x s x cm⁻⁵; normal value 1100 ± 200) x cardiac output (l/min) : 80). The cardiac outputs measured in sepsis and septic shock (———), however, are normally lower than the calculated values, probably due to the cardiodepressant effects of catecholamines, bacterial toxins, sepsis mediators and cardiodepressant factor CDF. "CO" = cardiac output; "C" = catecholamines necessary to stabilize blood pressure.

REFERENCES

1. Romberg E. Die septische akute Myokarditis. In: Romberg E, ed. Lehrbuch der Krankheiten des Herzens und der Blutgefässe. 3rd ed. Stuttgart: Ferdinand Enke, 1921:494.

2. Parrillo JE. Pathogenetic mechanisms of septic shock. N Engl J Med 1993; 328:1471-1477.

3. Goldfarb RD, Tambolini W, Wiener SM et al. Canine left ventricular performance during LD_{50} endotoxemia. Am J Physiol 1983; 244:H370-H377.

4. Hayes MA, Timmins AC, Yau EHS et al. Elevation of systemic oxygen delivery in the treatment of critically ill patients. N Engl J Med 1994; 330:1717-1722.

CHAPTER 2

SEPTIC CARDIOMYOPATHY

A SECONDARY FORM OF CARDIOMYOPATHY

The classification of secondary cardiomyopathies is based on "myocardial damage within the scope of a systemic disease". In view of this definition, myocardial impairment in sepsis, septic shock and septic multiple organ dysfunction syndrome (MODS) might be reckoned as "septic cardiomyopathy", a term proposed by H.P. Schuster in our workshop "Sepsis: Toxinwirkung, Herzschädigung, Quantifizierung, supportive Therapie mit Immunglobulinen" held at Rottach-Egern (01.06. – 03.06.1989);[1] various infectious disease entities and myocardial virulence factors may trigger common mediator pathways. Thereby, a complex pattern of myocardial depression with different grades of severity may result, characterized, on the one hand, by common principles, e.g., catecholamine desensitization and the effects of TNF-α, (see chapter 4), and, on the other hand, by toxin-specific and therefore infectious agent-specific pathways, e.g., inhibition of protein synthesis by Pseudomonas exotoxin A, (see chapter 4).

THE CHARACTERISTIC PATTERN

The case report of Figure 2.1 illustrates the typical cardiovascular changes seen in Gram-negative, but also in Gram-positive septic shock. Characteristically, a fall in blood pressure due to an extensive vasodilatation comes about with lowering of the systemic vascular resistance (SVR) down to 30% of the normal value. To a certain degree, blood pressure can be kept within physiological ranges by an increase in cardiac output. However, a full compensation as seen in Figures 2.1 and 2.2, with a 2- to 3-fold rise in cardiac output, is only rarely encountered in patients with septic shock. The only inadequate rise is explained by the reversible, multifactorial myocardial depression in sepsis (Fig. 1.3 in chapter 1). It is the merit of Parrillo and his group to have contributed a major part to featuring the clinical findings of cardiac dysfunction in sepsis[2-7] (Table 2.1), characterized by a dilatation of both ventricles, reduced ejection fractions, and global as well as regional, and systolic pump as well as diastolic relaxation failure. A surprising finding moreover is an increase in ventricular compliance

Table 2.1. The clinical picture of septic cardiomyopathy

Inadequate rise in cardiac index, taking the lowered systemic vascular resistance
    into account
No increase in stroke volume (LV, RV)
Ejection fraction (LV, RV) decreased
Regional and global cardiac dysfunction
Considerable dilation of the heart
Increase in ventricular compliance
Contraction and relaxation abnormalities
Coronary arteries dilated, high coronary sinus blood flow

Right ventricular failure due to ARDS–induced pulmonary hypertension

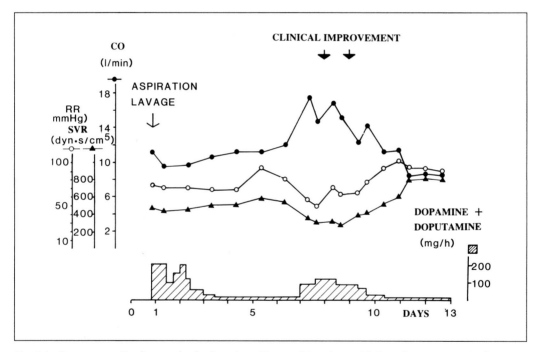

Fig. 2.1. Case report: Cardiovascular findings in a 47-year-old patient with Pseudomonas sepsis due to an aspiration pneumonia which had occurred on October 19. After initial improvement, the clinical course worsens until October 26, with the development of shock requiring catecholamine support. Beginning with October 27, sustained clinical improvement of the patient is evidenced. Adapted from Werdan K. Therapie der akuten septischen Kardiomyopathie. In: Schuster H-P, ed. Intensivtherapie bei Sepsis und Multiorganversagen. Berlin, Heidelberg: Springer-Verlag, 1993:164-197.

Fig. 2.2. Opposite page: Cardiac function of two patients with septic shock—Influence of pathologic afterload reduction. In both patients, parameters of heart function have been monitored over a period of 20 days (patient no. 1, ○) and 8 days (patient no. 2, [ ]), respectively, during the recovery phase from septic shock. Data are given in relation to the respective systemic vascular resistance. For comparison, values of healthy individuals with a normal vascular resistance of 1100 dynes x s x cm^{-5} are given (◆). (Adapted from Werdan K. Therapie der akuten septischen Kardiomyopathie. In: Schuster H-P, ed. Intensivtherapie bei Sepsis und Multiorganversagen. Berlin, Heidelberg: Springer-Verlag, 1993:164-197.)

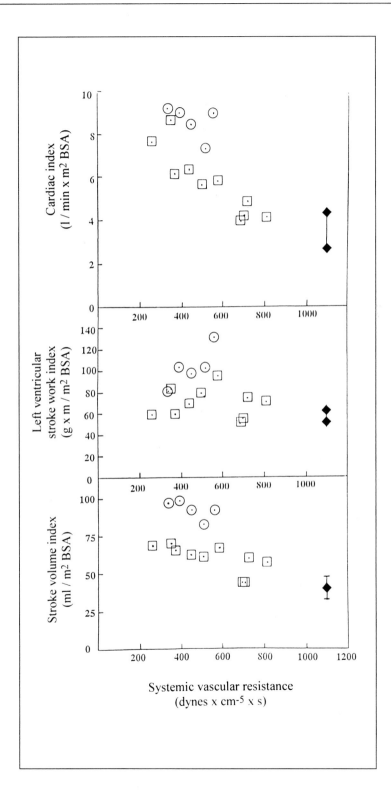

which is responsible for the pathological expansion in heart size after volume substitution; finally, coronary arteries are dilated and coronary blood flow is high.

The impressive impact of the pathologically reduced afterload due to vascular impairment in sepsis on heart function is documented in Figure 2.2, exhibiting the changes in cardiac output, left ventricular stroke work index and stroke volume index of two patients recovering from septic shock. In both patients, myocardial function was at most slightly depressed, as can be seen from the high values at low SVR, which were even considerably higher than the reference values of healthy individuals with their normal SVRs of about 1100 dynes x s x cm[-5]. Therefore, in estimating myocardial depression in sepsis, only values from healthy individuals with a dramatically lowered SVR could serve as reference values, but not those obtained with a SVR of 1100. As these results are not available, data from septic patients as described in Figure 2.2 may yield approximative reference values. On the basis of these considerations septic cardiomyopathy is evidenced not only in the late phase of hypodynamic, but also in the hyperdynamic phase of septic shock (Fig. 1.3 in chapter 1) and even in septic patients with normal blood pressure.[8]

OCCURRENCE IN GRAM-NEGATIVE AND GRAM-POSITIVE SEPSIS

There has been some suggestion from clinical studies that hemodynamic impairment in sepsis may vary depending on the type of organism invading.[9,10] In experimental work, this possibility has been substantiated, particularly in the case of Pseudomonas infections; in a canine model of septic shock[11] *Pseudomonas aeruginosa* produced more cardiovascular dysfunction than another Gram-negative organism (*E. coli*).

However, these and other experimental findings of an infectious agent-specific severity of cardiac depression could not be confirmed in 128 patients with similar disease and sepsis profiles.[12] Patients with various forms of Gram-negative (Pseudomonas, *E. coli*, other Gram-negative), of Gram-positive and of fungal sepsis suffered from similar degrees of septic cardiomyopathy, as measured by a reduction in left ventricular stroke work index (Fig. 2.3). Neither were infectious agent-specific differences discerned for some sepsis-subgroups, e.g., septic patients with or without culture-proven bacteremia, with or without septic shock and also with and without pre-existing cardiovascular disease.[12] Interpreting these results one may hypothesize that not the specific virulence factors, but rather the mediators of the common final pathway determine the occurrence and severity of septic cardiomyopathy.

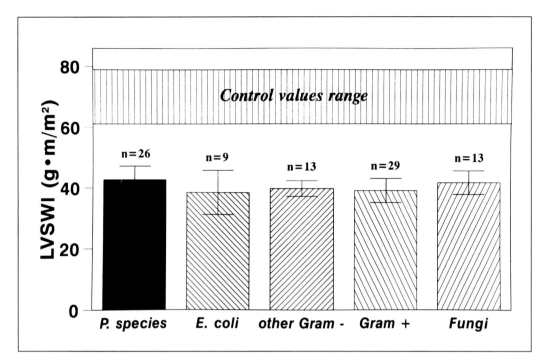

Fig. 2.3. Decreased left ventricular stroke work indices in various forms of Gram-negative, Gram-positive and fungal sepsis. (Adapted from Pilz G, McGinn P, Boekstegers P et al. Pseudomonas sepsis does not cause more severe cardiovascular dysfunction in patients than non-Pseudomonas sepsis. Circ Shock 1994; 42:174-182.)

REFERENCES

1. Werdan K, Müller U, Reithmann C et al. Mechanisms in acute septic cardiomyopathy: evidence from isolated myocytes. Basic Res Cardiol 1991; 86:411-421.
2. Kumar A, Parrillo JE. Clinical manifestations of cardiovascular dysfunction in sepsis. In: Schlag G, Redl H, eds. Pathophysiology of Shock, Sepsis, and Organ Failure. Berlin, Heidelberg: Springer-Verlag, 1993:859-881.
3. Parrillo JE. Pathogenetic mechanisms of septic shock. N Engl J Med 1993; 328:1471-1477.
4. Conrad SA, Finkelstein JL, Madden MR et al. Cardiovascular dysfunction in multiple organ failure. In: Deitch EA, ed. Multiple Organ Failure—Pathophysiology and Basic Concepts of Therapy. New York: Thieme, 1990:172-191.
5. Vincent JL, Berlot G. Cardiac effects of the mediators of sepsis. In: Lamy M, Thijs LG, eds. Mediators of Sepsis (Update in Intensive Care and Emergency Medicine 16). Berlin, Heidelberg, New York: Springer-Verlag, 1992:255-266.

6. Dhainaut J-F, Dall'Ava J, Mira JP. Coronary hemodynamics and myocardial metabolism in sepsis and septic shock. In: Schlag G, Redl H, eds. Pathophysiology of Shock, Sepsis, and Organ Failure. Berlin, Heidelberg: Springer-Verlag, 1993: 882-892.

7. Ellrodt AG, Riedinger MS, Kimchi A et al. Left ventricular performance in septic shock: Reversible segmental and global abnormalities. Amer Heart J 1985; 110:402-409.

8. Raper R, Sibbald WJ, Driedger AA et al. Relative myocardial depression in normotensive sepsis. J Crit Care 1989; 4:9-18.

9. Kwaan HM, Weil MH. Differences in the mechanism of shock caused by bacterial infections. Surg Gynec Obstet 1969; 128:37-45.

10. Blain CM, Anderson TO, Pietras RJ et al. Immediate hemodynamic effects of Gram-negative versus Gram-positive bacteremia in man. Arch Intern Med 1970; 126:260-265.

11. Danner RL, Natanson C, Elin RJ et al. *Pseudomonas aeruginosa* compared with *Escherichia coli* produces less endotoxemia but more cardiovascular dysfunction and mortality in a canine model of septic shock. Chest 1990; 98:1480-1487.

12. Pilz G, McGinn P, Boekstegers P et al. Pseudomonas sepsis does not cause more severe cardiovascular dysfunction in patients than non-Pseudomonas sepsis. Circ Shock 1994; 42:174-182.

13. Werdan K. Therapie der akuten septischen Kardiomyopathie. In: Schuster H-P, ed. Intensivtherapie bei Sepsis und Multiorganversagen. Berlin, Heidelberg: Springer-Verlag, 1993:164-197.

CHAPTER 3

RESEARCHING MECHANISMS OF SEPTIC CARDIOMYOPATHY: EXPERIMENTAL MODELS, WITH SPECIAL EMPHASIS ON CARDIOMYOCYTES

THE PROBLEM

Clinical observations, animal models and work with isolated heart preparations have undoubtedly revealed the existence of myocardial depression in sepsis and make up a valuable mosaic of phenomenological information about this topic.[1] However, this kind of collecting data about septic cardiomyopathy nevertheless has its limitations, especially when looking for the underlying molecular mechanisms; In animal experiments as well as in studies with isolated heart preparations, direct effects of bacterial toxins and sepsis mediators on heart function interfere with indirect ones and are often difficult to discern; primary effects on the coronary circulation and stimulation of local mediator cells often superimpose direct negative inotropic and cytotoxic effects of toxins and mediators in the heart. Although the methodological limitations are conspicuous, experiments with isolated heart muscle cells may circumvent many of these problems and represent a suitable model to study direct cardiodepressive effects of these substances.[2]

ADULT AND NEONATAL CARDIOMYOCYTES

Isolated cardiomyocytes (CMs) can be obtained from hearts of either adult or neonatal/embryonic species including man (Figs. 3.1- 3.3).[3,4] The basic principle of most preparation methods in use is the exposure of heart tissue to a dissociating medium low in Ca^{2+} and

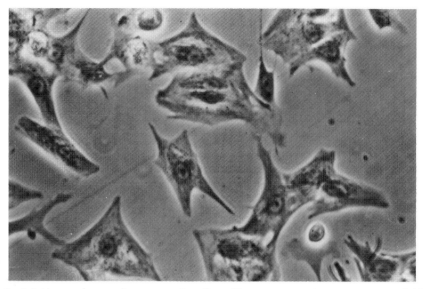

Fig. 3.1. Neonatal rat cardiomyocytes in culture. Phase contrast microscopy, 2 x 300-fold magnification.

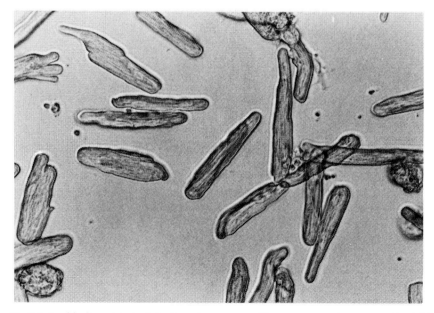

Fig. 3.2. Freshly dissociated adult rat cardiomyocytes. Phase contrast microscopy, 300-fold magnification.

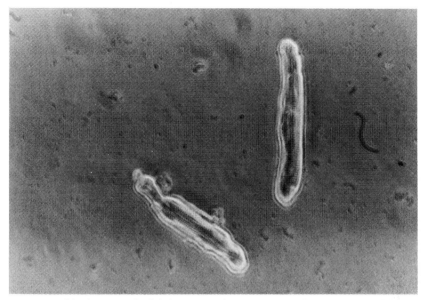

Fig. 3.3. Freshly dissociated adult human cardiomyocytes. Cells were obtained from an explanted heart of a cardiac allograft recipient with dilative cardiomyopathy. Phase contrast microscopy, 300-fold magnification.

supplemented with proteolytic enzymes. By this procedure, a low Ca^{2+} concentration is achieved in myocardial tissue (20-100 μM),[3] and Ca^{2+} dissociates from the Ca^{2+}-dependent desmosome structures in the intercalated discs. The proteolytic enzymes cleave the connections of the individual cells with the extracellular matrix network. For preparations of CMs of adult species, e.g., guinea pigs or rats, whole hearts are perfused in the Langendorff mode, or small pieces of myocardial tissue are immersed in the dissociating medium. For preparation of CMs of neonatal/embryonic species, e.g., 1- to 3-day-old rats or 12- to 13-day-old chicken embryos, the hearts are cut into small pieces and incubated in the dissociation medium. These procedures result in suspensions of isolated heart muscle cells, with several techniques available to produce relatively pure myocyte preparations. Adult CMs differ from neonatal ones by their rod-shaped morphology and their regular sarcomeric structure. They can be investigated upon as cell suspensions immediately after preparation or be cultured as monolayers for up to several weeks. Neonatal/embryonic CMs attach to the culture flask within hours and can be kept in culture as monolayers for several weeks. In contrast to the quiescent adult CMs, neonatal/embryonic CMs within several hours after attachment take up spontaneous, synchronous beating. Both cell types can be electrically driven, too.

Recently, a system has been developed that allows the continual electric field stimulation of adult CMs in culture for several days

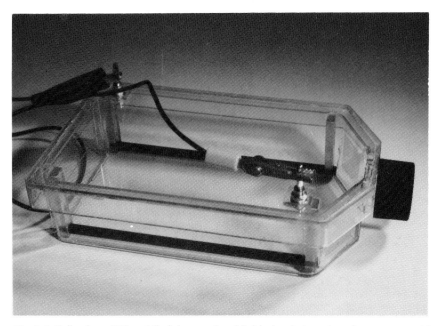

Fig. 3.4. Cell culture 175 cm²-flask for continual field stimulation of cardiomyocytes with parallel graphite electrodes.

(Fig. 3.4).[5] It has been demonstrated that the abrupt decline in contractile function typical for quiescent CMs can be attenuated by continual uniform electric field stimulation. Furthermore, it appears that regular gene expression is preserved in these continuously contracting cells.

The use of serum-free, well-defined culture medium often is of great advantage, especially when the long-term effects of hormones, toxins and cytokines are studied. Preparation and cultivation procedures have also been established for the different nonmuscle cell types of the heart, e.g., for endothelial cells, vascular smooth muscle cells, pericytes and fibroblasts.[3,4] To study the more complex interaction of different cell types (e.g. paracrine effects) coculture systems have been developed (Fig. 4.33 in chapter 4).

Limitations of isolated CMs in culture include the extensive phenotypic changes that occur during adaptation to primary culture, especially in adult CMs after approximately four to five days in culture. The velocity of phenotype changes depends on a variety of factors including type of culture medium (trophic factors, serum), cell densities, cell attachment factors (e.g. laminin, fibronectin) and rate of contraction. The underlying mechanisms are not well understood and are under intensive investigation.

Both for adult and neonatal/embryonic CMs methods are available for monitoring contractility and measuring chronotropic, "inotropic" and "lusitropic" (increase/decrease in pulsation amplitude/contraction and relaxation velocity) as well as bathmotropic effects of substances of interest (Fig. 3.5).[4,6] A number of processes have been very thoroughly characterized in these cells by well established methods, including gene expression[7] and protein synthesis,[8] metabolism, cell membrane transport, trans-sarcolemmal ion movement and cellular ion homeostasis,[5,9] as well as mechanisms and regulation of signal transduction by membrane receptors and intracellular second messengers (see chapter 4). For measurement of intracellular ion concentrations a variety of methods has been developed. In recent years ionic-sensitive dyes (e.g. fura-2, fluo-3 for Ca^{2+}, BCECF for pH) have been applied that emit light of different wavelengths and intensities depending on the cellular free ion concentration (Fig. 3.6).[6] By adding them to the culture medium, these dyes can be loaded into the cell. Figure 3.7 demonstrates the rapid changes of intracellular Ca^{2+} as the result of cell contraction. In situ calibration ascertains the intracellular ion concentration.

The choice of the suitable CM model depends on the question under investigation; in certain cases, like substrate utilization, the adult

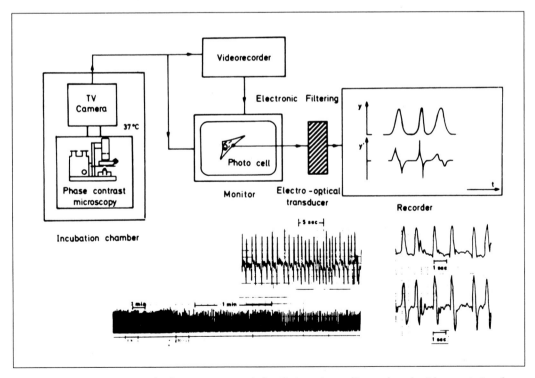

Fig. 3.5. Monitoring system for beating myocardial cells in culture. (Reproduced with permission from: Werdan K, Erdmann E. Preparation and culture of embryonic and neonatal heart muscle cells: modification of transport activity. Methods Enzymol 1989; 173:634-662.)

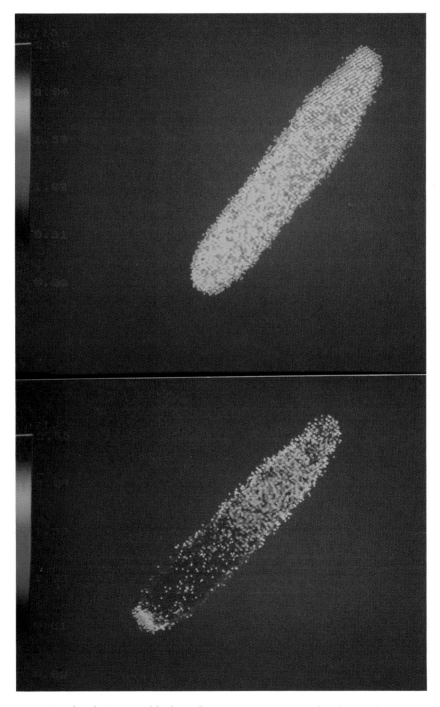

Fig. 3.6. Pseudocolor images of the fura-2 fluorescence ratio in an isolated rat cardiomyocyte. Increasing ratio emission intensities, coded in spectrum from blue, green, yellow (upper graph) to red (lower graph), were associated with increasing intracellular Ca^{2+} concentration.

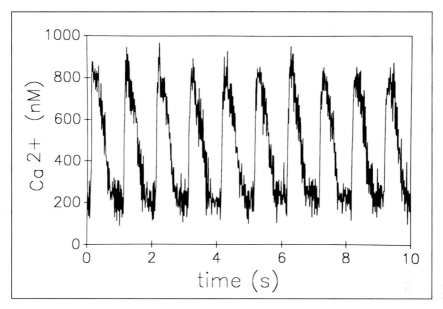

Fig. 3.7. Measurement of intracellular Ca^{2+} concentration by in situ calibration of the fura-2 fluorescence signal (ratio of the excitation wavelengths 340 and 380 nm) in an isolated cardiomyocyte from an adult guinea pig. The cardiomyocyte was electrically stimulated with 1 Hz.

CM offers the advantage of a better comparability with results obtained in adult animal experiments. Neonatal/embryonic CMs in culture, on the other hand, are good candidates for studies requiring several days of cell incubation, for instance regulation of gene expression and protein synthesis-dependent phenomena.

THE PLACE OF ISOLATED CARDIOMYOCYTES IN RESEARCHING MECHANISMS OF MYOCARDIAL DEPRESSION IN SEPSIS

In view of the complexity of "acute septic cardiomyopathy", research activities must range from observations in humans and in animal sepsis models to isolated heart preparations and molecular biology. What is the role of the isolated cardiomyocyte in this arena of research? In the opinion of the authors, several facets are apparent:

DISCRIMINATION BETWEEN DIRECT AND INDIRECT CARDIODEPRESSANT EFFECTS OF BACTERIAL TOXINS AND SEPSIS MEDIATORS

The lack of a direct effect of a toxin on the CM can give a clue either to the mediator cascade as a missing link or focus attention to another cell type in the heart as primary target for the toxin.

LOOKING NOT ONLY FOR ACUTE, BUT ALSO FOR CHRONIC TOXIN- AND MEDIATOR-INDUCED CARDIODEPRESSION

Cardiodepressant effects based on protein synthesis-dependent processes (e.g. by Pseudomonas exotoxin A; see chapter 4) require several hours to days to become manifest. Cytokines (chapter 4) are especially thought to act predominantly in this manner. Heart muscle cells, cultured under serum-free conditions, are an ideal model to study these events.

CLARIFICATION OF THE MECHANISMS OF ACTION OF CARDIODEPRESSANT BACTERIAL TOXINS AND SEPSIS MEDIATORS

Heart cell cultures and isolated heart cells are structurally simple enough to allow measurement and quantification of cellular components (e.g. receptors) and of cell metabolism. On the other hand, complexity is high enough so that contractile function is preserved and can be measured in a semiquantitative manner. These combined properties are a good basis for clarifying the mechanism of action of a cardiodepressant substance. The described blockage of transsarcolemmal Ca^{2+}-flux by the cardiodepressant factor CDF (chapter 4) is a typical example of that kind of research, carried out with minute amounts of the substance under investigation.

ESTABLISHING IN VITRO MODELS OF CELL-MEDIATED CARDIODEPRESSION IN SEPSIS

The finding that contractile function of cultured heart cells is compromised by activated leukocytes (chapter 4) gives the incentive for in vitro models to study leukocyte-mediated cardiodepression in sepsis. These studies will enlarge our knowledge in two respects: first, the mechanisms of action by which leukocytes can damage heart cells can be clarified; and second, the potency of a variety of bacterial toxins, not only from Gram-negative but also from Gram-positive bacteria, can be tested with respect to their possible indirect cardiodepressant effects via leukocyte activation.

REFERENCES

1. Schlag G, Redl H, eds. Pathophysiology of Shock, Sepsis, and Organ Failure. Berlin, Heidelberg: Springer-Verlag, 1993:
   Taylor FB Jr, Kosanke SD. Three clinical presentations of *E. coli* sepsis studied in the baboon model, 676-688.
   Abel FL. Myocardial dysfunction in experimental shock, 772-786.
   Krösl PE, Pretorius JP. Myocardial dysfunction in septic shock, 835-852.
   Bahrami S, Redl H, Schlag G. Models of endotoxemia in rodents, 1019-1030.
   Traber DL, Traber LD, Redl H et al. Models of endotoxemia in sheep, 1031-1047.

Chaudry IH, Ayala A, Singh G et al. Rodent models of endotoxemia and sepsis, 1048-1059.

Dehring DJ. Sheep and pigs as animal models of bacteremia, 1060-1075.

Schlag G, Redl H, Davies J et al. Live *Escherichia coli* sepsis models in baboons, 1076-1107.

Spitzer JA. Animal models of endotoxemia and sepsis, 1108-1118.

Martin CM, Neal A, Sibbald WJ. Models of sepsis: subacute peritonitis in sheep and rats, 1119-1131.

Dixon AC, Parrillo JE. Chronic models of endotoxemia and sepsis: lessons from both a canine peritonitis and a human endotoxemia model, 1132-1142.

2. Werdan K, Müller U, Reithmann C. "Negative inotropic cascades" in cardiomyocytes triggered by substances relevant to sepsis. In: Schlag G, Redl H, eds. Pathophysiology of Shock, Sepsis, and Organ Failure. Berlin, Heidelberg: Springer-Verlag, 1993:787-834.

3. Piper HM, ed. Cell Culture Techniques in Heart and Vessel Research. Berlin, Heidelberg, New York: Springer-Verlag, 1990.

4. Werdan K, Erdmann E. Preparation and culture of embryonic and neonatal heart muscle cells: modification of transport activity. Methods Enzymol 1989; 173:634-662.

5. Berger H-J, Prasad SK, Davidoff AJ et al. Continual electric field stimulation preserves contractile function of adult ventricular myocytes in primary culture. Am J Physiol 1994; 266:H341-H349.

6. Berger H-J, Taratuska A, Smith TW et al. Activated complement directly modifies the performance of isolated heart muscle cells from guinea pig and rat. Am J Physiol 1993; 265:H267- H272.

7. Springhorn JP, Ellingsen O, Berger H-J et al. Transcriptional regulation in cardiac muscle. Coordinate expression of Id with a neonatal phenotype during development and following a hypertrophic stimulus in adult rat ventricular myocytes in vitro. J Biol Chem 1992; 267:14360-14365.

8. Reithmann C, Gierschik P, Müller U et al. Pseudomonas exotoxin A prevents β-adrenoceptor-induced upregulation of G_i protein α-subunits and adenylyl cyclase desensitization in rat heart muscle cells. Mol Pharmacol 1990; 37:631-638.

9. Hallström S, Koidl B, Müller U et al. A cardiodepressant factor isolated from blood blocks Ca^{2+} current in cardiomyocytes. Am J Physiol 1991; 260:H869-H876.

============== CHAPTER 4 ==============

RELEVANT SUBSTANCES AND CONDITIONS TRIGGERING "NEGATIVE INOTROPIC CASCADES" IN CARDIOMYOCYTES

The main emphasis of this chapter will be on the description of alterations of cardiomyocyte (CM) function by substances and pathophysiological conditions relevant to sepsis; Based on clinical data and animal experiments, some "rationale" of a conceivable alteration of myocardial function in sepsis will be proposed for each substance. Available data concerning its effects on CMs are discussed. In "conclusions", the authors then try to evaluate whether the presently available data obtained with isolated heart cells may add some information concerning the relevance of the respective substance in acute septic cardiomyopathy. With these data in mind, a scenario of "negative inotropic cascades" in CMs is composed (cf. chapter 8), speculating about the most likely candidates responsible for contractile dysfunction of the heart cell in sepsis.

To avoid repetitions, original data presented in chapters 8 to 10 are omitted in chapter 4; therefore the reader is asked to complement the information of chapter 4 with that of chapters 8 to 10.

CATECHOLAMINES

RATIONALE

In sepsis and endotoxemia, plasma catecholamine levels are increased up to 100-fold,[1-4] while the adrenergic responsiveness of the heart seems to be markedly depressed.[3,6-8] These results give rise to the concept of a catecholamine-induced desensitization of the β-adrenergic inotropic pathway,[9] as it is well established for nonseptic heart failure.[10] Several experimental findings support this concept: (a) endotoxin treatment of rats induces a decrease in β-adrenoceptor agonist-stimulated adenylyl cyclase activity without any change in the number of β-adrenoceptors, suggesting a functional uncoupling of the β-adrenoceptors from the stimulatory G_s protein,[11] (b) In *E. coli*-infected rats, the distribution of myocardial β-adrenoceptors between sarcolemma and cytosol is shifted to the cytosolic pool, consistent with a bacteremia-provoked internalization of β-adrenoceptors,[12] (c) CMs prepared from endotoxin-treated rats show a decrease (down-regulation) of β-adrenoceptors by 25% compared to myocytes from the respective controls,[3] (d) Incubation of neonatal rat CMs in vitro with plasma of patients in septic shock induces a decrease in adrenaline-mediated cAMP-formation, in comparison to CMs treated with control plasma.[13]

THE RECEPTOR/G PROTEIN/ADENYLYL CYCLASE SYSTEM OF CARDIOMYOCYTES

The adenylyl cyclase system is composed of stimulatory and inhibitory receptors, the stimulatory and inhibitory G proteins (G_s and G_i) and the catalytic subunit of adenylyl cyclase (Fig. 4.1 "control").[10]

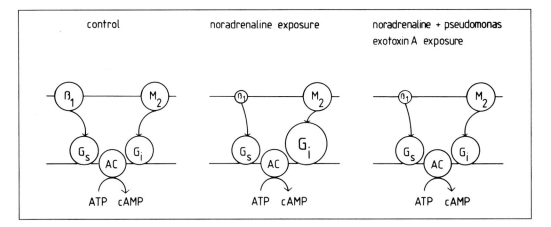

Fig. 4.1. Noradrenaline-induced desensitization of the β-adrenoceptor/G protein/adenylyl cyclase axis in cardiomyocytes—influence of P. exotoxin A. The scheme describes the reduction in the number of $β_1$-adrenoceptors("$β_1$") and the increase in the number of inhibitory G proteins("G_i"), induced by 48-hour-incubation of neonatal rat CMs in the presence of 10^{-6}M noradrenaline ("noradrenaline exposure"). P. exotoxin A (1 ng/ml), when present during this incubation period, suppresses the increase in the number of G_i, without affecting the reduction in the number of $β_1$-adrenoceptors ("noradrenaline + pseudomonas exotoxin A exposure"). "G_s": stimulatory G protein; "AC": adenylyl cyclase; "M_2": M_2-muscarinic receptor. (Reproduced with permission from: Werdan K, Müller U, Reithmann C. "Negative inotropic cascades" in cardiomyocytes triggered by substances relevant to sepsis. In: Schlag G, Redl H, eds. Pathophysiology of Shock, Sepsis, and Organ Failure. Berlin, Heidelberg: Springer-Verlag, 1993: 787-832.)

Table 4.1. Components of the receptor/G protein/adenylyl cyclase system in cardiomyocytes

Receptors	Cell type	Method	K_D	B_{max}	Functional response	Ref.
β-Adrenoceptor	Embryonic chick cardiomyocytes	[125I]-labled HYP	150 pM	23 fmol/mg protein	cAMP formation	18
β-Adrenoceptor	Embryonic chick cardiomyocytes	[125I]-labled CYP	243pM	62 fmol/mg protein	cAMP formation	19
β₁-Adrenoceptor	Embryonic chick cardiomyocytes	[³H]CGP12177	410pM	41 fmol/mg protein	Positive "inotropy" EC_{50}(Iso):6nM	339
β₁-Adrenoceptor	Embryonic chick cardiomyocytes	[³H]CGP12177	580pM	44 fmol/mg protein; 5000 sites/cell	Positive "inotropy" EC_{50}(Iso):20nM	340
β₂-Adrenoceptor	Embryonic chick cardiac nonmuscle cells	[³H]CGP12177	740pM	24 fmol/mg protein 3000 sites/cell	–	340
β-Adrenoceptor	Neonatal rat cardiomyocytes	[³H]CGP12177	300pM	103 fmol/mg protein	cAMP formation	341
β-Adrenoceptor	Neonatal rat cardiomyocytes	[125I]-labeled CYP	167pM	84 fmol/mg protein	cAMP formation	20
β₁-Adrenoceptor	Neonatal rat cardiomyocytes	[³H]CGP12177	430pM	60 fmol/mg protein 24000 sites/cell	Positive "inotropy" EC_{50}(Iso):60nM	337
β₂-Adrenoceptor	Neonatal rat cardiac nonmuscle cells	[³H]CGP12177	280pM	24 fmol/mg protein 10000 sites/cell	cAMP formation	337
β₁-Adrenoceptor β₂-Adrenoceptor	Neonatal rat cardiomyocytes	–			Positive chronotropy EC_{50}(Iso):670nM	342
β₁-Adrenoceptor	Neonatal rat cardiomyocytes	[125I]-labled CYP	24pM	12000 sites/cell	cAMP formation	343

Table 4.1. Components of the receptor/G protein/adenylyl cyclase system in cardiomyocytes (continued)

Receptors	Cell type	Method	K_D	B_{max}	Functional response	Ref.
β_1-Adrenoceptor	Neonatal rat cardiomyocytes	^{125}I-labled HYP	88pM	7600 sites/cell	cAMP formation	344
β_2-Adrenoceptor	Neonatal rat cardiac fibroblasts	^{125}I-labled HYP	71pM	9000 sites/cell	cAMP formation	344
β-Adrenoceptor	Adult rat cardiomyocytes	^{125}I-labled CYP	4nM	228 fmol/mg protein	Positive chronotropy EC_{50}(Iso):0.4nM	345
β_1-Adrenoceptor β_2-Adrenoceptor	Adult rat cardiomyocytes				cAMP formation	346
β_1-Adrenoceptor	Adult rat and guinea pig cardiomyocytes	^{125}I-labled CYP	15–30pM			347
β_2-Adrenoceptor	Adult guinea pig coronary endothelial cells	^{125}I-labled CYP				347
β_1-Adrenoceptor	Adult rat cardiomyocytes	[^{3}H]CGP12177	0.3nM	68 fmol/mg protein 20000 sites/cell		348
β-Adrenoceptor	Adult rat cardiomyocytes; subendocardial subepicardial arterioles	[^{3}H]DHA Autoradiography	1.57nM 1.71nM 0.26nM	(grains/0.9 $\times 10^{-2}$mm^2) 911 936 986		349
β_1-Adrenoceptor	Adult rat cardiomyocytes	[^{3}H]CGP12177	1.4nM	26fmol/mg protein	cAMP formation	21
Prostaglandin E_1 receptor	Embryonic chick cardiomyocytes				Positive "inotropy"	14
Prostaglandin E_1 receptor	Adult rabbit cardiomyocytes				cAMP formation	350
Muscarinic M_2 receptor	Embryonic chick cardiomyocytes	[^{3}H]QNB	0.1nM	150 fmol/mg protein	Adenylyl cyclase inhibition	351

Table 4.1. Components of the receptor/G protein/adenylyl cyclase system in cardiomyocytes (continued)

Receptors	Cell type	Method	K_D	B_{max}	Functional response	Ref.
Adenosine A_1 receptor	Embryonic chick cardiomyocytes	[³H]CPX	2.1nM	26 fmol/mg protein	Negative "inotropy" EC_{50} (R-PIA): 310nM	352
G protein subunits						
$G_{s\alpha45}$, $G_{s\alpha52}$	Neonatal rat cardiomyocytes	Cholera toxin-catalyzed ADP-ribosylation			—	68
$G_{s\alpha45}$, $G_{s\alpha52}$	Neonatal rat cardiomyocytes	Immunoblotting			—	353
$G_{i\alpha40}$, ($G_{i\alpha2}$)	Neonatal rat cardiomyocytes	Pertussis toxin-catalyzed ADP-ribosylation Immunoblotting			—	110
$G_{i\alpha40}$, ($G_{i\alpha2}$)	Neonatal rat cardiomyocytes	Immunoblotting			—	354
$G_{i\alpha41}$, ($G_{i\alpha3}$)	Neonatal rat cardiomyocytes	Pertussis toxin-catalyzed ADP-ribosylation Immunoblotting			—	110
$G_{i\alpha41}$, ($G_{i\alpha1,3}$)	Neonatal rat cardiomyocytes	Immunoblotting			—	353
$G_{o\alpha39}$	Neonatal rat cardiac fibroblasts	Immunoblotting			—	354
$G_{\alpha39}$ ($G_{i\alpha39}$?)	Embryonic chick cardiomyocytes	Pertussis toxin-catalyzed ADP-ribosylation			—	351
$G_{\alpha39}$ ($G_{o\alpha39}$?)	Embryonic chick cardiomyocytes	Pertussis toxin-catalyzed ADP-ribosylation			—	355
$G_{i\alpha41}$ ($G_{i\alpha3}$?)	Embryonic chick cardiomyocytes	Pertussis toxin-catalyzed ADP-ribosylation			—	351 355
$G_{\beta36}$ ($G_{\beta1}$)	Adult guinea pig coronary endothelial cells	Immunoblotting			—	68

Available data in heart cells are shown in Table 4.1; CMs possess about 5000-20,000 β-adrenoceptors predominantly of the β_1-subtype, while heart nonmuscle cells are characterized by β_2-adrenoceptors. Binding of a β-adrenergic agonist, like isoprenaline, to this receptor results in cellular cAMP production (Table 4.1) and in a positive "inotropic"

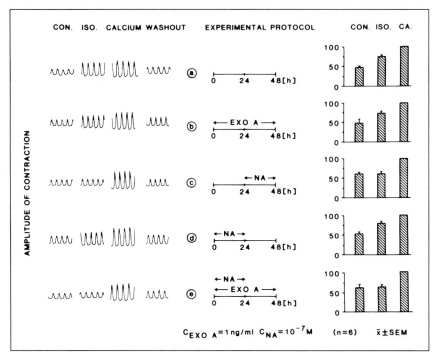

Fig. 4.2. *Catecholamine response of beating neonatal rat cardiomyocytes—influence of pre-exposure of the cells to noradrenaline and/or P. exotoxin A. After cultivation for 48 hours under the conditions given below (a-e), electrically driven (102/min) CMs have been successively incubated for periods of 3 minutes each, in saline ("CON"), 10^{-5}M isoprenaline ("ISO") and high Ca^{2+} ("CALCIUM", 2.4mM). Amplitude of contraction has been monitored with an electrooptical system[115] during these incubation periods and the following washout period ("WASHOUT", about 5 minutes). On the left, original registrations are given; on the right, mean values of these amplitude measurements are plotted. Data are given as % of maximal amplitude, measured in the presence of 2.4 mM Ca^{2+} instead of 0.3 mM. Experiments have been carried out after a culture period of 48 hours in serum-free medium:[115]*

(a) control: serum-free medium (0-48 h); (b) serum-free medium supplemented with P. exotoxin A (1 ng/ml; 0-48 h); (c) serum-free medium supplemented with noradrenaline (10^{-7}M; 24-48 h); (d) serum-free medium supplemented with noradrenaline (10^{-7}M; 0-24 h); (e) serum-free medium supplemented with noradrenaline (10^{-7}M; 0-24 h) and P. exotoxin A (1 ng/ml; 0-48 h). Before measurement of contractility, noradrenaline and/or P. exotoxin A have been removed from the surface of the cells by several washings. (Reproduced with permission from: Werdan K, Müller U, Reithmann C. "Negative inotropic cascades" in cardiomyocytes triggered by substances relevant to sepsis. In: Schlag G, Redl H, eds. Pathophysiology of Shock, Sepsis, and Organ Failure. Berlin, Heidelberg: Springer-Verlag, 1993: 787-832.)

effect (Fig. 4.2a). Concerning adenylyl cyclase-mediated positive inotropy, stimulation of the β_1-adrenoceptors plays the very prominent role; with histamine as another receptor-coupled agonist, only small effects in embryonic chicken CMs[14] and even less in neonatal rat CMs can be achieved.

In neonatal rat CMs, the α-adrenergic agonist phenylephrine exerts a frequency-dependent positive "inotropic effect", mediated by adenylyl cyclase independent α_1-adrenoceptors (about 8000/cell), while α_2-adrenoceptors with inhibitory action on adenylyl cyclase are absent in these cells.[15]

CATECHOLAMINE-INDUCED DESENSITIZATION OF CARDIOMYOCYTE ADENYLYL CYCLASE IN VITRO

Isolated CMs have been used to study the mechanism and time course of catecholamine-induced desensitization of adenylyl cyclase stimulation (Table 4.2). Incubation of chicken CMs with 1 μM isoproterenol for 30 minutes leads to a marked depression of the β-adrenoceptor agonist-induced increase in contraction velocity in these cells; concomitantly, the isoproterenol exposure (for 30 minutes) produces a loss of high-affinity state of the receptor, but no reduction in total receptor number.[16,17] More prolonged agonist exposure of chicken CMs leads to a concentration-dependent decrease in the number of β-adrenoceptors, associated with a desensitization of β-adrenoceptor-mediated adenylyl cyclase stimulation.[17,18] This down-regulation of β-adrenoceptors is apparently dependent on cyclic AMP formation and not on the occupation of β-adrenoceptors per se;[19] it is suppressed by colchicine, an inhibitor of microtubule function, and appears, therefore, to be modulated by microfilaments.[17]

Similar as shown for chicken CMs, a dissociation between the loss of adenylyl cyclase activity and β-adrenoceptor density after 30 minutes of β-adrenoceptor agonist exposure was also observed in neonatal rat CMs.[20] The authors suggested that during the early desensitization phase, alterations in agonist affinity for the β-adrenoceptor could be responsible for the β-adrenoceptor desensitization in mammalian CMs, whereas subsequent long-term desensitization is associated with both changes in agonist affinity and a redistribution of β-adrenoceptors from the plasma membrane into the cytosol. As shown in Figure 4.2c, long-term β-adrenoceptor agonist exposure (24 hours) leads to a marked reduction in β-adrenoceptor agonist-mediated increase in pulsation amplitude (suppression of the positive "inotropic" effect) of neonatal rat CMs, which is unaffected by the concomitant presence of the protein synthesis inhibitor Pseudomonas (P.) exotoxin A (see also Table 4.3).

Following short-term β-adrenoceptor agonist exposure (15-30 minutes), the high affinity state of the receptor as well as the functional response to isoproterenol stimulation recover rapidly (within 20-60 minutes).[17,21] On the other hand, receptor recovery after β-adrenoceptor

Table 4.2. Adenylyl cyclase sensitization in cardiomyocytes

Time	Cell type	Mechanism	Protein synthesis dependence	Recovery	Ref.
15 min	Adult rat cardiomyocytes	Internalization of β-adrenoceptors	No (cycloheximide)	Within 20 min	21
30 min	Embryonic chick cardiomyocytes	Loss of high affinity state of β-adrenoceptors	No (colchicine)[a]	Within 60 min	17
30 min	Neonatal rat cardiomyocytes	Loss of high affinity state of β-adrenoceptors	–	–	20
4 h	Neonatal rat cardiomyocytes	Internalization of β-adrenoceptors	–	–	20
4 h	Embryonic chick cardiomyocytes	Decrease in the number of β-adrenoceptors	Yes (colchicine)[a]	Within 72 h	17
16 h	Neonatal rat cardiomyocytes	Decrease in the number of β-adrenoceptors	–	Within 72 h	20
16 h	Embryonic chick cardiomyocytes	Decrease in the number of β-adrenoceptors	–	Within 24 h	18
3 days	Neonatal rat cardiomyocytes	Decrease in the number of β-adrenoceptors; increase in inhibitory G protein α-subunits	No (*Pseudomonas* exotoxin A) Yes (*Pseudomonas* exotoxin A)	– –	67 67
3 days	Embryonic chick cardiomyocytes	Decrease in the number of β-adrenoceptors; increase in inhibitory G protein α-subunits	– –	– –	351
5 days	Neonatal rat cardiomyocytes	Decrease in the number of β-adrenoceptors	–	–	356

agonist exposure of the cells for 4 hours is a protein synthesis-dependent process and is only completed within 72 hours.[17] Consequently, the cells remain refractory to catecholamines when protein synthesis is inhibited by Pseudomonas exotoxin A during the recovery period (Fig. 4.2d,e).

In addition to the catecholamine-induced, agonist-specific (homologous) desensitization of adenylyl cyclase stimulation, agonist-nonspecific (heterologous) desensitization affecting various receptor-coupled hormones and direct adenylyl cyclase stimulators (e.g. forskolin) have been shown to occur in CMs, following long-term catecholamine exposure. Noradrenaline treatment of chicken CMs for 3 days leads, in addition to a decrease in β-adrenoceptor agonist stimulation, to a reduction in cAMP formation by prostaglandin E_1 and forskolin.[14] While β-adrenoceptor down-regulation occurs at relatively low concentrations of noradrenaline (10^{-9} M), much higher noradrenaline concentrations ($\geq 10^{-7}$ M) are necessary to induce heterologous desensitization.[14] In neonatal rat CMs, noradrenaline treatment leads to a marked depression of the contractile response to the β-adrenoceptor agonist isoproterenol and to the phosphodiesterase inhibitor isobutylmethylxanthine.[22] This heterologous desensitization of adenylyl cyclase stimulation in rat CMs is due to an increase—about 2- to 3-fold—in the level of two inhibitory G-protein α-subunits, most probably the α-subunits of G_{i2} and G_{i3}.[23] On the other hand, the $β_1$-subunit of G proteins and the $G_{sα}$ protein are apparently unaffected by the β-adrenoceptor agonist exposure (Table 4.1).

Taken together, the presently available data indicate that the desensitization of β-adrenoceptor-coupled adenylyl cyclase stimulation in CMs following short-term exposure is mediated by uncoupling of the receptors from the $G_{sα}$ protein, probably by phosphorylation of the receptor, whereas desensitization following long-term treatment is due to down-regulation of β-adrenoceptors and an increase in the level of inhibitory G-protein α-subunits (Fig. 4.1, "noradrenaline exposure").

CATECHOLAMINE-INDUCED DESENSITIZATION OF ADENYLYL CYCLASE IN AN EXPERIMENTAL "EX VIVO-IN VITRO" SYSTEM

Using an experimental "ex vivo – in vitro" system it has recently been studied whether the mechanisms of catecholamine-induced desensitization of cardiac β-adrenoceptor stimulation are modified in septic shock.[24] Exposure of neonatal rat CMs for 48 hours to plasma of noradrenaline-treated patients with septic shock (group IV, Fig. 4.3) led to a down-regulation of β-adrenoceptors by 35%, an increase in the level of inhibitory G protein α-subunits by 60% and a decrease in isoproterenol-stimulated adenylyl cyclase activity by 50% in membranes prepared from the rat CMs (Fig. 4.3). Similar alterations were observed following pretreatment of the cells with plasma of adrenaline-treated patients with cardiogenic shock (group II). In contrast, exposure of

Table 4.3. Catecholamine desensitization of β₁-adrenoceptor/G protein/adenylyl cyclase axis in neonatal rat cardiomyocytes—influence of P. exotoxin A.

	Control	Noradrenaline	*Pseudomonas* exotoxin A	Noradrenaline + exotoxin A
β_1-Adrenoceptors (%)	100	55	101	64
Adenylyl cyclase activity				
β_1-Adrenoceptor stimulation by isoproterenol (%)	100	41	98	63
Direct adenylyl cyclase stimulation by forskolin (%)	100	78	109	99
G-proteins				
$G_{i\alpha2}$, $G_{i\alpha3}$ (%)	100	200–300	70–100	120
$G_{s\alpha45}$, $G_{s\alpha52}$ (%)	100	No change		
$G_{\beta1}$ (%)	100	No change		

Neonatal rat CMs have been incubated for 48 hours in the absence or presence of 10^{-6}M noradrenaline, 1 ng/ml P. exotoxin A, or both; thereafter, crude membranes have been prepared: with these membranes, adenylyl cyclase activities have been measured in the presence of either 10^{-4}M isoprenaline or 10^{-4}M forskolin; the number of β-adrenoceptors characterized as $β_1$-adrenoceptors[337] has been evaluated by (^{3}H)(-)CGP 12177-binding; G proteins have been measured by cholera toxin (G_s)- and by pertussis toxin (G_i)-catalyzed ADP-ribosylation and immunoblotting respectively. For experimental details see refs. 22, 23, 67. The table summarizes results from refs. 67, 68, 338.
(Reproduced with permission from: Werdan K, Müller U, Reithmann C. "Negative inotropic cascades" in cardiomyocytes triggered by substances relevant to sepsis. In: Schlag G, Redl H, eds. Pathophysiology of Shock, Sepsis, and Organ Failure. Berlin, Heidelberg: Springer-Verlag,\ 1993: 787-832.)

the CMs to plasma of intensive care patients without shock (group I), and to plasma of dopamine-treated patients with septic shock (group III) did not induce alterations of the CM adenylyl cyclase system (Fig. 4.3).

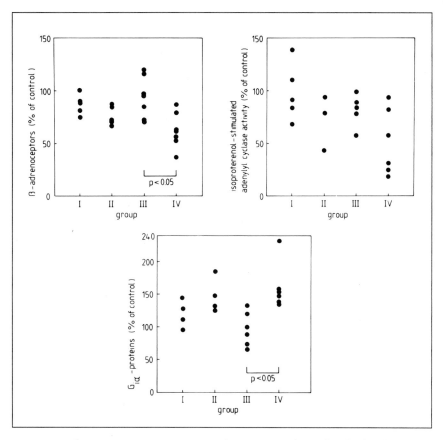

Fig. 4.3. β-Adrenoceptors, $G_{i\alpha}$ proteins, and isoproterenol-stimulated adenylyl cyclase activity in rat cardiomyocyte membranes following treatment of the intact cardiomyocytes with plasma of intensive care patients. Group I: Patients with cardiac diseases without shock treated with dopamine at a "dopaminergic dose" (200 µg/min). Group II: Patients with cardiogenic shock treated with adrenaline plus dopamine (200 µg/min). Group III: Patients with septic shock treated with dopamine at doses ≥ 400 µg/min (mean dosage 671 ± 237 µg/min) suggested to activate α- as well as β-adrenoceptors. Group IV: Patients with septic shock treated with noradrenaline (plus adrenaline) plus dopamine (200 µg/min). Following pretreatment of the cardiomyocytes with plasma of the patients of Groups I-IV for 48 hours, membranes were prepared. β-Adrenoceptors ((^{3}H)CGP 12177-binding), $G_{i\alpha}$ proteins (pertussis toxin-catalyzed (^{32}P)ADP-ribosylation), and isoproterenol (100µM)-stimulated adenylyl cyclase activity were determined as described.[24] All values are calculated in percentages of the control values obtained from cardiomyocytes exposed to the respective patient's plasma in the presence of 10^{-7}M timolol. The effect of group IV plasma on β-adrenoceptors and $G_{i\alpha}$ proteins was statistically significantly different from the effect of group III plasma (p < 0.05). (Reprinted with permission from: Reithmann C, Hallström S, Pilz G et al. Circ Shock 1993; 41:48-59.)

The relation between plasma noradrenaline levels of the patients with septic shock and the β-adrenoceptor number in the CM membranes following treatment of the cells with these plasma samples for 48 hours (in percentage to the respective betablocker-containing plasma) is shown in Figure 4.4. At plasma noradrenaline levels below 200 pg/ml, the β-adrenoceptor number of CMs was apparently unchanged. However, at higher noradrenaline concentrations in the plasma of patients with septic shock, the CM β-adrenoceptors were increasingly down-regulated. Maximal β-adrenoceptor down-regulation occurred at 10,000 pg/ml (about 5×10^{-8} M) noradrenaline and amounted to about 40-50% of the control level. As demonstrated in Figure 4.5 pretreatment of the CMs with the plasma of the patients without shock (cardiogenic, DOPA) and with the plasma of the dopamine-treated patients with septic shock did not significantly alter the level of $G_{i\alpha}$ proteins

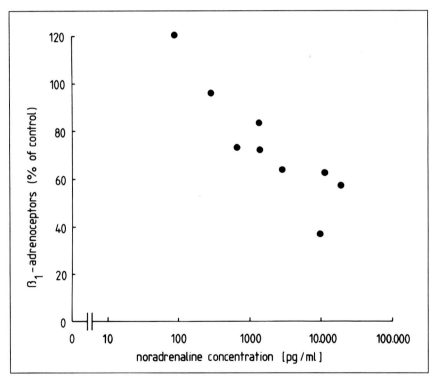

Fig. 4.4. Scatter diagram of β-adrenoceptor regulation in rat cardiomyocytes by plasma noradrenaline levels of patients with sepsis. Rat cardiomyocytes were treated for 48 hours with plasma obtained from patients with septic shock in the presence and absence of 10^{-7} M timolol. Thereafter, β-adrenoceptors in rat cardiomyocyte membranes were quantified by (^{3}H)CGP 12177-binding. β-Adrenoceptor-binding (measured in the absence of timolol) is given as percent of the β-adrenoceptor binding in the presence of timolol (control). Plasma noradrenaline levels of patients were measured by HPLC with electrochemical detection. (Reproduced with permission from: Reithmann C, Hallström S, Pilz G et al. Desensitization of rat cardiomyocyte adenylyl cyclase stimulation by plasma of noradrenaline-treated patients with septic shock. Circ Shock 1993; 41:48-59.)

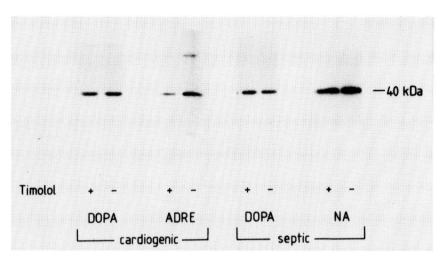

Fig. 4.5. Rat cardiomyocyte $G_{i\alpha}$ proteins following exposure of the cells to plasma of patients with cardiogenic and septic shock. Rat cardiomyocytes were treated for 48 hours with plasma of dopamine (DOPA)-treated patients with cardiac diseases without shock, with plasma of adrenaline (ADRE)-treated patients with cardiogenic shock and with plasma of dopamine (DOPA)- or noradrenaline (NA)-treated patients with septic shock, in the absence or presence of 10^{-7} M timolol. Thereafter, cardiomyocyte $G_{i\alpha}$ proteins were determined. Representative experiments are shown for each "treatment condition". The molecular weight (40 kDa) of rat cardiomyocyte $G_{i\alpha}$ proteins is indicated. (Reproduced with permission from: Reithmann C, Hallström S, Pilz G et al. Desensitization of rat cardiomyocyte adenylyl cyclase stimulation by plasma of noradrenaline-treated patients with septic shock. Circ Shock 1993; 41:48-59.)

(40 kDa) in membranes of the rat CMs. In contrast, the exposure of the CMs to plasma of the adrenaline-treated patients with cardiogenic shock and to the plasma of the noradrenaline-treated patients with septic shock led to increases by 48% and 61%, respectively, in the level of $G_{i\alpha}$ proteins (Fig. 4.5).

To study whether the increases in $G_{i\alpha}$ proteins induced by the plasma of the septic shock patients are associated with the decreases in β-adrenoceptors, the levels of β-adrenoceptors were plotted versus the $G_{i\alpha}$ protein levels. The data showed a negative correlation (r = -0.79) (Fig. 4.6).

To investigate the hemodynamic effects of noradrenaline in the patients with septic shock included in the study, the effects of noradrenaline on mean arterial blood pressure (MAP) and left ventricular stroke work index (LVSWI) (n = 5) during the first 4 days of treatment (days 1-4) in comparison to the pretreatment with dopamine (day 0) are shown in Figure 4.7. The onset of the noradrenaline therapy (mean dosage 6.6 ± 3.0 µg/min) led to a statistically significant increase in MAP from 52.2 ± 7.8 to 72 ± 7.7 mm Hg (p < 0.05) and in LVSWI from 22.2 ± 6.8 to 34.9 ± 1.9 g x m/m^2 (p < 0.05) in the patients with septic shock pretreated with dopamine (mean dosage 760 ± 686 µg/min). MAP and LVSWI remained high during the following three days (Fig. 4.7). To analyze whether the effect of the catecholamines may increase during the long-term treatment, the mean dosage of noradrenaline and adrenaline (n = 8) and the mean dosage of dopamine necessary to maintain MAP at levels of about 65 mm Hg were calculated from day 1 to day 4 of the catecholamine therapy. The catecholamine dosage (noradrenaline + adrenaline) significantly increased from 9.7 ± 6.5 to 24.9 ± 14.4 µg/min ($p < 0.05$) from day 1 to day 2 of the catecholamine therapy. In contrast, no increase in the dosage of dopamine from day 1 to day 4 was required in the dopamine-treated patients with septic shock to maintain arterial blood pressure. Thus, the observed tolerance to noradrenaline in the treatment of septic shock may, in part, be due to a desensitization of cardiac β-adrenoceptor stimulation induced by the β-adrenoceptor-stimulatory effect of noradrenaline.

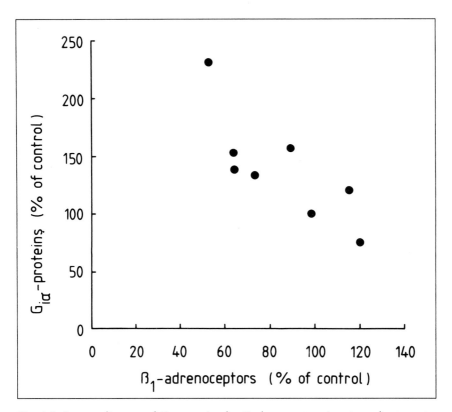

Fig. 4.6. Scatter diagram of $G_{i\alpha}$ proteins by β-adrenoceptors in rat cardiomyocytes following pretreatment with plasma of patients with septic shock. After treatment of rat cardiomyocytes for 48 hours with plasma of patients with septic shock in the absence and presence of 10^{-7} M timolol, β-adrenoceptors and $G_{i\alpha}$ proteins were determined as described. The values (obtained in the absence of timolol) are given in percentages of the values obtained in the presence of timolol (control). The correlation between the two variables is -0.79. (Reproduced with permission from: Reithmann C, Hallström S, Pilz G et al. Desensitization of rat cardiomyocyte adenylyl cyclase stimulation by plasma of noradrenaline-treated patients with septic shock. Circ Shock 1993; 41:48-59.)

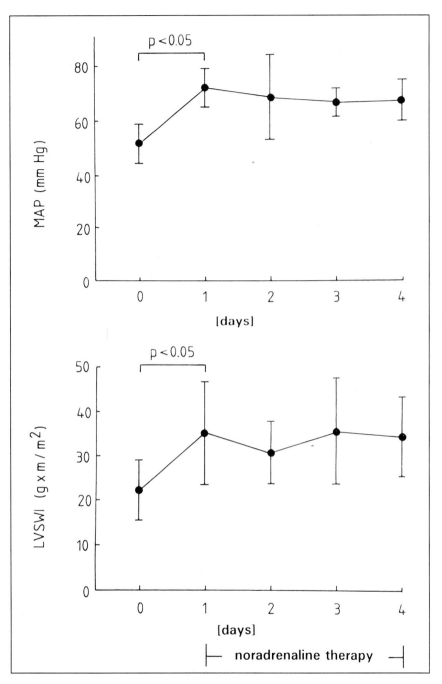

Fig. 4.7. Effect of noradrenaline therapy on mean arterial blood pressure (MAP) and left ventricular stroke work index (LVSWI) in patients with septic shock. Patients were pretreated with dopamine (760 ± 686 μg/min) at day 0, and were treated with noradrenaline (6.6 ± 3.0 μg/min at day 1) from day 1 to day 4. Values are given as mean ± SD, n = 5. MAP and LVSWI were significantly higher at day 1 than at day 0 (p < 0.05). For further information see text. (Reproduced with permission from: Reithmann C, Hallström S, Pilz G et al. Desensitization of rat cardiomyocyte adenylyl cyclase stimulation by plasma of noradrenaline-treated patients with septic shock. Circ Shock 1993; 41:48-59.)

CATECHOLAMINE-INDUCED DESENSITIZATION
OF CARDIOMYOCYTE ADENYLYL CYCLASE IN VIVO

As could be expected from the in vitro data, catecholamine infusion into rats desensitizes adenylyl cyclase of the heart in vivo, and ventricular CMs isolated from these animals consequently show less cAMP production in response to catecholamines than cells from untreated control rats.[25]

Catecholamine desensitization can also be found in experimental heart failure with increased plasma catecholamine levels; a decrease in the contractile response to isoproterenol has been described in CMs prepared from rats with monocrotaline-induced right-sided hypertrophy and heart failure[26] and in CMs from rabbits with adriamycin-induced cardiomyopathy.[25] Recently, atrial cells from hearts of patients with severe heart failure have been shown to be less sensitive to isoproterenol (contractile response) than cells from hearts of patients with mild heart failure.[27] It is interesting to note in this context that also CMs from rats treated with endotoxin in vivo have a markedly decreased sensitivity to cAMP formation by isoproterenol and forskolin and show about a 25% decrease in the number of surface β-adrenoceptors.[3]

POSSIBLE ROLE OF AUTOANTIBODIES AGAINST β-ADRENOCEPTORS

The presence of anti-β-adrenoceptor autoantibodies in patients with dilated cardiomyopathy was first demonstrated by Limas et al (1989).[28] The anti-β-adrenoceptor-autoantibodies apparently induce a down-regulation of β-adrenoceptors by interfering at several steps in the cycling of β-adrenoceptors; therefore it has been suggested that these autoantibodies may contribute to the decline in β-adrenoceptor responsiveness in cardiomyopathic myocardium.[29]

In neonatal rat CMs, anti-β-receptor-autoantibodies from patients with myocarditis and dilated cardiomyopathy increase the frequency of spontaneous beating.[30] Furthermore, anti-β$_2$-receptor-autoantibodies from patients with allergic asthma bronchiale inhibit the β$_2$-adrenoceptor-mediated positive chronotropic action in neonatal rat CMs.[31] At present it is unknown whether autoimmune mechanisms involving β-adrenoceptors or other components of the adenylyl cyclase system may play a role in the decreased adrenergic sensitivity of the heart in endotoxemia and sepsis.

CONCLUSIONS

Similarly as shown for nonseptic heart failure, the responsiveness to β-adrenergic stimulation has also been demonstrated to be markedly reduced in various experimental models of endotoxinemia and sepsis. This decrease in β-adrenoceptor-mediated adenylyl cyclase stimulation in sepsis has been attributed to a desensitization by high concentrations of circulating catecholamines. In (nonseptic) heart failure, the refractoriness to β-adrenergic stimulation is mainly due to a decrease in the number of β-adrenoceptors.[10] However, in experimental endotoxinemia the mechanism of the desensitization of adenylyl cylcase stimulation is much less clear.

In contrast to the alterations which were found in hearts from patients with severe (nonseptic) heart failure, none or only a relatively low-grade down-regulation of β-adrenoceptors, inadequately low for the excessively high catecholamine plasma levels, has been found in cardiac preparations obtained from experimental endotoxemia and sepsis. As a possible explanation, it has to be taken into account, that in most of the current experimental models of sepsis the cardiac β-adrenoceptors are exposed to catecholamines for a relatively short period of time (several hours at maximum). Several studies concerning the time course of adenylyl cyclase desensitization by catecholamines have shown that short exposure (for up to 60 minutes) leads to an uncoupling but not to a down-regulation of the β-adrenoceptors whereas longer exposure decreases the number of cell surface receptors. It can therefore be speculated that in the current models of endotoxinemia and sepsis the cardiac β-adrenoceptors are uncoupled from the G_s protein but that the number of receptors is not yet reduced. To confirm this hypothesis, experimental studies with a prolonged exposure to endotoxin or other bacterial toxins more closely mimicking the situation of human sepsis are necessary.

Another possible explanation for the discrepancy between the pronounced decrease in β-adrenergic stimulation and the relatively low extent of receptor down-regulation may be that mechanisms other than the catecholamine-induced desensitization may be involved in the refractoriness to β-adrenoceptor stimulation. Alterations in the coupling between β-adrenoceptors and the adenylyl cyclase by cytokines such as tumor necrosis factor α (TNF-α) and interleukin 1 (IL-1) have recently been suggested to be mechanisms which may contribute to the decreased effects of catecholamines in sepsis. In addition to a decrease in the number of β-adrenoceptors, other mechanisms such as changes in the level or activity of G protein subunits or of the adenylyl cyclase catalytic subunit could be involved in the relative refractoriness of β-adrenergic stimulation in sepsis.

As described it has been shown in an experimental ex vivo (plasma of patients with sepsis and septic shock) – in vitro (rat CMs) model that exposure of CMs to plasma of noradrenaline-treated patients with septic shock can induce the same alterations of the adenylyl cyclase system as plasma of catecholamine-treated patients with cardiogenic shock.

Thus the mechanisms of β-adrenoceptor agonist-induced β-adrenoceptor down-regulation and $G_{i\alpha}$-up-regulation are apparently not altered by factors present in the plasma of patients with septic shock.

BACTERIAL AND FUNGAL TOXINS

ENDOTOXIN

Rationale

Bacterial endotoxin is believed to be one of the principal mediators of cardiovascular dysfunction in human septic shock. In healthy human beings, an intravenous bolus dose of *Escherichia (E.) coli* endotoxin (4 ng/kg of body weight) mimics within hours the cardiac impairment seen in septic shock: an increase in volume indices, a decrease in ejection fraction and a depression of performance (ratio of peak systolic pressure to the end-systolic volume index) of the left ventricle.[32] Endotoxin injection in dogs clearly impairs cardiac function, with the maximum reduction in ejection fraction occurring 48 hours after endotoxin clot implantation.[33] In isolated hearts from endotoxemic dogs, a vasoconstriction of coronary arteries has been observed.[34]

Acute Effects of Endotoxin on Beating of Cardiomyocytes

Acute exposure of neonatal rat CMs to endotoxin (*E. coli, Pseudomonas (P.) aeruginosa*) produces no depression of CM contraction and amplitude of pulsation, even in concentrations substantially higher (1 up to 200 µg/ml) than those measured during human septic shock.[35-41] Also, beating frequency of these cells is neither impaired during acute exposure with 0.001-10 µg/ml endotoxin (*P. aeruginosa* lipopolysaccharide, Fisher types I, II and VII) in serum-free medium[40] nor with *E. coli* endotoxin in rat serum.[35]

Chronic Effects of Endotoxin on Cultured Cardiomyocytes

In cell cultures of neonatal rat CMs, even high concentrations (0.001-10 µg/ml) of endotoxin (*P. aeruginosa* lipopolysaccharides, Fisher types I, II and VII) in serum-free medium neither impair spontaneous beating and beating frequency of the cells during a 72-hour incubation period nor influence in concentrations up to 100 µg/ml gross morphology and cell viability (cell potassium, cell protein/well, lactate dehydrogenase release) of these CMs,[38-40] suggesting that this toxin exerts its detrimental effects on the heart mainly by indirect action, with TNF-α and IL-1 liberated from endotoxin-activated mediator cells being the most likely candidates (Table 4.4).

However, at least under one experimental condition in the absence of glucocorticoids, endotoxin suppresses "positive inotropy" of the β-adrenoceptor agonist isoproterenol; when neonatal rat CMs are cultured in a well-defined, serum free medium in the absence of dexamethasone, with which it is regularly supplemented, addition of endotoxin (10 µg/ml) for 24 hours suppresses the "positive inotropic" effect of isoproterenol (Fig. 4.8, upper graph). The enhanced production of nitrite, an end product of nitric oxide (NO) formation, by the cells under the very same conditions (Table 4.6) strongly argues for a NO-mediated depression of this catecholamine "inotropy" by endotoxin in the absence of glucocorticoids.[42] When, however, dexamethasone (10^{-7} mol/l), which suppresses the formation of the inducible NO synthase, is added to the culture medium, the endotoxin effect is clearly abolished (Fig. 4.8, lower graph). It remains to be clarified, whether only the β-adrenoceptor agonist-triggered positive inotropy is impaired by endotoxin in a specific manner or, as in the case of TNF-α (see below), also other inotropic pathways are altered, like Na^+/K^+-ATPase inhibition by ouabain, α-adrenoceptor stimulation or high calcium. This direct effect on CM's contractility is at present merely an experimental finding. It remains to be clarified whether it also plays a role in vivo.

Table 4.4. Myocardial depression in sepsis—"negative inotropic" cascades documented in cardiomyocytes

Endotoxin ---→	**Catecholamines** **TNFα, IL 1** **Reactive oxygen species**	→	**Impairment of α-** **and ß- adrenoceptor** **pathways**
	P. exotoxin A	→	**Inhibition of** **protein synthesis**
	CDF **TNFα**	→ →	**Impairment of cellular** **calcium homeostasis by** **Calcium channel blockage,** **lowering of Ca^{2+}- transient** **(due to SR dysfunction?)**
S. α- Toxin ---→ **Endotoxin** ---→ **Mediators** ---→	**Activated neutrophils**	→	**Predominantly via reactive** **oxygen species**
TNFα, IL - 1 → **Endotoxin** → **?** ---→	**NO**	→	**cGMP ↑ (?)**

The dashed lines indicate possible—still not yet experimentally proven—indirect "negative inotropic" effects triggered by stimulated mediator cells. "S.α-Toxin" = staphylococcal α-toxin; "CDF" = cardiodepressant factor; "SR" = sarcoplasmic reticulum. For further explanation see text and ref. 103.

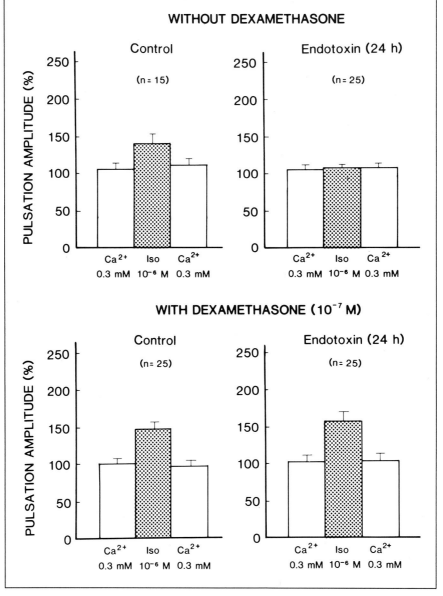

Fig. 4.8. Endotoxin-induced depression of the "positive inotropic" effect of isoproterenol in neonatal rat cardiomyocytes: effect of dexamethasone. Neonatal rat cardiomyocytes were cultured for 24 hours in serum-free medium, in the presence or in the absence of endotoxin (10 μg/ml) and dexamethasone (0.1 μmol/ml). After the incubation period, the "positive inotropic" effect of isoproterenol (10^{-6} M, "Iso") was measured. For further details see legend to Figure 4.2 and ref. 42.

Acute Effects of Serum from Endotoxin-Treated Rats in Cardiomyocytes

In neonatal rat CMs serum from rats treated with a sublethal dose of *E. coli* endotoxin depresses contractile activity (decrease in deflection amplitude of about 35%) and induces arrhythmias when perfusion is prolonged. It also attenuates the chronotropic effect of isoprenaline (10^{-7}M) by 40% (25°C). These effects are only seen when the sera are collected within 2-16 hours after endotoxin administration to the rats.[35]

This depression of contractility is, however, not a direct effect of endotoxin itself nor of nonesterified fatty acids, but is attributed to an endotoxin-induced early and prolonged (up to 14-16 hours) induction of one or more humoral lipid soluble cardiodepressant factors.[35]

Adrenergic Responsiveness of Cardiomyocytes from Endotoxin-Treated Rats (Ex Vivo – In Vitro)

Isoproterenol- and forskolin-stimulated cAMP accumulation is decreased in CMs prepared from hearts of rats pretreated with endotoxin 4 hours before. The extent of this suppression depends on the endotoxin-dose applied (10-100 μg), isoproterenol-stimulated cAMP production being more sensitive to the endotoxin effect than forskolin-stimulated cAMP production. Catecholamine desensitization is accompanied by a reduction of β-adrenoceptor density of the cells by 25%.[3] The authors conclude that the blunted CM hormonal responsiveness following endotoxin challenge appears to be related to the decreased activity of the adenylyl cyclase system that may be attributed to alterations in both receptor density and in the adenylyl cyclase itself.

Adrenergic Responsiveness of Adult Rat Cardiomyocytes and Isolated Rat Heart Preparation after In Vitro Exposure to Endotoxin or Endotoxin-Activated Macrophage-Conditioned Medium

Following infusion of endotoxin, basal rate pressure product, rate of contraction, rate of relaxation and cAMP concentrations in isolated rat heart preparation were unaffected by endotoxin infusion. Endotoxin impaired increases in rate pressure product, rate of contraction and relaxation, and cAMP to isoproterenol, but the response to the direct adenylyl cyclase activator forskolin was unaffected by endotoxin.[43] As a possible mechanism of the disruption of β-adrenergic signal transduction by endotoxin in the heart it was shown recently[44] that the depression of contractile response of adult rat ventricular CMs to β-adrenergic agonists by exposure to soluble inflammatory mediators is mediated at least in part by induction of an autocrine NO signaling pathway. Following preincubation of ventricular CMs from adult rat hearts for 24 hours in medium conditioned by endotoxin-activated rat alveolar macrophages, the subsequent inotropic response to isoproterenol was reduced from 225% to 155% of baseline amplitude of shortening.

Addition of the L-arginine analog N^G-monomethyl-L-arginine (L-NMMA) completely restored the positive inotropic response to isoproterenol in CMs preincubated in activated macrophage medium, while the response of control CMs to isoproterenol was unaffected. Release of NO by ventricular CMs following exposure to activated macrophage medium was detected as an increase in cGMP content in a reporter-cell bioassay and also as increased nitrite content in macrophage-conditioned medium.[44] In neonatal rat CMs the negative chronotropic effect of the muscarinic cholinoceptor agonist carbachol was inhibited by L-NMMA and by methylene blue, an inhibitor of guanylyl cyclase, suggesting that the physiologic response to muscarinic cholinergic stimuli is also mediated, at least in part, by products of an endogenous NO synthase.[45]

Baseline contraction of guinea pig cardiac ventricular CMs was reduced by 46% after endotoxin pretreatment of the animals.[46] This effect of endotoxin was abolished by pretreatment with the NO synthase inhibitor N-nitro-L-arginine methyl ester (L-NAME), with dexamethasone and with methylene blue.[46]

In endothelium-myocyte coculture experiments, 10^{-7} M bradykinin reduced guinea pig CM shortening by 11%. This effect was inhibited in the presence of L-NMMA. Sodium nitroprusside (3 x 10^{-5} M) reduced CM shortening by 23% (reversal by methylene blue). Superfusion with NO solution and 8-bromo-guanosine 3'5' cyclic monophosphate had an effect similar to sodium nitroprusside. These experiments showed that CM contractility can be attenuated by NO, which appears to act via production of guanosine 3'5'-cyclic monophosphate (cGMP) within the cells.[47]

Depressed Contractility in Cardiac Myocytes from Endotoxin-Exposed Animals

In endotoxin-treated rabbits, both hearts in vivo and CMs ex vivo – in vitro exhibit depressed contractility.[48] Moreover, endotoxin results in a shortening of the action potential of the CM,[48] an impaired sarcoplasmic reticulum Ca^{2+}-ATPase activity, a reduced Ca^{2+}-induced Ca^{2+} release of the sarcoplasmic reticulum, an altered Na^{2+}-Ca^{2+} exchange and an inhibition of (Na^++K^+)-ATPase, the latter two effects probably being due to changes in the cell membrane microenvironment in response to phospholipase A activation.[48,49]

Conclusion

Endotoxin treatment of rats depresses contractility and attenuates catecholamine responsiveness of CMs. However, the results of several groups exclude to a high degree a direct depressive or cytotoxic effect of *E. coli* and *P. aeruginosa* endotoxin in cultured neonatal rat CMs, concerning concentrations relevant to produce an endotoxin shock in this species with concomitant myocardial depression. These cell culture data therefore confirm reports with isolated heart preparations from various species, most of them failing to demonstrate a direct negative inotropic effect of endotoxin.[50,51] Even keeping species differences in mind, the results favor the concept not of a direct, but of an indirect, cytokine- and catecholamine-mediated myocardial depression by endotoxin in vivo.[33,52,53] These data are in agreement with the concept that induction of NO synthase by cytokines and endotoxin reduces myocardial contractility in endotoxemia.[44,46]

However, in the absence of dexamethasone, endotoxin turns out to be a strong stimulus for NO production, going along with depressed adrenergic responsiveness. Recent data obtained in adult rat ventricular CMs and isolated rat heart preparations demonstrated a disruption of β-adrenergic signal transduction by endotoxin or endotoxin-activated macrophage-conditioned medium.[43,44] As a possible mechanism of this decrease in β-adrenoceptor responsiveness the induction of an endogenous NO signaling pathway was suggested,[44] as at least part of these effects can be overcome by inhibition of NO synthase induction and/or activity,[46,54,55] arguing for an indirect, NO-mediated effect of endotoxin on the heart. The crucial role of NO as potential mediator of endotoxin-induced myocardial depression is furthermore strongly supported by the expression of a constitutive as well as an endotoxin- and cytokine-inducible NO synthase in the heart, the latter with a maximum of its activity 6 hours after induction,[44,45,56-59] by high plasma levels of NO_2^-/NO_3^-—the stable end products of NO—in septic patients[60] and also by the detrimental effects of exogenously produced NO on CMs.[47] The negative inotropic effect of NO has been proposed to be due to elevated intracellular levels of cGMP as a possible "second messenger".[47]

It remains to be clarified to which proportion the cardiodepressive effect of endotoxin in vivo is mediated by direct or indirect impact on the CM.

PSEUDOMONAS EXOTOXIN A

Rationale

Pseudomonas (P.) exotoxin A has been recognized as one of the main virulence factors in Pseudomonas sepsis.[61,62] As mechanism of virulence, the toxin inhibits protein synthesis via ADP-ribosylation of elongation factor 2 in various cell species.[63] In keeping with this, about 20% of the protein synthesis rate is inhibited in the hearts of mice burned and infected with Pseudomonas rods.[64] In Langendorff heart preparations of P. exotoxin A treated rats, no impairment of basal contractility is observed, but the hearts are more susceptible to the arrhythmogenic and contractile-suppressive effects of hypoxia.[65]

Cytotoxicity in Cardiomyocytes

Incubation of neonatal rat CMs in the presence of P. exotoxin A for up to 72 hours results in time- and concentration-dependent cytotoxicity: even at the high concentration of 100 ng/ml, detrimental effects become manifest only after several hours; within 24 to 72 hours, extensive arrhythmias and standstill of the cells are evident, accompanied and followed by potassium loss, gross morphological changes, rounding up and detachment of the cells from the culture well with subsequent cell death.[38-40,66] Electron microscopic pictures demonstrate an extensive damage of the cells, after an incubation period of 72 hours at 100 ng/ml toxin, involving numerous intracytoplasmic neutral lipid bodies, scarce or completely deranged myofibrils and swelling of mitochondria with radiopaque inclusion bodies.[66] At the lower concentrations of 1-10 ng/ml exotoxin A, cytotoxicity is less marked: although in an irregular manner, at least part of the cells continue beating. After a 72-hour-culture period with 1 ng/ml, the cellular ATP content is normal, and the cellular potassium content is reduced to about 80% of control; with 10 ng/ml, the ATP content falls to 65%, and the potassium content is lowered to 30-40% of control cells.[40] Within 72 hours, the global protein content of the cells is not significantly lowered by 1-100 ng/ml exotoxin A.[40]

In comparison to cultured CMs from neonatal rats, cultured nonmuscle cells from the same neonatal rat hearts document cytotoxic effects in response to P. exotoxin A earlier and at lower toxin concentrations.[40]

Inhibition of Protein Synthesis in Cardiomyocytes

When neonatal rat CMs are cultured in the presence of P. exotoxin A, the incorporation of (^{3}H)-leucine into acid-insoluble cell precipitate, as a measure of global cellular protein synthesis, is inhibited in a time-dependent (at 10 ng/ml: about 50% inhibition after 24 hours and complete inhibition after 48 hours) and concentration-dependent (half maximal inhibition at about 10 ng/ml, incubation period 24 hours) manner.[66] This block in the protein synthesis pathway can be localized at the level of elongation factor 2; functional elongation factor 2, i.e., accessible to ADP-ribosylation, was drastically reduced after incubating the cells for 72 hours in the presence of 1 ng/ml P. exotoxin A.[38,67] This indicates that elongation factor 2 has been ADP-ribosylated and thereby inactivated by the toxin to a high degree, or that the cells have been depleted from the factor during toxin incubation. As a consequence of both, inhibition of protein synthesis must ensue.

In the tested range of concentrations of up to 10 ng/ml P. exotoxin A, after 24 hours the inhibition was at least partially reversible within the next 48 hours, either by washout of the toxin, or by neutralization of extracellular P. exotoxin A with a Pseudomonas hyperimmunoglobulin G (1 mg/ml).[66]

Protective Effects of Pseudomonas Hyperimmunoglobulin in Cardiomyocytes

The cytotoxic effect of P. exotoxin can be prevented by simultaneous addition of immunoglobulin G to the culture medium;[38-40] a Pseudomonas hyperimmunoglobulin G, about 5-fold enriched in antibodies to P. exotoxin A, yields a better protection than a polyvalent immunoglobulin G. The protective effect is concentration-dependent and superior to simply washing out the toxin. Even when the Pseudomonas hyperimmunoglobulin G is given 24 hours after the toxin, protection is on the whole preserved. This finding is in good agreement with the reversal of toxin-inhibited protein synthesis by this immunoglobulin. The beneficial effect is lost after a time delay of 36 hours or longer.

Impairment of Catecholamine-Triggered Regulation of β-Adrenoceptor/G Protein/Adenylyl Cyclase Axis, of Recovery from Catecholamine Desensitization and of Catecholamine-Induced Myosin Isoenzyme Shift in Cardiomyocytes

Incubation of neonatal rat CMs for 48-72 hours in the presence of a low concentration (1 ng/ml) by P. exotoxin A results in inhibition of global protein synthesis of about 20%. Neither spontaneous beating nor the positive "inotropic" effect of isoprenaline (Fig. 4.2b) are grossly impaired by this low toxin concentration. Also the number of β_1-adrenoceptors and the β_1-adrenoceptor-dependent as well as receptor-independent stimulation of adenylyl cyclase remain unaltered (Table 4.3); with respect to the G_i protein, only a small inhibitory effect of maximally 30% can be observed (Table 4.3).

The same toxin concentration, however, completely inhibits heterologous catecholamine desensitization in these cells (Fig. 4.1); while the protein synthesis-independent β_1-adrenoceptor down-regulation ("homologous desensitization") is not influenced by the toxin,[66,67] the increase in functional $G_{i\alpha2,3}$ protein by 10^{-6}M noradrenaline is completely suppressed (Table 4.3)[67,68] despite an only 20% inhibition of global cellular protein synthesis. As a consequence, heterologous desensitization of the system is abolished; P. exotoxin A completely prevents the noradrenaline-induced decrease in adenylyl cyclase stimulation by forskolin (100 μM) (prevention of heterologous desensitization pathway) and considerably reduces the noradrenaline-mediated decrease in isoprenaline-stimulated adenylyl cyclase activity in rat heart cell membranes from about 60% to about 35% (prevention of heterologous desensitization component on total desensitization pathway)(Table 4.3).[67] Though not yet experimentally proven, the consequence of this toxin effect should be a less severe depression of "inotropic" response to catecholamines after catecholamine desensitization of these cells.

The toxin also interferes with recovery of the cells from catecholamine desensitization; after replacement of the desensitizing noradrenaline

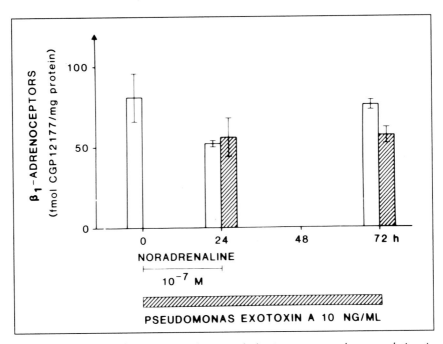

Fig. 4.9. β_1-adrenoceptor recovery after catecholamine receptor down-regulation in neonatal rat heart muscle cells cultured in the presence of Pseudomonas exotoxin A. The cells were cultured for 72 hours in serum-free CMRL medium, either in the absence or the presence of 10 ng/ml exotoxin A. The culture medium was supplemented with noradrenaline (0.1 µmol/l), during the initial 24 hours, with a subsequent washout of norepinephrine and cultivation in a norepinephrine-free medium for additional 48 hours. Thereafter, the specific (^{3}H)-CGP 12177-binding to β-adrenoceptors was determined, which was significantly reduced in the exotoxin A-treated cells (P < 0.05).

in incubation medium, neonatal rat CMs regain their regular catecholamine responsiveness (positive "inotropic" effect) within 24-48 hours (Fig. 4.2d), mainly due to synthesis of new β_1-adrenoceptors.[66] In the presence of 1-10 ng/ml P. exotoxin, receptor synthesis is blocked,[66] and the CMs remain catecholamine-insensitive (Fig. 4.2e, Fig. 4.9) as long as the toxin is present.

β-adrenoceptor agonists shift the myosin isoenzyme pattern of neonatal rat from V_3 to V_1,[69] correlating with an increase in speed of shortening of maximally activating isoprenaline concentrations.[70] This isoenzyme shift, again, can be completely prevented by 5 ng/ml Pseudomonas exotoxin A.[66] In contrast, the increase in V_1 induced by T_3 was not suppressed by concentrations of exotoxin A up to 10 ng/ml (Fig. 4.10). These results demonstrate that inhibition of protein synthesis at the translational level can affect T_3- and catecholamine-induced synthesis of cellular proteins in a differential manner. The observed difference could be due to the fact that T_3, but not isoproterenol, stimulates the expression of elongation factor 2 (Fig. 4.11) and thereby overcomes the inhibitory action of exotoxin A.

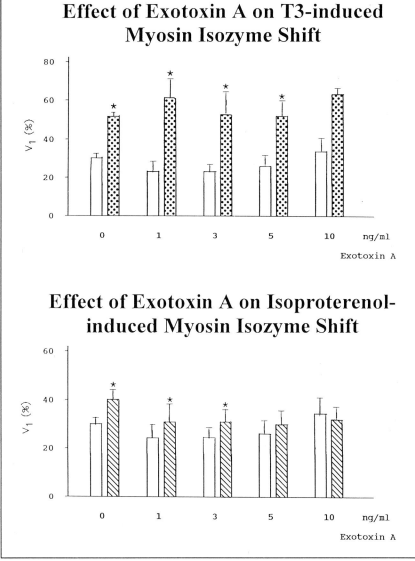

Fig. 4.10. Effect of Pseudomonas exotoxin A on T_3- or isoproterenol-induced changes in myosin isoenzyme populations in rat heart myocytes. The myocytes were cultured in serum-free CMRL medium in the absence or in the presence of T_3 (30 nmol/l; dotted columns, upper graph) or isoproterenol (10 nmol/l; hatched columns, lower graph) and/or Pseudomonas exotoxin A for 4 days. Values are mean ± SD, n = 3-9; *P < 0.05 vs control (absence of exotoxin A).

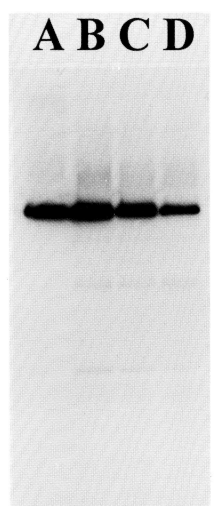

Fig. 4.11. Pseudomonas (P.) Exotoxin A-catalyzed ADP-ribosylation of elongation factor 2. After culturing the cardiomyocytes for 2 days in serum-free CMRL medium without additives (A) or in the presence of 30 nM T_3 (B) or with 10 nM isoproterenol (C) or with 1 ng/ml exotoxin A (D), cytoplasmic fractions were prepared. P. exotoxin A-catalyzed [^{32}P]ADP-ribosylation of the cytosols was followed by SDS-polyacrylamide gel electrophoresis, Coomassie-blue staining and autoradiography. Thereafter, the bands were cut out and liquid scintillation counting was performed. Relative to control, (B) amounted to 169%, (C) to 96%, (D) to 57% in this experiment. The results were reproduced with three independent preparations.

Conclusions

Neonatal rat CMs are sensitive to the cytotoxic effects of P. exotoxin A in the ng/ml concentration range. The mechanism of toxin uptake, in other cell types described as receptor-mediated endocytosis,[71] remains to be established. Like in other cell species, also in rat CMs inhibition of protein synthesis via ADP-ribosylation of elongation factor 2 was demonstrated to be the most likely mechanism of cytotoxicity. Neutralization of extracellular toxin by antibody-enriched immunoglobulin can restore partially suppressed protein synthesis.

Applied for several days, low toxin concentrations with only partial inhibition of global protein synthesis interfere neither with the spontaneous activity of the cells nor with their positive "inotropic" acute response to catecholamines, but profoundly derange the regulation of the "inotropic state" by catecholamines (Fig. 4.12); the loss of heterologous catecholamine desensitization might attenuate myocardial depression by catecholamines, but the lack of recovery from catecholamine desensitization should prolong a catecholamine refractory state. The relevance of these P. exotoxin A effects in Pseudomonas sepsis remains unclear yet; in a canine sepsis model, myocardial depression was more profound in Pseudomonas sepsis than in *E. coli* sepsis; however, the Pseudomonas strain did not produce exotoxin A.[72] In patients with Pseudomonas sepsis, myocardial impairment, as measured by left ventricular stroke work index, is not worse than in patients with non-Pseudomonas sepsis[73,74] (Figs. 2.3, 4.13).

STREPTOLYSIN O

Rationale

Streptolysin O has profound effects on the heart,[75] and it might play a role in the toxic shock-like syndrome due to *Streptococcus pyogenes.*[76]

Effects of Streptolysin O in Cardiomyocytes

Neonatal rat CMs in culture are highly susceptible to rapid destruction by streptolysin O, prepared from group A and group C-streptococcal culture supernatants; ≥ 100 hemolytic units of the pore forming toxin[77] lead, from within minutes up to almost immediately, to cessation of beating (in principle reversible), followed within minutes by multiple cell membrane bleb formation.[75] In parallel to these changes, the cytoplasm becomes intensely granular and the nuclear membrane apparently thickened. At the ultrastructural level, the cell membrane blebs are found to contain relatively small numbers of granular fragments; the endoplasmic reticulum is quite swollen, and its contents

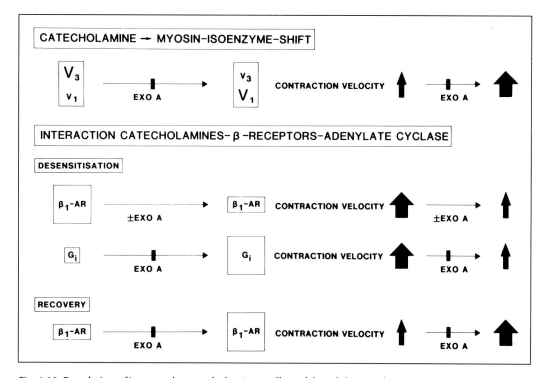

Fig. 4.12. Regulation of inotropy by catecholamines—effect of the inhibition of protein synthesis by P. exotoxin A. The scheme describes the influence of P. exotoxin A (EXO A) on catecholamine-triggered regulatory processes in neonatal rat cardiomyocytes. V_3, V_1: myosin isozyme V_3, V_1. (Reproduced with permission from: Werdan K, Müller U, Reithmann C. "Negative inotropic cascades" in cardiomyocytes triggered by substances relevant to sepsis. In: Schlag G, Redl H, eds. Pathophysiology of Shock, Sepsis, and Organ Failure. Berlin, Heidelberg: Springer-Verlag, 1993: 787-832.)

Fig. 4.13. Cardiac dysfunction in Pseudomonas (P.) versus non-Pseudomonas sepsis. Cardiac dysfunction is represented by a lowering in left ventricular stroke work index (LVSWI); results are expressed as means ± SEM. For all LVSWI, P. versus non-P. comparisons, p was not significant. Pulmonary capillary wedge pressure values (mm Hg) for P. versus non-P. comparisons (all p = n.s.). Total study population: 15.0 ± 1.2 versus 16.3 ± 0.7; culture-proven bacteremia: 10.3 ± 0.3 versus 15.3 ± 1.5; no pre-existing cardiovascular disease: 15.5 ± 1.3 versus 13.3 ± 1.0; pre-existing cardiovasular disease: 14.6 ± 1.8 versus 18.3 ± 0.8; no septic shock: 12.0 ± 2.5 versus 17.3 ± 2.0; septic shock: 15.4 ± 1.3 versus 16.1 ± 0.7. (Reproduced with permission from: Pilz G, McGinn P, Boekstegers P et al. Pseudomonas sepsis does not cause more severe cardiovascular dysfunction in patients than non-Pseudomonas sepsis. Circ Shock 1994; 42:174-182.)

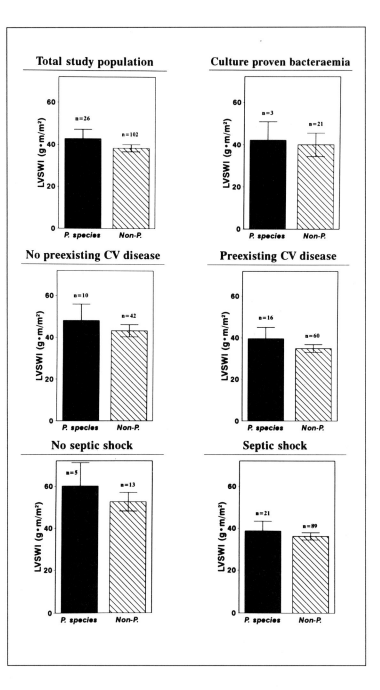

are considerably condensed. The myofibrils are not strikingly altered, but cytoplasmic and mitochondrial vacuoles are rather abundant.[75] Pulsating fetal rabbit CMs are equally susceptible to the toxicity of streptolysin O.[75] Cardiac endothelial and fibroblast cells are also susceptible to lysis by this toxin, but the reactions occur more slowly or bleb formation is less evident.[40,75]

The influence of streptolysin O (0.01-100 µg/ml) on contraction velocity and beating frequency of neonatal rat CMs has also been studied.[40] The results document a negative "inotropic" effect, arrhythmias and final standstill of the cells within minutes by streptolysin O concentrations of 1-10 µg/ml; a reduction in beating frequency of about 30% is evident even at lower concentrations (0.01 µg/ml); the cytotoxic effect, measured as potassium loss after a 4-hour-incubation period, emerges at 10 µg/ml streptolysin, while at 1 µg/ml toxin, potassium loss is still absent.

Conclusions

The occurrence of a toxic shock-like syndrome due to *Streptococcus pyogenes* gave rise to a renewed interest in streptococcal toxins.[76]

In case of the pore-forming streptolysin O,[77,78] acute cytotoxic effects are clearly demonstrable in cultured heart cells. One can suggest that a disturbance of active and passive ion fluxes across the cell membrane may be responsible for this cytotoxicity, but experiments clarifying this respect are still lacking.

STAPHYLOCOCCAL α TOXIN

Rationale

In cynomolgus monkeys, injection of 100-200 µg/kg staphylococcal α-toxin results in marked cardiac alterations (e.g. arrhythmias, prolongation of QRS complex and ST segment depression in ECG) during development of septic shock.[79] This pore-forming toxin[77] is produced by most pathogenic strains of *Staphylococcus aureus*. In animal models there is consensus regarding its pathogenetic relevance (ref. 16 in 79). Also, human platelets and peripheral blood monocytes have been identified as highly susceptible targets,[79] suggesting a role of this toxin in staphylococcal pathogenicity in man as well.[79]

Effects on Beating and on Ion Fluxes in Cardiomyocytes

In CM cultures from neonatal rats and chicken embryos, α-toxin induces a time- and concentration-dependent decrease in beating frequency, a lowering of automaticity and a "negative inotropic" effect. At high toxin concentrations (100 µg/ml), beating ceases within 15 minutes; no cell contracture or detachment of the cells occurs.[80]

Both ouabain-sensitive (EC_{50} 5 µg/ml) and ouabain-insensitive potassium influx is inhibited by the toxin, with a consecutive decrease in cell potassium of 80% and an increase in cell sodium to 200%. This documents not only a relatively unspecific damage of the cell membrane by the toxin, but also an inhibition of active Na^+/K^+-transport.[80]

Conclusions

Alpha-toxin attacks virtually all mammalian cells, albeit with greatly varying efficiency, due to the presence of specific binding sites occupied already at low toxin concentrations as well as nonspecific adsorption to target cell membranes at higher concentrations.[81] In the case of CMs, the mechanism of binding remains to be established. In comparison to the relatively toxin-sensitive human platelets and monocytes,[79,81] CMs from rats and chicken seem to be at least 10-fold more resistant.

The role of α-toxin and other staphylococcal toxins in cardiac impairment of various forms of staphylococcal sepsis yet remains to be determined.[82,83] The availability of monoclonal antibodies and an efficient human hyperimmune globulin against the cytotoxic action of staphylococcal α-toxin in vitro and in vivo[79] may help clarify the pathogenetic role of this toxin.

T-2 Toxin

Rationale

Cardiovascular failure following exposure to T-2 toxin, the most lethal component of several strains of Fusarium fungi, has repeatedly been reported (for review see ref. 84).

Effects of T-2 Toxin in Neonatal Rat Cardiomyocytes

In neonatal rat CMs, only very high toxin concentrations (500 μg/ml) produce cytotoxic effects during acute cell exposure, with rounding up, swelling, blebbing and fragmentation of the cells after one hour. At concentrations less than 50 μg/ml, beating is almost completely unaffected. Higher concentrations cause slowing of the beating rate and a decrease in pulsation amplitude; an increasing dose-related proportion of cells stop beating after 7-30 minutes, and in spite of the preserved structural integrity the resting cells do not resume the contractions after washout of the toxin.[84]

Conclusions

It is as yet not clear whether the myocardium is damaged directly in fusarium toxicity or the injury is secondary to a cascade of extracardiac events. The results obtained with CMs from the T-2 toxin-sensitive rat argue for an indirect cardiotoxic effect of this toxin.

CYTOKINES

Tumor Necrosis Factor α

Rationale
Plasma-/serum-levels of tumor necrosis factor α (TNF-α) are not only increased in sepsis and septic shock,[85,86] but also in various forms of non-septic cardiac diseases (see also chapter 9 and Fig. 9.1), like severe heart failure,[87-89] acute myocardial infarction,[90-92] ischemia-reperfusion injury,[93] Kawasaki disease,[94] acute viral myocarditis[95] and heart allograft rejection.[96,97] After infusion of TNF-α in man, impairment of heart function has been documented.[98-101] In humans, the occurrence of a TNF-α-induced cardiomyopathy has been reported.[101] In animal studies the infusion of TNF-α induces all of the changes in cardiovascular function seen in sepsis in man.[33,53]

Experimental evidence argues for a persistent negative inotropic effect of TNF-α,[33,102-104] as well as for an attenuation of the positive inotropic catecholamine effect,[105,106] but also for an early positive inotropic effect and for a decrease in resting membrane potential.[107] Nitric oxide (NO) seems to be a mediator of this cardiodepressant action of TNF-α,[108] with the induction of a Ca^{2+}-independent NO synthase in heart muscle cells.[58]

Table 4.5. Contractile-depressant effects of TNF-α in cardiomyocytes—nitric oxide dependence

Species	Preparation	Contractile depressant effect on	TNF-α U/ml	Latency	Reversibility	NO dependence	Refs
Rat, neonatal	Cardiomyocytes	Basal activity → standstill	10,000	11 min	Rapid	?	357
Hamster	Papillary muscle	Basal activity	1,000	5 min	40 min	Yes	108
Cat	Cardiomyocytes	Basal activity	100	10-20 min	45 min	No	111
Rat, neonatal	Cardiomyocytes	Basal activity	64-512	15-30 min	?	?	358
Rat, neonatal	Cardiomyocytes	"positive inotropic" effect of α_1- and β_1-adrenoceptor stimulation, of Ca^{2+} and of digitalis	0.1-10	> 2h ≤ 12h	> 2h ≤ 12h	No	42

Cardiodepressant effects of TNF-α were documented by several groups, their experimental set-ups considerably differing with respect to the measured impairment of the contractile state, the TNF-α concentrations necessary, the kinetics of the process and the nitric oxide dependence.

Acute Versus Chronic TNF-α effects

In CMs depression of contractility and impairment of cellular signal transduction by cytokines—especially by TNF-α—has been described by several groups[43-45,58,103,105,106,109-112] (Table 4.5). However, looking at the reported TNF-α effects in the heart in more detail, it emerges that the cardiodepressant effects obtained (Table 4.5) differ considerably with respect to the measured impairment of the contractile state, the TNF-α concentrations necessary, the kinetics of the process and, most important, the NO dependence. We therefore wondered which of these effects are NO-dependent or NO-independent. For further elucidation we characterized the "negative inotropic" effect of low TNF-α concentrations in neonatal rat CMs in culture, investigated into the probably underlying signal transduction pathways and the pathophysiological conditions for which NO might play a role, with the ensuing consequences on beating.

Acute Effects of TNF-α on Cardiomyocyte's Contractility

In neonatal rat CMs, recombinant TNF-α (5 ng/ml) decreases amplitude of contraction by about 25%, whereas endotoxin, interleukin 1 and interleukin 2 had no effect.[37] This negative "inotropic" effect of TNF-α is most probably not mediated by a direct inhibition of adenylyl cyclase by the cytokine, as TNF-α has no acute effect on adenylyl cyclase activity in rat CM membranes.[109] In fetal mouse CMs, TNF-α (10,000 U/ml) induces arrhythmias and standstill of the cells, being reversible after washout of TNF-α.[113,357]

In adult rat CMs an acute negative inotropic effect of TNF-α (200 U/ml) was demonstrated that was paralleled by decreased levels of peak intracellular calcium.[111]

Chronic Effects of TNF-α on Cardiomyocyte's Contractility

Incubation of the CMs for 24 hours in the presence of TNF-α abolishes the positive inotropic effect of isoproterenol as well as that of high calcium (Fig. 4.14). This effect is concentration-dependent; while 0.01 U/ml TNF-α is ineffective, a clear-cut depression is seen at 0.1 U/ml. Most of the experiments presented were carried out at 1-10 U/ml TNF-α.

The TNF-α effect is time-dependent; it is conspicuous after an incubation period of 12 hours, but not after 2 hours (Fig. 4.14). It is reversible, either by washing of the cells, or by the presence of an anti-TNF-α antibody; in less than 12 hours but more than 2 hours, the TNF-α effect is reversed. Focusing on the role of NO in this TNF-α-induced contractile depression, TNF-α exposure of the cells was carried out in the presence as well as in the absence of dexamethasone, which suppresses the expression of the inducible form of NO synthase and of N^G-monomethyl-L-arginine (L-NMMA), an inhibitor of NO synthase. Neither dexamethasone nor L-NMMA can prevent the

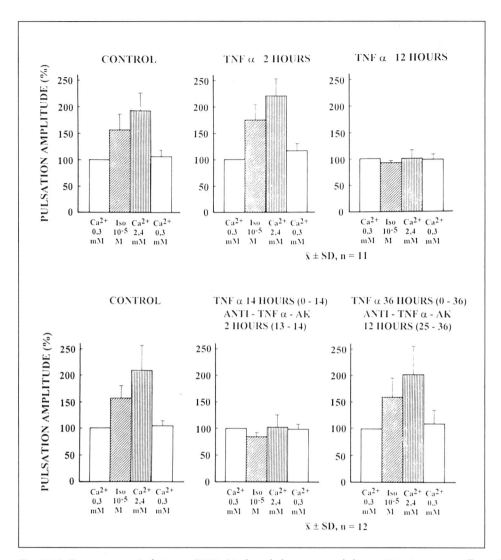

Fig. 4.14. Tumor necrosis factor α (TNF-α)-induced depression of the positive inotropic effect of isoproterenol and high Ca²⁺ in neonatal rat cardiomyocytes: kinetics (upper graph) and reversibility by anti-TNF-α antibodies (lower graph). Neonatal rat cardiomyocytes were cultured in serum-free medium supplemented with dexamethasone (0.1 μM) in the presence of recombinant human TNF-α (1 U/ml) for the times indicated; in the experiments concerning TNF-α antibody treatment, a sufficient amount of murine anti-TNF-α antibodies for neutralization of extracellular TNF-α was added to the medium during the last 2 and 12 hours, respectively. By the end of the incubation period, the positive inotropic effects of isoproterenol (10⁻⁵ M; Iso) and of high Ca (2.4 mM) were measured. (Reproduced with permission from: Werdan K, Müller-Werdan U, Reithmann C et al. Nitric oxide-dependent and nitric-oxide-independent effects of tumor necrosis factor α on cardiomyocyte's beating activity and signal transduction pathways. In: Schlag G, Redl H, eds: 4th Wiggers Bernard Conference. Springer, Berlin Heidelberg, 1995:286-309.)

TNF-α-induced impairment of isoproterenol and of high calcium positive inotropy in these cells (Fig. 4.15). These results strongly argue against the involvement of NO in the depressant effects of TNF-α in rat CMs under the experimental conditions described. Not only are the positive inotropic effects of β_1-adrenoceptor stimulation by isoproterenol and of high calcium abolished, but also that of α_1-adrenoceptor stimu-

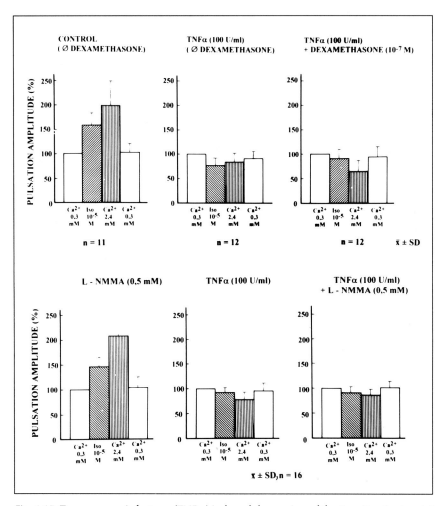

Fig. 4.15. Tumor necrosis factor α (TNF-α)-induced depression of the "positive inotropic" effects of isoproterenol and high Ca²⁺ in neonatal rat cardiomyocytes: effect of dexamethasone and N^G-monomethyl-L-arginine (L-NMMA). Neonatal rat cardiomyocytes were cultured for 24 hours in serum-free medium, in the presence of 100 U/ml recombinant human TNF-α. As indicated, dexamethasone (0.1 µM; a) or L-NMMA (0.5 mM; b) were added to the medium. After the incubation period, the "positive inotropic" effects of isoproterenol (10⁻⁵ M; Iso) and of high Ca²⁺ 2.4 mM) were measured. (Reproduced with permission from: Werdan K, Müller-Werdan U, Reithmann C et al. Nitric oxide-dependent and nitric-oxide-independent effects of tumor necrosis factor α on cardiomyocyte's beating activity and signal transduction pathways. In: Schlag G, Redl H, eds: 4th Wiggers Bernard Conference. Springer, Berlin Heidelberg, 1995:286-309.)

lation,[112] or forskolin (10^{-5} M), a direct activator of adenylyl cyclase, and of the digitalis glycoside ouabain (10^{-6} M) by prior 24-hour-exposure of the cells to TNF-α (1 U/ml) (I. Kainz, P. Boekstegers, K. Werdan, unpublished results). Therefore, we assume that TNF-α exerts its depressant effects, at least in part, by interfering with a common final step in the inotropic cascade of the CM, shared by α_1- and β-adrenoceptor agonists, activators of the adenylyl cyclase and inhibitors of Na$^+$/K$^+$-ATPase (ouabain).

Chronic Effects of TNF-α on Nitric Oxide Production and Consequences on Contractility

CMs express a constitutive as well as an inducible NO synthase.[44,45,58] Formation of NO can be determined by measurement of nitrite production with the Grieß reaction, as NO is degraded to nitrite and nitrate in a relatively stable 1:1 stoichiometry under these cell culture conditions. In the absence of dexamethasone, endotoxin was the strongest stimulus of nitrite production during a 24-hour-incubation period among the substances tested (Table 4.6). Both dexamethasone and L-NMMA suppressed the endotoxin-triggered nitrite production down to the baseline or even lower.

In contrast to endotoxin, TNF-α, up to the high concentration of 100 U/ml, did not induce any measurable nitrite production above the basal level (Table 4.6). Interferon γ (recombinant human, Sigma I

Table 4.6. Nitrite production by cultured muscle and nonmuscle cells from neonatal rat hearts

Incubation (24 h)	Nitrite Production (nmol/mg protein/24 h)				
	Cardiomyocytes		Nonmuscle cells		
Basal	30.5	± 5.8	30.2	± 20.8
TNF 10 U/ml	25.7	± 3.3	18.5	± 0.7
TNF 100 U/ml	20.2	± 2.4	22.1	± 4.8
IL-1 20 U/ml	36.8	± 4.5	32.3	± 5.0
LPS 10 μg/ml	139.0	± 15.0	180.9	± 39.4
LPS 10 μg/ml + TNF 100 U/ml	153.8	± 44.7	208.9	± 46.5
LPS 10 μg/ml + IL-1 20 U/ml	253.8	± 80.9		

Neonatal rat heart muscle cells ("Cardiomyocytes") were cultured in serum-free medium without dexamethasone; in case of nonmuscle cells, the medium was supplemented with 10% calf serum. Recombinant human TNF-α, recombinant human IL-1α, *E. coli* endotoxin (lipopolysaccharide, LPS), or the combination of these substances indicated were added to the medium. After the incubation period, the accumulated nitrite was determined photometrically by the Grieß reaction, with the nitrite accumulated being a measure of NO produced during the incubation period. Data are given as mean ± SD, n = 3. (Reproduced with permission from Werdan K, Müller-Werdan U, Reithmann C et al. Nitric oxide-dependent and nitric-oxide-independent effects of tumor necrosis factor α on cardiomyocyte's beating activity and signal transduction pathways. In: Schlag G, Redl H, eds: 4th Wiggers Bernard Conference. Springer, Berlin Heidelberg, 1995:286-309.)

3265, 100 U/ml) was of no additional value in the induction of nitrite production (data not shown).

Primary cultures of neonatal rat CMs are contaminated by about 10-20% with nonmuscle cells,[114] which also are likely candidates for NO production in the heart. These non muscle cells can be cultured and investigated separately from the muscle cells.[115] Measurement of nitrite production in both primary CM cultures and pure cultures of cardiac non muscle cells[115] reveals similar production rates (Table 4.6). Therefore one may assume that in primary cultures of neonatal rat CMs NO is produced mainly by the muscle cells, with some additional amount released from the contaminating non muscle cells. In both cell types, endotoxin is a strong stimulus, while TNF-α and interleukin 1 in the concentrations chosen are not. However, combinations of endotoxin plus TNF-α and interleukin 1, respectively, boost nitrite production (Table 4.6).

Nitric Oxide-Independent Effects of TNF-α in Neonatal Rat Cardiomyocytes

In neonatal rat CMs cultured in serum-free medium in the presence of dexamethasone, low concentrations of TNF-α, after a 24-hour-incubation period, abolish the positive inotropic effects of catechola-

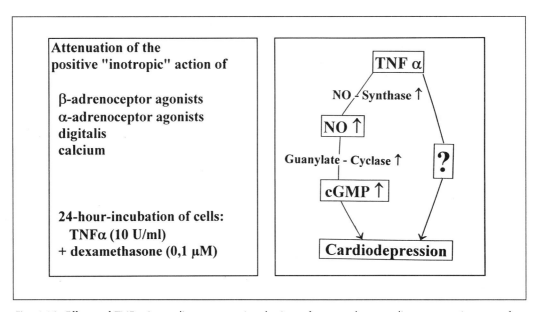

Fig. 4.16. Effects of TNF-α in cardiomyocytes. Incubation of neonatal rat cardiomyocytes in serum-free, dexamethasone supplemented medium for 24 hours in the presence of very low (≥ 0.1 U/ml) concentrations of TNF-α depresses the "positive inotropic" effects of α_1- and β_1-adrenergic agonists, digitalis and Ca^{2+}. These TNF-α effects are unlikely to be mediated by the nitric oxide pathway. Though TNF-α under the very same experimental conditions lowers cellular ATP content and modifies the β-adrenoceptor/G protein/adenylyl cyclase system, both mechanisms probably are not responsible for the depressive effects of TNF-α. Thus some other metabolic pathway probably is involved.

mines, digitalis and high calcium (see above). Under the very same conditions, no enhanced nitrite production is induced by TNF-α (Table 4.6). Therefore, experimental evidence is strongly in favor of a NO-independent "negative inotropic" effect of chronically applied TNF-α at very low concentrations, under the experimental conditions described (Fig. 4.16). This conclusion is supported by findings of a direct acute negative inotropic effect of TNF-α (200 U/ml) in adult rat CMs not significantly attenuated by preincubation with L-NMMA,[111] and by recent data concerning chronotropic effects of cytokines in CMs independent of NO (see chapter 8 and ref. 52 in chapter 8).

TNF-α and Cellular Protein Pattern

In view of the powerful interplay of TNF-α with the protein expression machinery, rather the chronic TNF-α effects at low, clinically relevant concentrations and not the acute TNF-α effects seem the likely mode of action. In agreement with this hypothesis, interaction with protein expression of the inotropic machinery was documented for TNF-α in CMs, including NO synthase,[58] the β_1-adrenoceptor/G proteins/ adenylyl cyclase pathway[42] and the α_1-adrenoceptor/phosphoinositide cascade.[112]

This NO-independent "negative inotropic" effect of TNF-α is, however, not accompanied by a gross disturbance of cellular protein pattern; By high-resolution two-dimensional polyacrylamide gel-electrophoresis, which combines isoelectric focusing and polyacrylamide gel electrophoresis, followed by silver staining, a map of cellular proteins can be visualized.[116-119] This method was applied to cultured neonatal rat CMs, and about 500 protein spots could be characterized by isoelectric point and molecular weight.[120,121] By adding single substances to the culture medium, a "finger print" of the individual substance on cellular protein pattern can be obtained.[120,121] In comparison to control cells, chronic exposure (48 hours) of the cells to TNF-α at low concentrations (10 and 100 U/ml) does not measurably alter the protein pattern (Fig. 4.17). The modification of cellular metabolism by TNF-α to yield contractile disturbance seems to be rather discrete.

TNF-α and Energy Metabolism

Yet incubation of the cells for 24 hours in the presence of 1-10 U/ml TNF-α results in a fall in cellular ATP by about 20-30%, which is even augmented in the presence of isoproterenol; this ATP-depletion can be overcome by a 24-hour-application of anti-TNF-α-antibodies. It is, however, questionable, whether this ATP-depletion is indeed responsible for the "negative inotropic" TNF-α-effects; ATP-depletion in these cells by 2-deoxy-D-glucose to a similar degree does not impair the "positive inotropic" effects of isoproterenol and high calcium (I. Kainz, P. Boeksteegers, K. Werdan, unpublished results), while TNF-α does. However, additional experiments revealed effects of TNF-α on second messenger pathways (see below), which might account for the contractile disturbance.

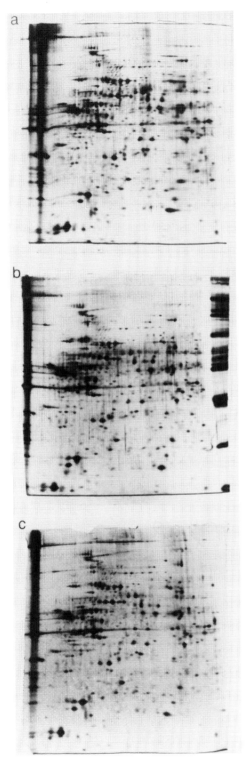

Chronic Effects of TNF-α on Cardiomyocytes' Adenylyl Cyclase Activity

Long-term (3 days) treatment of neonatal rat CMs with immune cell supernatants induces a marked depression of β-adrenoceptor-mediated increase in contractility and intracellular cAMP accumulation of the cells. By chromatographic separation of the supernatant fractions, the cAMP suppressive activity has been attributed to the cytokines IL-1 and TNF-α.[105] Exposure of the cells to recombinant TNF-α (100 U/ml) leads to similar effects on isoproterenol-stimulated cAMP formation as the exposure to the immune cell medium. In addition to the decrease in β-adrenoceptor agonist-stimulated cAMP-formation, the long-term treatment of the rat CMs with the immune cell conditioned media induces an increase in direct stimulation of the adenylyl cyclase catalytic subunit by forskolin. Parameters of β-adrenoceptor binding and affinity are unaffected. Most interestingly, pretreatment of the CMs with pertussis toxin completely abolishes the cytokine-induced inhibition of cAMP-

Fig. 4.17. Effects of TNF-α on protein pattern of cardiomyocytes. Neonatal rat cardiomyocytes were cultured for 48 hours in serum-free medium without additives (a) or in the presence of 1 U/ml TNF-α (b) or 10 U/ml TNF-α (c). After the culture period the cells were harvested, lysed and the proteins separated according to the isoelectric point in the first dimension (pI 4-7; horizontally in the figure) and according to molecular weight (340-14.3 kDa; vertically in the figure) as described in refs. 120 and 121. After silver staining, protein spots were characterized by molecular weight and isoelectric point, and the gels compared. The 2DE maps shown are representative of three independent experiments. For further details see text.

formation; this argues for an involvement of the inhibitory G protein (G_i) in the depressant effect of the cytokine containing immune cell supernatant on cAMP production.[106]

Using the same cell type (neonatal rat CMs), we have recently studied the effects of TNF-α on several components of the adenylyl cyclase system in membrane preparations of these cells (Fig. 4.18). Treatment of the CMs in a serum-free, hormonally defined medium with rTNF-α for 2-3 days induces a marked increase in the level of two inhibitory G protein α-subunits, most probably the α-subunits of G_{i2} and G_{i3}. The effect is concentration-dependent, and the maximal effect occurs at 10 U/ml. In addition to its effect on the level of $G_{i\alpha}$ proteins, the cytokine treatment also increases the level of the stimulatory G protein (G_s) and the level of the β_1-subunit of G proteins. In contrast to the data of Gulick et al,[105] demonstrating a decrease in isoprenaline-stimulated cAMP-formation by TNF-α,[105] we have found that treatment of the cells with TNF-α induces an increase in adenylyl cyclase stimulation by isoproterenol and forskolin by about 30% (Figs. 4.18, 4.19). While number and affinity of β-adrenoceptors are unchanged by TNF-α in the experiments of Gulick et al,[105] in our experiments we found a decrease in the number of β_1-adrenoceptors by the TNF-α treatment of about 40% (Fig. 4.18).

At present, we cannot provide an obvious explanation for the discrepancy between the results reported by Gulick et al[105] and ours.[109] However, we suspect that the conflicting results could be due to differences in culture medium, as myocytes were cultured either in a defined serum free-medium (our study)[109] or in a medium containing 10% fetal calf serum.[105] The hypothesis that serum factors (which may be present in the fetal calf serum) may interact with the effects of TNF-α on CMs is substantiated by the finding that concomitant treatment of the cells with noradrenaline completely abolishes the effects of TNF-α on adenylyl cyclase activity (Fig. 4.19).[110]

Chronic Effects of TNF-α on the Phosphoinositide Pathway in Rat Cardiomyocytes[112]

Treatment of neonatal rat CMs for 72 hours in the presence of TNF-α (10 U/ml) leads to a decrease in basal and α_1-adrenoceptor-induced formation of the calcium-mobilizing second messenger inositol triphosphate (IP_3) and its metabolites, IP_2 and IP_1, by 35% and 26%, respectively (Fig. 4.20). The synthesis of phosphatidylinositol bisphosphate (PIP_2), the substrate of PI-specific phospholipase C, was decreased by 45% following the TNF-α (10 U/ml) exposure (Fig. 4.21). As the TNF-α-induced decrease of PIP_2 was associated with a decreased synthesis of the phospholipid phosphatidylinositol (PI), the precursor of PIP_2 by 33%, the decreased availability of PIP_2 is apparently, at least in part, the result of the decreased synthesis of PI (Fig. 4.21).

Time courses of TNF-α (10 U/ml)-induced alterations in rat CMs showed a parallel decline of basal inositol phosphate formation and

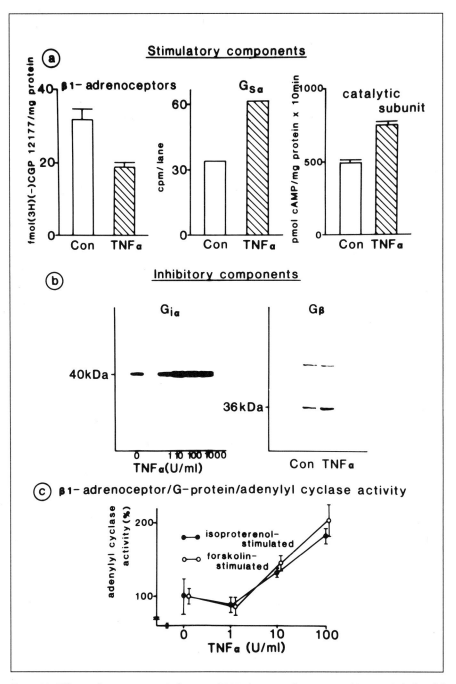

Fig. 4.18. Effects of tumor necrosis factor α (TNF-α) on β₁-adrenoceptor/G protein/adenylyl cyclase system in neonatal rat cardiomyocytes. Spontaneously beating neonatal rat CMs have been cultured for 48 hours in a serum-free medium, supplemented with various concentrations of TNF-α. Thereafter, the following measurements have been carried out with membrane preparations of these cells:[109] (a) Stimulatory components of β-adrenoceptor/G protein/adenylyl cyclase system: the number of β₁-adrenoceptors has been determined by radioligand binding of the β-adrenoceptor antagonist (³H)(-)CGP 12177 (2.5x10⁻⁹M). The

(continued on facing page)

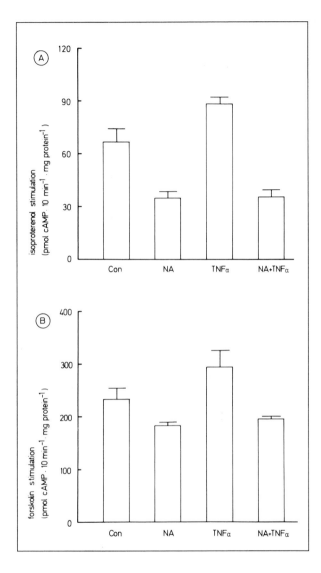

Fig. 4.19. Effect of noradrenaline, TNF-α and noradrenaline plus TNF-α on β-adrenoceptor-dependent and receptor-independent stimulation of adenylyl cyclase activity in neonatal rat cardiomyocytes. After cultivation of CMs for 48 hours in serum-free medium in the presence of 1 μM noradrenaline ("NA"), 10 U/ml TNF-α ("TNF-α") or 1 μM noradrenaline plus 10 U/ml TNF-α ("NA+TNF-α") or in the absence of any additions ("Con"), crude membranes were prepared. Adenylyl cyclase activities were determined in the presence of 100 μM isoproterenol (isoprenaline) for measurement of β-adrenoceptor-stimulated activity, and in the presence of 100μM forskolin for measurement of receptor-independent activity. (Reproduced with permission from: Werdan K, Müller U, Reithmann C. "Negative inotropic cascades" in cardiomyocytes triggered by substances relevant to sepsis. In: Schlag G, Redl H, eds. Pathophysiology of Shock, Sepsis, and Organ Failure. Berlin, Heidelberg: Springer-Verlag, 1993: 787-832.)

amount of $G_{s\alpha}$ has been quantified by choleratoxin-catalyzed (^{32}P)-ADP-ribosylation of $G_{s\alpha}$ by means of SDS-polyacrylamide gel electrophoresis and autoradiography. The activity of the catalytic subunit of adenylyl cyclase has been measured in the presence of 100 μM forskolin and 10 mM Mn^{2+}. TNF-concentration 10 U/ml ("β$_1$-adrenoceptors"; "$G_{s\alpha}$") and 100 U/ml ("catalytic subunit"), respectively. "Con": cultivation of the cells in the absence of TNF-α. (b) Components with assumed inhibitory effects: SDS-polyacrylamide gel electrophoresis and autoradiography of the α-subunit of G_i and the common β-subunit of G proteins. The amount of $G_{i\alpha}$ (40 kDa protein) has been measured by pertussis toxin-catalyzed (^{32}P)-ADP-ribosylation of $G_{i\alpha}$. The amount of β-subunits of G proteins (G_β, 36 kDa protein) has been determined by immunoblotting with antibodies reactive against G_β, after pretreatment of the cells in the absence ("Con") and in the presence of 10 U/ml TNF-α, [resp. (c)] β$_1$-adrenoceptor/G protein/adenylyl cyclase activity: β-adrenoceptor-stimulated as well as receptor-independent adenylyl cyclase activity has been measured in membrane preparations, in the presence of either 100 μM isoproterenol or 100 μM forskolin. For further explanation see ref. 109. (Reproduced with permission from: Werdan K, Müller U, Reithmann C. "Negative inotropic cascades" in cardiomyocytes triggered by substances relevant to sepsis. In: Schlag G, Redl H, eds. Pathophysiology of Shock, Sepsis, and Organ Failure. Berlin, Heidelberg: Springer-Verlag, 1993: 787-832.)

PIP$_2$ synthesis suggesting that the decrease in inositol phosphate formation was due to the reduction in PIP$_2$ synthesis (Fig. 4.22).

As an apparent functional consequence of the decrease in IP$_3$ formation following the TNF-α exposure the α_1-adrenoceptor-mediated increase in contraction velocity (by 10 μM noradrenaline + 10 μM timolol) was abolished in TNF-α-pretreated rat CM (Fig. 4.23).

Similarly, the TNF-α pretreatment completely inhibited the α_1-adrenoceptor-mediated induction of arrhythmias (by 100 μM noradrenaline + 10 μM timolol) (Fig. 4.24).

To investigate one of the possible mechanisms of the TNF-α-induced derangement of the phosphoinositide pathway, the effect of TNF-α pretreatment on the cellular level of glycerol-3-phosphate was studied. Glycerol-3-phosphate is an important substrate of phospholipid synthesis which has to be channeled constantly into the phosphoinositide pathway. Chronic TNF-α (10 U/ml) exposure decreased the level of glycerol-3-phosphate in rat cardiomyocytes by 80% (experiments not shown).

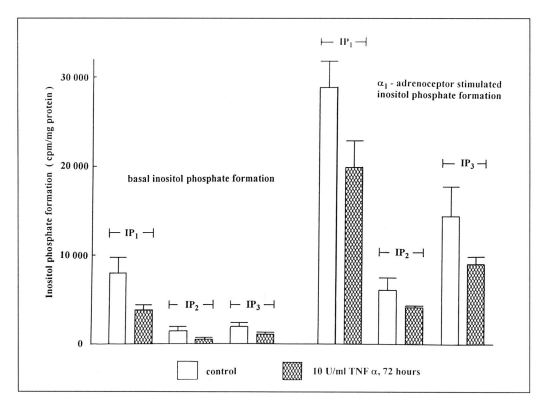

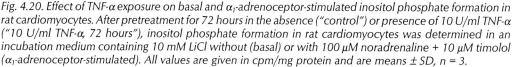

Fig. 4.20. Effect of TNF-α exposure on basal and α_1-adrenoceptor-stimulated inositol phosphate formation in rat cardiomyocytes. After pretreatment for 72 hours in the absence ("control") or presence of 10 U/ml TNF-α ("10 U/ml TNF-α, 72 hours"), inositol phosphate formation in rat cardiomyocytes was determined in an incubation medium containing 10 mM LiCl without (basal) or with 100 μM noradrenaline + 10 μM timolol (α_1-adrenoceptor-stimulated). All values are given in cpm/mg protein and are means ± SD, n = 3.

Glycerol-3-phosphate dehydrogenase (GDH) catalyzes the formation of glycerol-3-phosphate. To test the hypothesis that a decreased activity of the lipogenic enzyme GDH may be involved in the decreased synthesis of inositol phospholipids in TNF-α-treated rat cardiomyocytes, the effect of TNF-α exposure for 72 hours on GDH activity in rat CM cytoplasmic fractions was studied (Fig. 4.25). TNF-α treatment for 72 hours induced a concentration-dependent decrease in GDH activity by up to 55% (at 1000 U/ml TNF-α).

TNF-α concentrations necessary to impair rat CM GDH activity can be found in the plasma of patients with septic or cardiogenic shock; in the experiments illustrated in Figure 4.26, neonatal rat CMs were incubated for 72 hours with plasma (1:1 dilution) of patients with cardiogenic or septic shock or plasma (1:1 dilution) of patients with coronary artery disease, several hours after coronary angioplasty. After the incubation period, GDH activity of the cells was measured. A TNF-α-induced inhibition could be demonstrated for the plasma of about half of all patients. The decrease in CM GDH activity correlated well with the ratio of TNF-α and soluble TNF receptors (p55 and p75) in patient plasma. This ratio may be representative of free TNF-α activity.[122]

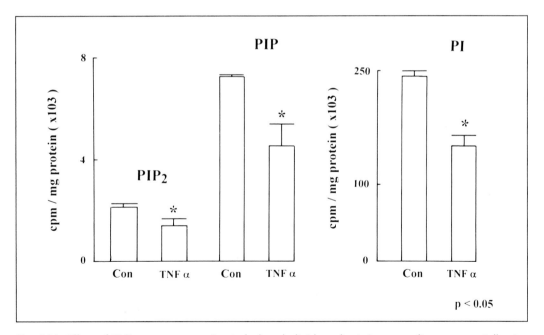

Fig. 4.21. Effect of TNF-α exposure on inositol phospholipid synthesis in rat cardiomyocytes. Following pretreatment for 72 hours in the absence ("control") or presence of 10 U/ml TNF-α ("TNF-α"), rat cardiomyocytes were incubated for 30 minutes with 10 mM LiCl. Thereafter, the reaction was stopped by the addition of 1000 μl of methanol/chloroform/HCl (1000:500:2) and inositol phospholipids were determined. Basal formation of IP$_1$, IP$_2$ and IP$_3$ was decreased in TNF-α-treated cells by 49%, 24% and 35%, respectively. Values (PI, PIP, PIP$_2$) are given as means ± SD, n = 3. *Values are significantly different from the respective control values, p < 0.05.

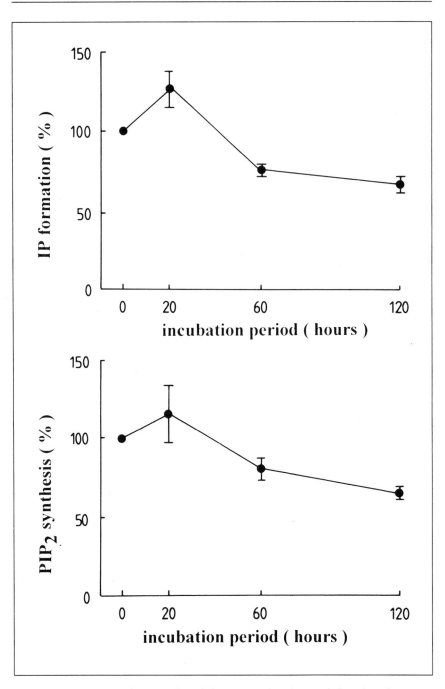

Fig. 4.22. Time courses of TNF-α-induced alterations in basal inositol phosphate formation and PIP₂ synthesis in rat cardiomyocytes. Rat cardiomyocytes were treated for up to 120 hours in the presence or absence of 10 U/ml TNF-α. At the indicated time points (20 h, 60 h, 120 h) basal inositol phosphate formation (IP₁ + IP₂ + IP₃) and PIP₂ synthesis were determined. The values of the TNF-α-treated cells are given in% of control cells. Values of basal IP formation and PIP₂ synthesis are means ± SD, n = 3. (Reproduced with permission from: Reithmann C, Werdan K. Tumor necrosis factor a decreases inositol phosphate formation and phosphatidiylinositol-bisphosphate (PIP₂) synthesis in rat cardiomyocytes. Naunyn-Schmiedeberg's Arch Pharmacol 1994; 349:175-182.)

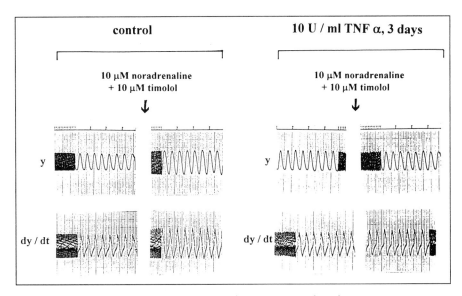

Fig. 4.23. Influence of TNF-α exposure on α₁-adrenoceptor-mediated increase in contraction velocity in rat cardiomyocytes. After pretreatment in the absence or presence of 10 U/ml TNF-α for 3 days, the rat cardiomyocytes were superfused with 10 μM noradrenaline + 10 μM timolol for 5 minutes. Contraction amplitude (y) and contraction/relaxation velocity (dy/dt) of electrically driven cells (120/min) is shown.

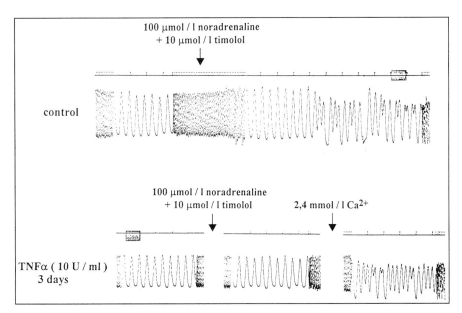

Fig. 4.24. Influence of TNF-α exposure on α₁-adrenoceptor-mediated induction of arrhythmias in rat cardiomyocytes. After pretreatment in the absence or presence of 10 U/ml TNF-α for 3 days the rat cardiomyocytes were superfused with 100 μM noradrenaline + 10 μM timolol for 3 minutes and subsequently (at the end of the experiment) with 2.4 mM Ca²⁺. Contraction amplitude of electically driven cells (120/min) is shown. For further explanation see text. (Reproduced with permission from: Reithmann C, Werdan K. Tumor necrosis factor α decreases inositol phosphate formation and phosphatidiylinositol-bisphosphate (PIP₂) synthesis in rat cardiomyocytes. Naunyn-Schmiedeberg's Arch Pharmacol 1994; 349:175-182.)

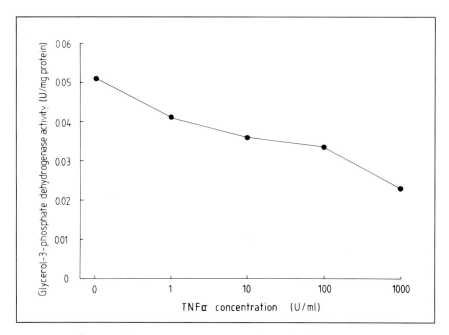

Fig. 4.25. Influence of TNF-α pretreatment on glycerol-3-phosphate dehydrogenase activity in rat cardiomyocyte cytoplasmic fractions. After incubation of rat cardiomyocytes for 72 hours in the presence of various TNF-α concentrations, cytoplasmic fractions were prepared. Glycerol-3-phosphate dehydrogenase (GDH) activities in rat cardiomyocyte cytoplasmic fractions (60 µl) were determined in a total reaction volume of 3110 µl; reaction period 10 min; 25°C. GDH activity was measured at different cytosol concentrations yielding very similar results. Values are means of very closely correlating duplicates (variations less than 5%). (Reproduced with permission from: Reithmann C, Werdan K. Tumor necrosis factor α decreases inositol phosphate formation and phosphatidiylinositol-bisphosphate (PIP$_2$) synthesis in rat cardiomyocytes. Naunyn-Schmiedeberg's Arch Pharmacol 1994; 349:175-182.)

TNF-α—Its Effect on the Action Potential and the Calcium Transient

This issue has been tackled and contributed to both with ex vivo-in vitro and with in vitro application of TNF-α.

In a rat model, papillary muscle for electrophysiological and mechanical analyses were obtained 4-5 hours after the animals had obtained an injection of TNF-α;[107] in the group having received 100 µg/kg TNF-α, resting membrane potentials were significantly depolarized and action potential durations increased, in parallel peak tension, development and velocity of contraction of these muscles were significantly increased. However, whole hearts perfused with serum from animals treated 18-22 hours earlier exhibited significant impairment of contractility, decreased rate of systolic pressure development and decreased rate of relaxation compared with controls.[107] These data suggest that an early beneficial effect of TNF-α on the heart is associated with cardiac impairment 18-22 hours later.

In isolated adult rat CMs, a 15-minute-treatment with 200 U/ml TNF-α did not change the magnitude of the inward calcium current or the current-voltage relationship.[111] However, a concentration- and time-dependent negative inotropic effect of TNF-α was demonstrated in vitro both for the left ventricle and for isolated CMs within the experimental phase lasting for 25 minutes, and these effects were paralleled by decreased levels of peak intracellular calcium during the systolic contractions (at 200 U/ml TNF-α).[111] Further analyses revealed that increased levels of NO, de novo protein synthesis and metabolites of the arachidonic acid pathway were unlikely to be responsible for the TNF-α-induced abnormalities in contractile function. The authors infer that the negative inotropic effects of TNF-α are the direct result of alterations in intracellular calcium homeostasis in the adult rat CM.[111]

Stress Protein Induction by TNF-α in Cardiomyocytes

In cultured fetal mouse CMs, TNF-α induces the synthesis of a 30 kDa stress protein.[113] This effect of TNF-α was suggested to be a relatively uniform "acute phase response" of the CM to various cytokines

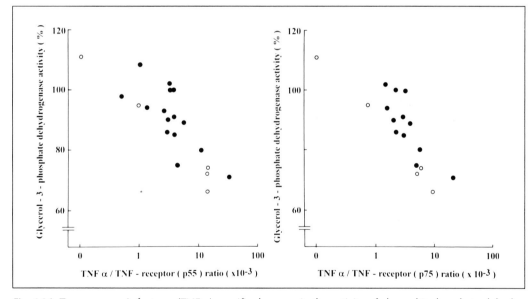

Fig. 4.26. Tumor necrosis factor α (TNF-α)-specific decrease in the activity of glycerol-3-phosphate dehydrogenase (GDH) in neonatal rat cardiomyocytes by plasma from patients with sepsis and heart diseases—correlation with the TNF-α/soluble TNF receptor (p55, p75) ratios in patient plasma. Neonatal rat cardiomyocytes were cultured for 72 hours in plasma of patients with septic or cardiogenic shock (filled circles) and of patients with coronary artery disease, several hours after coronary angioplasty (open circles). Plasma was diluted 1:2 with serum-free, dexamethasone (0.1 μM)-supplemented medium. To identify TNF-α-specific effects, incubation of the cells was carried out in the absence as well as in the presence of a saturating concentration of anti-TNF-α antibodies in the incubation medium. TNF-α-specific inhibition of GDH activity (ordinate) correlates with the ratios TNF-α/soluble TNF receptor p55 (r = -0.88) and TNF-α/soluble TNF receptor p75 (r = -0.86) (abscissa). Measurements of TNFα and TNF receptors by Dr. P. Fraunberger and Prof. Dr. A. Walli (Institute for Clinical Chemistry, University of Munich) are gratefully acknowledged.

such as interleukin 1, interleukin 3 and interleukin 6. In contrast to the effect of TNF-α on adenylyl cyclase in rat CMs, much higher concentrations of TNF-α (250-2000 U/ml) were necessary to induce the synthesis of this 30 kDa stress protein.

Conclusions

TNF-α has acute and chronic effects on isolated CMs. Taking into account the concentrations used and the effects achieved, the chronic effects of TNF-α seem to be of greater relevance than the acute actions of the cytokine. The current data suggest that the chronic effects of TNF-α may be mediated by interference with a common final step in the inotropic cascade of the cardiomyocyte. At present, the results concerning the functional consequences of this disturbance of the adenylyl cyclase multicomponent system by TNF-α are conflicting. However, the data suggest that the regulation of the β-adrenoceptor-coupled adenylyl cyclase system by TNF-α may be an important pathway by which the cytokine can modify myocardial contractility. In addition a chronic inhibition of the phosphoinositide pathway by TNF-α may lower intracellular Ca^{2+} and thereby impair the Ca^{2+} transient, a hypothesis that sufficiently explains the findings by Yokoyama et al.[111] Thereby, TNF-α exposure would not only impair $α_1$-adrenoceptor-mediated positive inotropy, but also the basal contractility and other inotropic pathways with the Ca^{2+} transient as the final step of contractile response. As this effect is seen under conditions, where TNF-α does not stimulate NO production, induction of NO synthase does not seem to be involved in TNF-α-induced impairment of phosphoinositide signaling. On the other hand, Ca^{2+} release from intracellular stores by IP_3 is a well-founded trigger mechanism of the constitutive NO synthase. Therefore one could speculate that TNF-α-induced lowering of IP_3-formation might reduce cellular Ca^{2+}-transients, with the consequence of a reduced activity of the constitutive NO synthase in CMs.

INTERLEUKIN 1 AND INTERLEUKIN 2

Rationale

There are data suggesting that interleukin 1 (IL-1) and interleukin 2 (IL-2), like TNF-α, possess the ability to induce hemodynamic and hematological changes typical of septic shock.[123-125] As IL-1 is known to induce similar effects on cell growth and differentiation in different cell types as TNF-α, it may be expected that IL-1 may produce similar effects on isolated CMs as TNF-α.

Acute Effects of Interleukins on Cardiomyocytes' Contractility

In the very same experimental model (neonatal rat CMs) where TNF decreases the amplitude of contraction (see above), IL-1 and IL-2 (1000 U/ml each) have apparently no effect on the contractile response of the cells.[37] In fetal mouse CMs, on the other hand, IL-1 (1000 U/ml) provokes arrhythmias, and IL-2 (100,000 U/ml) induces a complete standstill, and, comparable, results can be registered under perfusion with IL-3 (50,000-100,000 U/ml), all effects being reversible.[113]

Chronic Effects of IL-1 on Cardiomyocytes' Adenylyl Cyclase Activity

Long-term (3 days) treatment of neonatal rat CMs with immune cell supernatant induces a marked depression of the β-adrenoceptor-mediated increase in contractility.[105] As stated above, the cAMP-depressive activity of the immune cell supernatant in neonatal rat CMs has been attributed to both TNF-α and IL-1. Similar to the exposure to rTNF-α, treatment of rat CMs with recombinant IL-1β (5pM and 20 pM) for 3 days also decreased isoproterenol-stimulated cAMP formation by a maximum of 48%.[105] Experimental evidence points to a G_i-mediated depression of β-adrenoceptor-mediated cAMP production as a mechanism of action.[106]

Chronic Effects of IL-1 on Cardiomyocytes' Nitric Oxide Production

Both in cultured neonatal rat CMs and in nonmuscle cells, endotoxin is a strong stimulus of NO-production, while TNF-α and IL-1 in the concentrations chosen are not. However, combinations of endotoxin plus TNF-α and IL-1, respectively, boost nitrite production (Table 4.6).

Stress Protein Induction by Interleukins in Cardiomyocytes

In mouse fetal CMs, the synthesis of a 30 kDa stress protein is induced by IL-1 (500-5000 U/ml), IL-2 (6000-50,000 U/ml), IL-3 (300-10,000 U/ml) and IL-6 (2500-20,000 U/ml); besides the induction of this 30-kDa-stress protein, only IL-1 (500-5000 U/ml) also stimulates the formation of two stress proteins of the 70-kDa-molecular weight group.[113] This difference in the expression of the 70-kDa-stress proteins is a first hint on a specific action of the cytokines on cultured heart cells.

Conclusions

Interleukins induce marked alterations of the adenylyl cyclase system and stimulate stress protein formation in cultured CMs, yet, at least in rat heart cells, IL-1 seems to be only a weak stimulus of NO production.

INTERFERON

Interferon γ induces a reversible cardiomyopathy.[126] Experimental studies on a possible direct action of interferons on myocardial function are lacking. Interestingly, interferon γ has been shown to induce the expression of major histocompatibility complex (MHC) class I and

II antigens in human CMs in vitro. Other cytokines, such as interferon α, IL-1, IL-2, IL-3, IL-4 and TNF-α induce only MHC class I but not class II.[127] Also in fetal mouse CMs, interferon γ expresses marked levels of MHC class I.[128] The data suggest that CMs are sensitive to specific effects of interferon γ.

NITRIC OXIDE

RATIONALE

In patients with postoperative abdominal sepsis, serum levels of end products of NO synthesis were significantly increased.[129] There is abundant experimental and clinical evidence that the loss of vascular responsiveness in sepsis and endotoxemia involves activation of the L-arginine NO pathway.[130,131] Clinical studies on the application of inhibitors of the NO pathway in septic shock do not provide unequivocal results as to whether NO is involved in the pathogenesis of septic cardiomyopathy (also confer to chapter 10).[132]

EFFECT OF NITRIC OXIDE PROVIDED FROM EXOGENOUS SOURCES

Provided from exogenous sources (e.g. from sodium nitroprusside) clearly a negative chronotropic effect of NO on spontaneously beating neonatal rat CMs can be demonstrated[47] (own data not shown), which is prevented by the addition of hemoglobin (own data). In electrically triggered CMs, the contraction velocity is reduced by exogenous NO (data not shown), whereas in the presence of hemoglobin no effect is conspicuous.

NITRIC OXIDE PRODUCED ENDOGENOUSLY IN THE HEART AND ITS EFFECTS ON CONTRACTILITY AND cGMP

The heart contains a constitutive (Ca^{2+}-dependent) as well as an inducible (Ca^{2+}-independent) form of NO synthase, which form NO from arginine[44,45,58,133] (see also chapter 8 and ref. 5 in chapter 8). Among the reported intracellular effects of NO, the NO-induced stimulation of a soluble as well as of a particulate guanylyl cyclase with concomitant rise in intracellular cGMP plays the most important role in the heart, as a rise in cGMP counteracts the positive inotropic effect of cAMP,[44,45,47,134,135] with inhibition of a Ca^{2+} current probably being involved.[134,135] Although it could be demonstrated that NO from exogenous sources increases intracellular cGMP,[111] it is, however, still a matter of debate, whether the cardiodepressive effect of NO is mediated exclusively by an activation of the guanylyl cyclase.[44,45,47,134] The involvement of NO as an inhibitor of positive inotropic processes can be studied by means of NO synthase inhibitors,[136-139] e.g., N[G]-monomethyl-L-arginine (L-NMMA), or by preventing the expression of the inducible NO synthase by dexamethasone (Fig. 4.8).

EFFECTS OF NITRIC OXIDE PRODUCED
BY THE CONSTITUTIVE NO SYNTHASE

In rat CMs, both adult[44,58] and neonatal,[45] NO is produced by a constitutive as well as an inducible form of the NO synthase (see also chapter 8 and ref. 5 in chapter 8). The CM's potency for NO production is similar to that of cardiac non muscle cells (Table 4.6), the latter mainly consisting of fibroblasts and endothelial cells.

NO produced by the constitutive NO synthase mediates the negative chronotropic effect of the muscarinergic receptor agonist carbachol, and it partly inhibits the positive inotropic effect of β-adrenoceptor stimulation by isoproterenol.[45] With respect to basal contractility, a lack of effect of basal NO[44] as well as a reduction[47] by exogenous NO were described. Furthermore, the conductance of the coronary vascular bed and the resting myocardial blood flow are regulated physiologically by basal NO production, with inhibition of NO synthase resulting in an 30-50% reduction of coronary blood flow.[140]

EFFECTS OF NITRIC OXIDE PRODUCED BY THE INDUCIBLE NO
SYNTHASE (SEE ALSO CHAPTER 8 AND REF. 5 IN CHAPTER 8)

Induction of the inducible NO synthase in the heart comes about 6 hours after injecting endotoxin in rats and in adult rat CMs after a 24-hour incubation in the presence of TNF-α and IL-1,[58] or activated macrophage-conditioned medium.[44] NO produced by the inducible NO synthase partly reduces the positive inotropic effect of the β-adrenergic agonist isoproterenol.[45] Likewise a lack of effect of endotoxin-induced NO on basal contractility and the contractile response to high extracellular calcium was seen,[44] as well as a clear-cut reduction in basal contractility.[47]

In neonatal rat CMs cultured in serum-free medium under well-defined conditions, no significant NO production can be induced within a 24-hour incubation period with nonexcessive concentrations of TNF-α and IL-1, respectively (Table 4.6). The strongest trigger of NO production in these cells among the agents put to test is endotoxin, NO production being further enhanced by adding either TNF-α or IL-1 (Table 4.6). Endotoxin-induced NO production can be cut down, at least to the basal level, by adding dexamethasone (0.1 μM) to the incubation medium, or by 0.5 mM L-NMMA.[42] Only in cells cultured in the absence, but not in the presence of dexamethasone, exposure of the cells to endotoxin yields increased NO production (Table 4.6) and attenuates the "positive inotropic" effect of isoproterenol (Fig. 4.8). These findings argue for a NO-mediated endotoxin effect on contractility. On the other hand, the reported effects of TNF-α on β- and α-adrenoceptor-mediated contractility in these cells (Figs. 4.14, 4.23), on the components of the adenylyl cyclase system (Fig. 4.18) and on the phosphoinositide pathway (Fig. 4.20) do not seem to be mediated by NO, as these experiments were carried out in the presence of dexamethasone.

There is no doubt that NO attenuates β-adrenoceptor-mediated positive inotropy, probably by the increase in cGMP (see above). However, it is questionable whether NO interferes exclusively with the β-adrenoceptor/G proteins/adenylyl cyclase system; if this would be the case, then the reduction in basal contractility of CMs, either by exogenous NO[47] or by endotoxin-induced NO,[46] would be difficult to understand.

CONCLUSION

Inhibitors of the NO/guanylyl cyclase pathway like N[G]-monomethyl-L-arginine (L-NMMA), N[G]-nitro-L-arginine methyl ester (NAME) or methylene blue undoubtedly raise blood pressure by increasing systemic vascular resistance. With respect to the heart, however, the data available are in favor of deterioration (fall in cardiac output) rather than of improvement of heart function by these substances,[59] both in animal models[136-138] and in patients,[132,139,140] with the potential risk of coronary vasoconstriction[140] and pulmonary hypertension.[141] However, one cannot rule out that the induced rise in afterload achieved by NO inhibition may mask a potential benefit of these substances on myocardial function.

Clearly, effects of the constitutive NO synthase and the inducible NO synthase activity can be demonstrated for the CM in vitro both with respect to basal contractility and with regard to β-adrenergic and muscarinergic mediated inotropy and chronotropy. These contractile alterations have been ascribed to a stimulated production of cGMP. Yet, not all the NO effects are mediated by cGMP. Also, unequivocally endotoxin, TNF-α and IL-1 have a potential for inducing NO synthesis in the heart. Yet not all the cardiac effects of TNF-α and IL-1 are NO-dependent.

Current evidence is in favor of a dominant role of NO for vascular impairment in sepsis, whereas in the heart only part of the negative inotropy conveyed by the septic disease seems to be related to NO.

COMPLEMENT FACTORS

RATIONALE

In sepsis, increased plasma levels of terminal complement complexes as well as of anaphylatoxins C3a, C4a and C5a are found.[142,143] In isolated heart preparations from guinea pigs, components of the complement system can impair cardiac function[144] and amplify cardiac anaphylaxis;[145] on the other hand, zymosan-induced complement activation in human blood and plasma did not impair isometrically contracting human right atrial trabeculae in vitro, harvested from patients undergoing elective open heart surgery who had given informed consent.[146]

EFFECT OF COMPLEMENT ON ISOLATED CARDIOMYOCYTES

In electrically driven adult rat and guinea pig CMs, the membrane attack complex (C5b-9) of the terminal complement complex has profound effects on contractility and on calcium homeostasis;[147] sublethal C5b-9 concentrations (about 40 µg/ml C8 and C9 each) transiently augment, in a dose-dependent manner, both basal cytosolic Ca^{2+} concentrations and Ca^{2+} transients, resulting in a significant increase in contractility (amplitude of contraction). In the presence of lytic concentrations of the membrane attack complex (about 350 µg/ml C5b, C6, C7, about 50 µg/ml C8/C9 each), basal Ca^{2+}, Ca^{2+} transients and the amplitude of contraction gradually increase for about 1-2 minutes; then, the basal Ca^{2+} concentration sharply increases, in association with spontaneous beating, followed by sustained contracture without relaxation, until the cells round up and eventually lyse.[147]

CONCLUSIONS

As demonstrated in various cell types, insertion of the membrane attack complex (C5b-9) of the complement system into the cell membrane results in disruption of its functional impermeability to cations (for discussion see ref. 147). In consequence, this leads to colloidosmotic lysis of the target cell or, at sublytic complement concentrations, to reversible changes of membrane permeability, resulting, among other changes, in an increased cytosolic free calcium activity. This process is counteracted by various cellular repair mechanisms (for discussion see ref. 147). In the case of the CM, an increase in contractility results at sublethal concentrations; and contracture, rounding up and eventually lysis result at lethal complement concentrations. The effects of other potentially cardiotoxic complement factors, like the anaphylatoxins C3a and C5a, on isolated CMs remain to be elaborated.

PLATELET ACTIVATING FACTOR

RATIONALE

Platelet activating factor (PAF) is suggested to be one of the main mediators in septic and endotoxin shock.[148-152] A complex pattern of cardiovascular dysfunction can be induced by PAF, with attenuation by PAF-antagonists, in animal models and isolated heart preparations including human heart tissue: coronary vasoconstriction, myocardial ischemia, arrhythmias, as well as negative inotropy, chronotropy and dromotropy.[153-162] In view of this complex pattern, information about direct PAF-effects on the myocardium is difficult to obtain.

ACUTE EFFECTS OF PAF IN ISOLATED CARDIOMYOCYTES: "INOTROPY" AND PHOSPHOINOSITIDE METABOLISM

In electrically driven isolated adult and neonatal rat ventricular CMs, 1-200 nM PAF decreases, within several minutes, twitch amplitude and contraction as well as relaxation velocity, in a concentration-dependent manner; in spontaneously beating neonatal CMs, beating frequency is increased. These functional changes can be blocked by the PAF antagonist BN 50739, in a concentration-dependent manner; the biologically inactive analog of PAF, lyso-PAF, has no effect on contractile behavior. Nanomolar concentrations of PAF rapidly stimulate the phosphoinositide pathway in these cells, with similar potency, specificity and time course as described for the functional effects. Abolishment of the negative inotropic and positive chronotropic effects was accomplished by depleting the cells of protein kinase C, which demonstrates that stimulation of protein kinase C via the phosphoinositide pathway mediates the described PAF effects in these cells. Functional studies characterize a PAF receptor in CMs similar to that of platelets.[163]

EFFECT OF PAF IN ISOLATED CARDIOMYOCYTES: INFLUENCE ON MEMBRANE POTENTIAL

In adult guinea pig ventricular CMs, subnanomolar PAF concentrations (10^{-11} to 10^{-10} M) have substantial effects on inwardly-rectifying potassium channels, responsible for the macroscopic inwardly-rectifying background potassium current (I_{K1}) of cardiac cells. PAF initially causes flickering of the channels, followed by a gradual prolonged depression of channel activity, the mechanisms at present being unknown. These effects are at least partially reversible upon prolonged washout. Again, the biologically inactive analog of PAF, lyso-PAF, was without effect.[164]

Since these potassium channels play a major role in determining the resting potential and excitability of CMs, the effects of PAF on I_{k1} may play a major role in the deleterious electrophysiological actions of PAF on the heart.[164] No further data are available yet concerning the effects of PAF on other channel species in the plasma membrane of CMs.

CONCLUSIONS

The data described strongly argue for the existence of specific PAF receptors in rat CMs with a dissociation constant in the nanomolar range; they document a probably receptor-mediated "negative inotropic" and a positive chronotropic PAF action, mediated by protein kinase C via PAF stimulation of the phosphoinositide pathway; and they further on characterize an interaction of PAF with the inwardly-rectifying potassium current in the subnanomolar range, which might explain electrical instability of the CMs induced by PAF. So far, at least some of the described deleterious PAF effects on the heart can be explained at the cellular level.

The relevance of these data for the human heart, however, is unclear; reports describing a negative inotropic PAF action in human heart preparations[157,159] are contradicted by the finding that in human myocardium PAF receptors are absent.[165]

EICOSANOIDS: THROMBOXANES, PROSTAGLANDINS, LEUKOTRIENES

RATIONALE

In endotoxemia and sepsis, plasma levels of various eicosanoids, prostaglandins (PG), thromboxanes (Tx) and leukotrienes (LT), are elevated.[166-169] Their pathogenetic roles are investigated upon by blocking eicosanoid synthesis via enzyme inhibitors and by blocking eicosanoid action via receptor antagonists, but results are equivocal.[166,169,170-172] Evaluation of eicosanoids' role in cardiac dysfunction, which as yet is unclear, is further complicated by their complex reaction patterns with not only the myocardium, but also, and even preferentially, the coronary vasculature as target; after direct injection into sheep coronary arteries, LTB_4 was without effect on myocardial contractility, but LTC_4 (1.6×10^{-10} moles) produced impairment of contractility (decrease in systolic shortening of 18%), far more than that expected on the basis of the 27% reduction in coronary blood flow.[173] However, taken together, the data concerning the cardiodepressant effects of LT are controversial.[174-177] Further on, most of the studies, where eicosanoid synthesis and action was blocked in endotoxemia, favor the assumption that these mediators exert only a minor, if at all, direct cardiodepressive effect.[149,169,178-181]

ACUTE EFFECTS OF EICOSANOIDS IN CARDIOMYOCYTES

Free fatty acids and especially arachidonic acid and its metabolites exert distinct effects on cell membrane channels, receptors and gap junctions in CMs[182-185] (see also Table 4.1 for PGE_1), with hypoxia being an important stimulus to arachidonic acid metabolism.[186-188] Contractility, however, does not seem to be influenced by most of the eicosanoids to a considerable degree; by acute exposure of neonatal rat CMs, PG E_2, LT B_4, C_4, D_4 and 5,8,9 and 12-HETES do not impair contractile activity up to 5 µg/ml; also PG I_2 has no effect itself. PG $F_{2\alpha}$ (0.3-30 µg/ml), however, induces a dose-dependent decrease in contractility of up to 100% inhibition at concentrations of this substance theorized to occur in microcellular environments.[36]

CARDIOMYOCYTE SUPERSENSITIVITY TO ISOPRENALINE BY EICOSATETRENOIC ACIDS

Incubation of neonatal rat CMs with 3 mM L(+)-lactate for 50 minutes or longer sensitizes the cells to the chronotropic effect of isoprenaline.[189-191] This β-adrenergic supersensitivity is thought to be mediated by otherwise cryptic β_2-adrenergic receptors that apparently become unmasked in the course of lactate treatment via phospholipase A_2 and 15-lipoxygenase activation; the lactate effect can be mimicked by the phospholipase A_2 activator melittin, by the phospholipase A_2 product arachidonic acid, and by the 15-lipoxygenase products 15-S-HETE and 11-R/S-HETE in the nanomolar range.

The increase in lactate level as seen in ischemia may launch the formation of lipoxygenase products deleterious to the myocardium. Lowering the threshold concentration of catecholamines for the induction of automaticity and thereby arrhythmogenicity[189,190] could be the mechanisms of their toxicity.

CONCLUSIONS

Various eicosanoids relevant to sepsis exert distinct effects on CMs. Prostaglandin $F_{2\alpha}$, however, is the only member of the eicosanoid family to emerge as a potential candidate contributing to myocardial depression in sepsis.

CARDIODEPRESSANT FACTORS

For decades there have been reports about the occurrence of shock factors impairing myocardial function.[192-195] CMs have been widely used to document negative "inotropic" effects of plasma fractions from patients with sepsis and septic shock and of various myocardial depressant factors isolated and partially purified from blood of patients with sepsis and of animals with experimental sepsis or shock[195,196] (Fig. 4.27) (for review see refs. 197, 198).

CDF is one of the myocardial depressant factors described with yet nonidentified structure,[197-199] but the only one whose mechanism of action has been clarified (Table 4.7). Primarily isolated from blood of dogs in hypovolemic-traumatic shock, it also was found in hemofiltrates of patients with septic and/or cardiogenic shock; at our present knowledge, CDF represents a family of low molecular weight ($\leq$ 1000 Da) N-terminally blocked peptides, with plasma concentrations of $\leq$ 1 to

Table 4.7. Negative inotropic factors reported to occur in shock and sepsis

Substance	Abbreviation	Postulated nature	Mechanism of action	Refs.
Myocardial depressant factor(s)	MDF	Peptide	?	192
Pancreatic cardiodepressant factor	MDF	Peptide	?	193
Early lipid-soluble cardiodepressant factor	ECDF	Lipid-soluble	Inhibition by caffeine	194
Myocardial depressant substance	MDS	Water-soluble	?	195
Cardiodepressant factor	CDF	Peptide	Blockage of calcium inward current	196

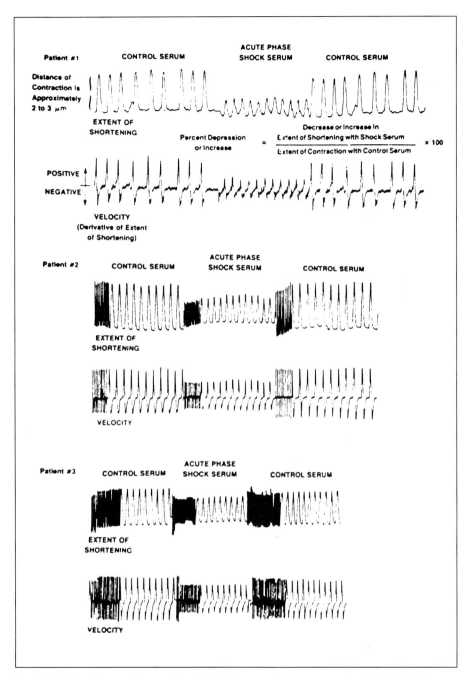

Fig. 4.27. Effect of serum from patients in shock on cardiomyocyte contractility. Diluted serum of three patients in the acute phase of septic shock was added to neonatal rat cardiomyocytes, resulting in a decrease in contraction amplitude and velocity of contraction/relaxation. (Reproduced with permission from: Parrillo JE, Burch C, Shelhamer JH et al. A circulating myocardial depressant substance in humans with septic shock. J Clin Invest 1985; 76:1539-1553.)

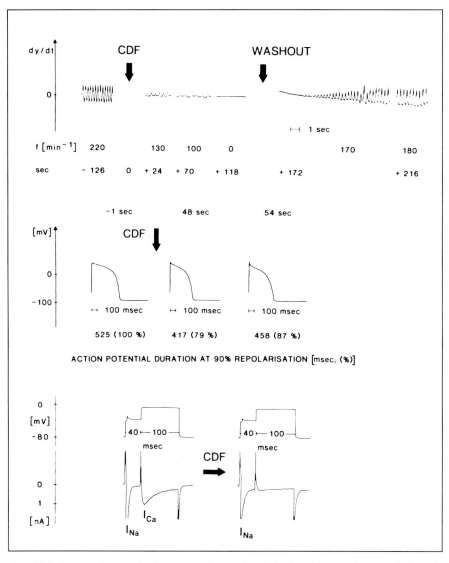

Fig. 4.28. Effect of a cardiodepressant factor (CDF) isolated from plasma of dogs in hypovolemic-traumatic shock in heart muscle cells. Upper graph: In spontaneously beating rat heart muscle cells in culture, CDF (60-fold enriched in comparison to shock plasma) decreases contraction/relaxation velocity (dy/dt) and beating frequency (f) within seconds, with a standstill of the cells coming about; upon washout, the effects are quickly reversible. Middle graph: In adult guinea pig cardiomyocytes, CDF reduces the duration and decreases the plateau of the action potential. Lower graph: Voltage-clamp measurement in single cardiomyocytes from adult guinea pigs. CDF completely blocks the calcium inward current. (Reproduced with permission from: Werdan K, Müller U, Reithmann C et al. Mechanisms in acute septic cardiomyopathy: evidence from isolated myocytes. Basic Res Cardiol 1991; 86:411-421.)

3 nmol/l.[200] Its documented negative inotropic and chronotropic effect is sufficiently explained by blockage of the calcium inward current seen in adult guinea pig CMs as well as in neonatal rat CMs (Fig. 4.28).[196] However, due to the calcium current blocking effect of CDF, not only the CM, but also the vascular smooth muscle cell might be a target of CDF, thereby possibly contributing to the refractory vasodilatation in septic shock.

REACTIVE OXYGEN SPECIES

RATIONALE
In myocardial reperfusion injury reactive oxygen species (ROS) are discussed to be one of the most important causative agents leading to contractile dysfunction, injury and eventually death of the CM.[201,202] Though these reperfusion data document the susceptibility of the CM to ROS, their relevance in acute septic cardiomyopathy remains to be determined.[203-205]

SYSTEMS GENERATING REACTIVE OXYGEN SPECIES APPLIED IN RESEARCH WITH CARDIOMYOCYTES
Several in vitro systems have been applied in studies with CMs to simulate the in vivo production of ROS by xanthine oxidase, polymorphonuclear leukocytes, macrophages, endothelial cells and CMs autochthonously:[206] xanthine(hypoxanthine)/xanthine oxidase for production of $O_2 \cdot^-$, H_2O_2 and $OH \cdot$,[207,208] either without or with iron-loaded transferrin (stimulation of $OH \cdot$-generation)[209] H_2O_2 and Fe^{3+}-nitriloacetate for generation of hydroxyl radicals;[210] dihydroxyfumaric acid for production of O_2^- radicals and H_2O_2,[211,212] and, in combination with Fe^{3+}-ADP, of $OH \cdot$; H_2O_2;[213-218] tert-butyl hydroperoxide;[219-222] $HOCl_2$;[215,218,222] $FeCl_2$;[214] ferryl myoglobin;[223] singlet oxygen by photoactivation of rose bengal.[224-226] Exemplarily, the xanthine/xanthine oxidase (X/XO) system applied in the experiments of Figures 4.29-4.32 shall be described in some detail; this system produces mainly superoxide radicals, hydrogen peroxide and hydroxyl radicals;[205,227,228] at 37°C, a standardized assay with 0.83 mM xanthine and xanthine oxidase (50 mU) in an incubation volume of 3 ml salt solution/cell culture flask produces sufficient amounts of $O_2 \cdot^-$-radicals (initial rate 13.4 nmol/min x 3 ml; after 75 minutes: 5.7 nmol/min x 3ml), H_2O_2 molecules (final concentration at 75 minutes about 400 µM) and $OH \cdot$-radicals, to induce a characteristic sequence of depressive and cytotoxic effects in CMs within 75 minutes (Fig. 4.29-4.32).[205,227,228] A similar system with 2 mM purine plus 20 mU/ml xanthine oxidase has been demonstrated to yield an amount of O_2^- radicals comparable to 670 PMN/mm³.[229]

IMPAIRMENT OF CONTRACTILITY AND CYTOTOXIC EFFECTS OF REACTIVE OXYGEN SPECIES IN CARDIOMYOCYTES

The effects of different ROS have been studied in various types of CMs. In neonatal rat CM cultures, a challenge of the cells with X/XO (see above) results in a characteristic sequence of contractile dysfunction and cytotoxicity (Figs. 4.29-4.31);[205,227,228] negative chronotropic ($T_{1/2}$ = 15 minutes), negative "inotropic" and arrhythmogenic effects (Figs. 4.29-4.30) are very early events; they correlate with a cellular decrease in reduced glutathione (oxidated glutathione 11% at t = 0 minutes and 68% at t = 15 minutes of total glutathione). The cardiotoxic effects are characterized by a fall in ATP-content ($T_{1/2}$: 20 minutes) to 15% of control; active Na^+/K^+-transport across the cell membrane goes down to 10% of control ($T_{1/2}$: 40 minutes), with a subsequent reduction of cell-K^+-content by 55% ($T_{1/2}$: 35 minutes) and an 8-fold rise in cell-Na^+ ($T_{1/2}$: 40 minutes). While ($^{86}Rb^+$)-efflux, as a measure of cell membrane leakiness, is not increased after 75 minutes, other specific transport processes of the cell membrane like glucose uptake are severely inhibited (the rate of 2-deoxy-D-(^3H)-glucose-uptake equals 10% of the control value, $T_{1/2}$:about 25 minutes). The 4-fold increase in cytosolic free calcium up to 1200 nM ($T_{1/2}$: 55 minutes) is a relatively late event, only shortly preceding ultrastructural alterations (loss of mitochondrial granula and swelling of mitochondria; hypercontracture of myofibrils and loss of cell contacts; Fig. 4.31) with subsequent cell death. These alterations are, in principle, reversible to some degree, and they are prevented (Fig. 4.32) by the application of catalase, but not by superoxide dismutase (SOD). Clearly hydrogen peroxide and/or successor products appear to be the causative agents, but not the superoxide anion.

Similar cascades of functional depression and cytotoxic effects have been described for various types of CMs after exposure to various ROS,[209,210,215,217,219,221,230] including documentation of lipid and protein oxidation under these conditions.[215,217,219,220,230] With regard to oxidation of proteins in heart tissue, H_2O_2 is approximately 20 times less effective than HOCl. Adult rat CMs are as sensitive to HOCl as rat heart tissue slices.[215] The rat heart has about the same susceptibility as the rat lung to H_2O_2, but is markedly more sensitive to HOCl than the lung.[215] Human ventricular myocytes are less resistant to free radical injury than human myocardial fibroblasts, but more resistant than human saphenous vein endothelial cells.[207]

In fetal mouse CMs, 10^{-3}M H_2O_2 induces the formation of a 30 kDa stress protein; it is worth mentioning that calcium antagonists as well are able to trigger the synthesis of this protein.[231]

IMPAIRMENT OF SUBSTRATE UTILIZATION AND MITOCHONDRIAL FUNCTION BY REACTIVE OXYGEN SPECIES IN CARDIOMYOCYTES

Morphological alterations of mitochondria are uniformly part of the ROS-induced damage in CMs (see Fig. 4.31). As a possible functional correlate, oxidation of the main substrates like glucose, lactate and octanoate was found to be inhibited to up to 70%;[232] furthermore, a mitochondrial key enzyme, pyruvate dehydrogenase, is inactivated in adult rat CMs by exposure to hydrogen peroxide.[221] Such disturbance of oxidative metabolism might explain the decrease in high-energy substrates observed under these circumstances (Fig. 4.29). On the other hand, the mitochondrion seems to be an organelle relatively resistant to ROS, as mitochondrial transmembrane potential collapses only after severe challenge with ROS.[218]

Glycolysis seems to be inhibited by ROS as well; this can be deduced from the finding of increased concentrations of sugar diphosphates in adult rat ventricular CMs exposed to hydroxyl radicals, accompanied by ATP depletion and cellular rigor.[210]

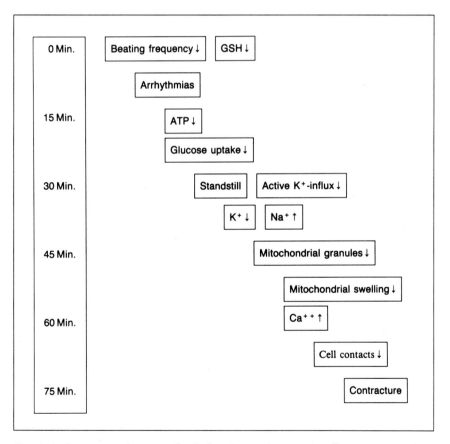

Fig. 4.29. Sequence of contractile dysfunction and cytotoxic effects in neonatal rat cardiomyocytes induced by reactive oxygen species (xanthine/xanthine oxidase system). For further explanation see refs. 205,227,228. (Reproduced with permission from: Werdan K, Müller U, Reithmann C. "Negative inotropic cascades" in cardiomyocytes triggered by substances relevant to sepsis. In: Schlag G, Redl H, eds. Pathophysiology of Shock, Sepsis, and Organ Failure. Berlin, Heidelberg: Springer-Verlag, 1993: 787-832.)

CELL MEMBRANE AND SARCOPLASMIC RETICULUM AS TARGETS FOR REACTIVE OXYGEN SPECIES IN CARDIOMYOCYTES

Irrespective of the cell type investigated (adult rabbit, rat, dog and guinea pig CMs, neonatal rat CMs) and the reactive oxygen species applied (X/XO and dihydroxyfumaric acid systems; H_2O_2; $FeCl_2$; rose bengal photoactivation), a concordant pattern of oxygen-radical-induced derangement of membrane potential emerges; initially, the voltage of the action potential becomes more positive,[233] and the duration of the action potential increases.[211,212,216,233] In this initial phase, an enhancement in contractility can be observed.[216] In the following, early and late after depolarizations occur[211,212,216,233] in combinations with after contractions.[216] Subsequently, a decrease in the duration of action potential duration ensues[211,214,216,233] in association with a decrease in con-

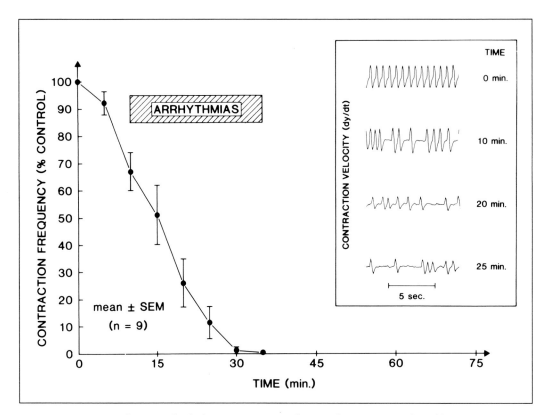

Fig. 4.30. Sequence of contractile dysfunction in neonatal rat cardiomyocytes induced by reactive oxygen species (xanthine/xanthine oxidase system). Starting at t = 0 minutes, neonatal rat CMs have been incubated with reactive oxygen species (X/XO system); during the following observation period, beating frequency and contraction velocity of the cells have been monitored with an electrooptical system.[115] For further explanantion see text and refs. 205,227,228. (Reproduced with permission from: Werdan K, Müller U, Reithmann C. "Negative inotropic cascades" in cardiomyocytes triggered by substances relevant to sepsis. In: Schlag G, Redl H, eds. Pathophysiology of Shock, Sepsis, and Organ Failure. Berlin, Heidelberg: Springer-Verlag, 1993: 787-832.)

tractility.[216] Finally, depolarization and inexcitability of the CM arises.[211,214,216,226,233] These membrane disturbances may fully account for the arrhythmias observed (Fig. 4.30).

So far, the mechanisms underlying these membrane disturbances are not fully recognized; some equivocal results concerning Na^+-, K^+ and Ca^{2+}-currents have been reported.[210-212,216,219,226,233] Flux measurements document inhibition of the sodium pump (Fig. 4.29) and the Na^+,Ca^{2+}-exchanger,[208] while L-type Ca^{2+} channels appear to be unaffected by ROS, at least by hydrogen peroxide.[216] This is in some contrast to findings in rat heart membranes, where a decrease in the number of calcium channels by ROS has been demonstrated.[234] Data on the effects of ROS on the β-adrenoceptor/G protein/adenylyl cyclase system are available for rat heart membranes,[235] but are scarce for isolated CMs. However, a reduction in adenylyl cyclase activity in neonatal rat CMs has been documented.[197] It remains to be clarified, which species of ROS account(s) for the detrimental effect on membrane potential, and to inquire into the contribution of $O_2\cdot^-$, H_2O_2 and $OH\cdot$.[208,211,212,216,233]

Uniformly, a rise of intracellular Ca^{2+} up to 3- to 7-fold in combination with a depression of Ca^{2+}-transients has been reported.[209,210,236,237] Calcium overload, preceding cellular depletion of ATP, and contractile dysfunction can be prevented by the calcium channel blocker nitrendipine.[210] The available data show that this cytoplasmic Ca^{2+} increase is either due to a stimulation of calcium influx through voltage-gated calcium channels[210] and/or an enhanced stimulation of Ca^{2+} release from the sarcoplasmic reticulum[237] in combination with an impairment in cellular Ca^{2+} extrusion mechanisms[237] and, as shown in the rat heart, an inhibition of sarcoplasmic Ca^{2+}-ATPase.[222] The occurrence of delayed aftercontractions early in the time-course of exposure to ROS has been attributed to a ryanodine-sensitive Ca^{2+} efflux from the sarcoplasmic reticulum.[216] Synoptically the question, whether this rise in cellular Ca^{2+} reflects indeed an early causative event, or merely an epiphenomenon of irreversible cell damage, awaits solution (Fig. 4.29).

SENSITIZATION OF CARDIOMYOCYTES TO REACTIVE OXYGEN SPECIES BY GLUTATHIONE DEPLETION

When spontaneously beating neonatal rat CMs are exposed to ROS produced by X/XO, a depletion in reduced glutathione (GSH) (fall of GSH from 23 to 8 nmol/mg cell protein) and increase in the percentage of oxidized glutathione (as GSH-equivalent: 3 vs 54)[238] is one of the early biochemical events[220] and shows a close temporal relationship with the impairment of contractility (Fig. 4.29). In order to establish a model for testing a possible protective action of GSH against oxygen reactive species, neonatal rat CMs were depleted of glutathione (23 vs 2 nmol/mg cell protein) by a 24-hour-incubation with 1 mM

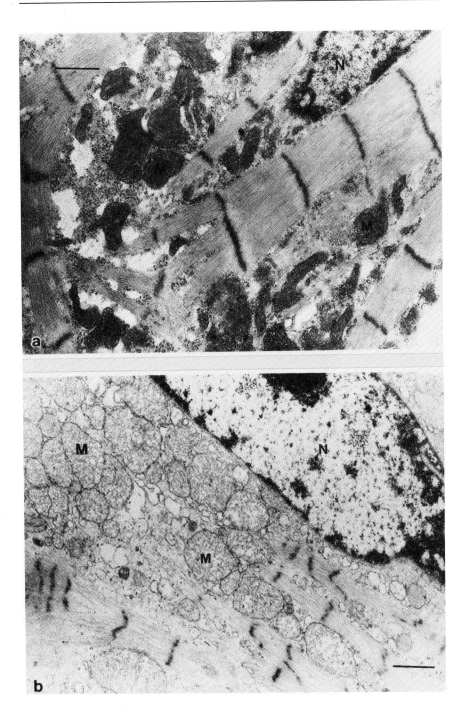

buthionine sulfoximine (BSO), an inhibitor of the τ-glutamyl-cysteinyl-synthetase;[238] in agreement with the findings obtained by Timerman et al (1990),[220] the depletion does not influence the ATP/ADP-ratio (10.5 vs 10.1) and the spontaneous contractile activity of the CMs. This depletion of cellular glutathione leads to a sensitization against ROS; arrhythmias (from 5 minutes) as well as a standstill of the cells (from 20 minutes) and the oxygen-radical induced fall in potassium contents (600 vs 400 nmol/mg protein after 30 minutes) occur earlier, and the decrease in GSH is even more pronounced. These data allow for the following conclusions to be drawn:[220,238] (a) A reduction of GSH to 10% of the control value even after 24 hours does not impair the spontaneous activity, the ATP/ADP-ratio and the potassium contents of neonatal rat CMs; (b) The depletion of GSH is not primarily responsible for the ROS-induced reduction of contractility; (c) The sensitization of rat CMs by BSO documents the protective effect of GSH towards ROS.

PROTECTION OF CARDIOMYOCYTES FROM REACTIVE OXYGEN SPECIES

Protection of CMs from detrimental effects of ROS can be accomplished at different steps of the cascade: prevention of nascent ROS, e.g., by allopurinol in the X/XO system,[208] inactivation of superoxide anion radicals by superoxide dismutase [207,208,212,214,233,239-241] and of hydrogen peroxide by catalase,[207,208,212,214,217,233,239] inactivation of hydroxyl radicals,[210,214,216,239] by antioxidants,[207,214,215,217,230,236,237] and also by other pharmacological agents like nitroxide stable radicals,[241] beta blockers[213] and calcium antagonists,[210,216,224,239] with yet not fully understood mechanisms of protection.

For example, the effects of allopurinol, superoxide dismutase and catalase on X/XO-generated ROS (Fig. 4.32) in neonatal rat CMs are shown; allopurinol as xanthine oxidase inhibitor and catalase, by degrading hydrogen peroxide, clearly demonstrate protection of ROS-induced cell depletion of ATP, while superoxide dismutase does not. By these data, hydrogen peroxide, the hydroxyl radical or other successor

---

Fig. 4.31. Opposite page: Ultrastructural alterations of neonatal rat cardiomyocytes induced by reactive oxygen species (xanthine/xanthine oxidase system) during an incubation period of 75 minutes (picture below); control (picture above). After the incubation period, CMs were fixed in 6.25% glutaraldehyde, washed in 0.2 M saccharose and embedded in epon resin. Electron microscopic observation was made with ultrathin sections contrasted with Pb- and uranyl acetate solution (G. Hübner, Institute of Pathology, University of Munich, Germany). Magnification: 8200 x 2.5 (a), 6800 x 2.5 (b). "M" = mitochondria, "N" = nucleus. The bar represents 1 μm. For further explanantion see text and refs. 205,228. (Reproduced with permission from: Werdan K, Müller U, Reithmann C. "Negative inotropic cascades" in cardiomyocytes triggered by substances relevant to sepsis. In: Schlag G, Redl H, eds. Pathophysiology of Shock, Sepsis, and Organ Failure. Berlin, Heidelberg: Springer-Verlag, 1993: 787-832.)

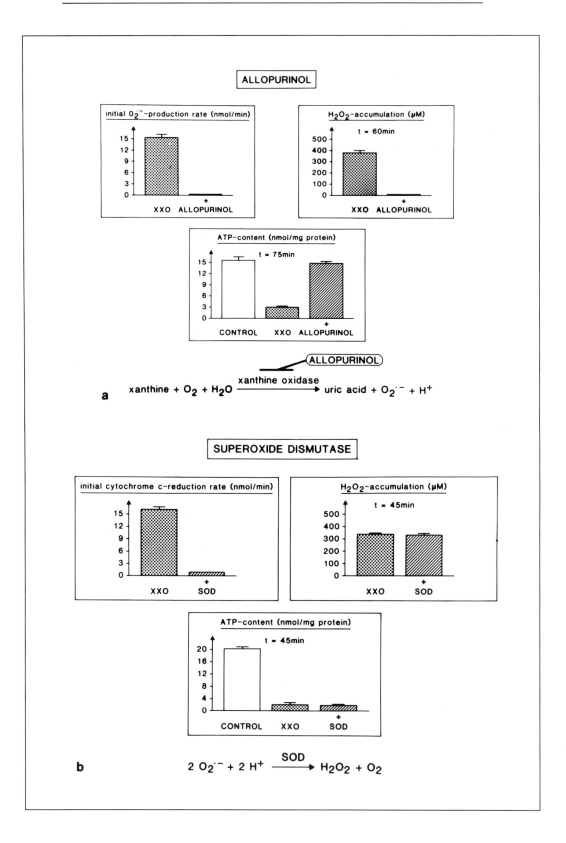

products, but not the superoxide anion radical per se, can be identified as the most relevant toxic ROS in this system.

Experiments like those described in Figure 4.32 might help identify the causative agent within the ROS-family and determine its mechanism of toxic action for a certain detrimental effect within the CM type tested; moreover, with an experimental setup of this kind protective agents can be examined with respect to their "therapeutic efficacy" at the cellular level.

CONCLUSIONS

ROS can impair heart function by direct effects on CMs. Phenomenologically, the cascade of contractility-depressant and cytotoxic events has been characterized in adult as well as in neonatal CMs of various species, a further discrimination between causal events and

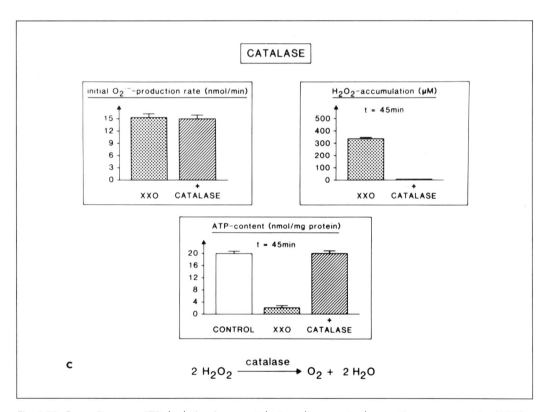

Fig. 4.32. Opposite page: ATP depletion in neonatal rat cardiomyocytes by reactive oxygen species (ROS)—protective effect of allopurinol, superoxide dismutase and catalase. Neonatal rat cardiomyocytes were exposed to the ROS creating xanthine/xanthine oxidase system, either in the absence or presence of allopurinol (1 mM), superoxide dismutase (100 U/ml) or catalase (100 U/ml). Under every condition, initial superoxide anion production was measured, as well as the final hydrogen peroxide concentration and cellular ATP content at the times indicated. For further experimental details see text and ref. 228. (Reproduced with permission from: Werdan K, Müller U, Reithmann C. "Negative inotropic cascades" in cardiomyocytes triggered by substances relevant to sepsis. In: Schlag G, Redl H, eds. Pathophysiology of Shock, Sepsis, and Organ Failure. Berlin, Heidelberg: Springer-Verlag, 1993: 787-832.)

epiphenomena being one of the tasks for the future. Up to now, little attention has been paid to the detrimental effects of ROS on nuclear acid metabolism and protein synthesis.[242,243]

In isolated CMs, hydrogen peroxide or successor products like the hydroxyl radical play a much more prominent role than the superoxide anion radical as causative agents, at least in adult and neonatal rat CMs (Fig. 4.32).[217] With isolated heart preparations, however, results are somewhat conflicting; findings supporting the primary pathogenetic importance of H_2O_2[244,245] are contradicted by data which argue for the superoxide anion as being the most relevant negative inotropic species.[246] This discrepancy may possibly point to the problem of direct versus indirect effects of ROS in the heart, taking into account different sensitivities of heart muscle cells, fibroblasts and endothelial cells for various ROS.[207]

In a dog model of myocardial reperfusion injury, quantitative measurements document the invasion of the myocardium by leukocytes amounting to about 2000-6000 neutrophils/mg myocardial tissue (about 6-fold of control).[202] The quantity of ROS produced by this accumulation of leukocytes should equal the amount of ROS necessary to produce the detrimental effects as described.[229] There are significant data arguing for a contribution of oxygen free radicals to the pathogenesis of organ dysfunction due to sepsis and septic shock.[247,248] However, a body of evidence allowing for a quantitative evaluation of ROS production in acute septic cardiomyopathy, analogous to myocardial reperfusion injury, is lacking, which limits the relevance of the in vitro findings presented for the in vivo situation.

ENDORPHINS

RATIONALE
In patients with sepsis, as well as in cynomolgus monkeys with endotoxic shock, plasma levels of β-endorphins are about 5-fold increased.[249] A pathogenic role of endogenous opiates (for discussion see ref. 250) is substantiated by data showing that the opiate receptor antagonist naloxone may increase lowered blood pressure and exert a positive inotropic effect both in septic patients[251] and in endotoxemic cynomolgus monkeys in a septic state (increase in LV dP/dt_{max} by 22%).[249] This finding, however, is discussed controversially. Likewise, in isolated heart preparations, contradictory results have been obtained concerning the inotropic effects of opiates and opioid peptides (for review see ref. 252). Also, the positive inotropic effect of the antagonist naloxone was found to be at best moderate.[249,250]

OPIATE RECEPTOR-MEDIATED EFFECTS IN CARDIOMYOCYTES
Binding experiments[252] with (^{3}H)naloxone in embryonic chicken CMs reveal the presence of about 10^4 opiate binding sites per cell (47 fmol/mg protein) with a dissociation constant (K_D) of 18 nM. Oc-

cupation of these opiate binding sites by enkephalins results in a positive "inotropic" effect of about 30%, the mechanism of action being unknown. Receptor displacement of enkephalins by naloxone abolishes this positive "inotropic" effect, naloxone itself being without intrinsic activity.

In cultured rat CMs, the μ-selective opioid antagonists naloxone and levallorphan induce positive "inotropic" effects, a modest increase in Ca^{2+}-transients and a calcium sensitization of the myofibrils; the μ-selective opioid agonists morphine and levorphanol decrease calcium sensitivity of the myofibrils, with a negative "inotropic" (levorphanol) or no effect (morphine) on contractility.[253]

In adult rat CMs, δ- and K-, but not μ-opioid agonists have negative "inotropic" effects and decrease Ca^{2+}-transients.[254] The stimulation of K opioid receptors increases inositol phosphate production, and the ensuing negative "inotropic" effect is, at least in part, due to Ca^{2+}-depletion of the sarcoplasmic reticulum.[255,256]

In cardiac membrane preparations, opioid peptides inhibit the sarcolemmal ouabain-sensitive Na^+-K^+-ATPase and Ca^+-dependent ATPase[257] and stimulate sarcolemmal NAD(P)H-vanadate dehydrogenase.[257] The relevance of these findings in the intact CMs remains to be clarified.

CONCLUSIONS

No direct negative "inotropic" effect of enkephalins and no direct positive "inotropic" effect of naloxone can be demonstrated in embryonic chicken CMs.[252] These findings are in agreement with the concept that increased plasma endorphin levels depress heart function in an indirect manner, namely by attenuation of the action of catecholamines,[249] and that also naloxone exerts its positive inotropic effect indirectly, by potentiating adrenergic stimuli in heart cells.[249,259]

At present it remains speculative, whether the direct opioid-receptor mediated effects described in some CM preparations necessitate a revision and extension of this concept.

ADDITIONAL ALTERATIONS OF NEUROHUMORAL, AUTOCRINE AND PARACRINE SYSTEMS

RATIONALE

Apart from the hormones and mediators discussed in the preceding chapters, modulation of inotropy is to be expected from the activation of several other neurohumoral axes and autocrine/paracrine systems in sepsis.

RENIN/ANGIOTENSIN II

Throughout the course of endotoxin shock, plasma concentrations of renin and angiotensin II are substantially elevated, as high as 12-fold in the case of renin.[260] This may eventually entail tachyphylaxis.[260-262]

The heart is one of the target organs of angiotensin II (for review see ref. 263).

In neonatal rat CMs, angiotensin II binds to high affinity receptors.[264] In the nanomolar range, it increases beating frequency with a concomitant decrease in pulsation amplitude and a decrease in contraction as well as in relaxation velocity.[265,266] In voltage-clamped cells, calcium current is augmented[265] and sodium channels are modulated.[267] Phosphoinositide hydrolysis is stimulated by angiotensin II, as opposed to basal and isoproterenol-stimulated adenylyl cyclase activity and cAMP accumulation, which are not affected.[265] Experimental evidence argues for protein kinase C as mediator of the action of angiotensin II in rat CMs,[266,267] while in embryonic chicken CMs receptor-coupling to phospholipase C has been documented.[263] A comparison of angiotensin II effects in CMs and isolated heart preparations reveals yet unexplained qualitative differences, for instance with respect to inotropy[265] and coupling to adenylyl cyclase.[268]

ATRIAL NATRIURETIC FACTOR FAMILY

In patients with severe heart failure, plasma atrial natriuretic factor is elevated several-fold (for review see ref. 269). In isolated heart preparations, members of the atriopeptin family depress myocardial performance (see ref. 270).

In neonatal rat CMs, 10 nM atriopeptin II does not affect the frequency of spontaneous contractions, but clearly depresses amplitude of pulsation as well as velocity of contraction and relaxation to about 65% of control.[270] This effect is attributed to receptor-mediated,[270] G_i protein-coupled inhibition of adenylyl cyclase, the resultant fall in cellular cAMP production decreasing Ca^{2+} influx, with consecutive depression of contractility.[270] Of note, the simultaneous stimulation of guanylyl cyclase, that is characteristic of the ANF group, is not the cause of the negative inotropic effect. In contrast to the data reported by McCall,[270] Brenner et al (1987)[36] did not find any effect of atrial natriuretic factor (1 and 5 µg/ml) on contractility.

CALCITONIN GENE-RELATED PEPTIDE

In patients with sepsis, an about 7-fold increase in plasma calcitonin gene-related peptide (CGRP) has been documented (see ref. 272), and in endotoxemic rat, plasma CGRP is raised 7- to 22-fold.[272]

Positive chronotropic and inotropic effects of CGRP have been described in isolated heart preparations,[273] though in dogs, ventricular contractility in vivo was not affected by CGRP.[274] Experiments with isolated CMs might help clarify the equivocal findings.

ENDOTHELIN

In patients with sepsis-syndrome, plasma endothelin levels were found to be 5-fold higher than in healthy volunteers (11.3 vs 2.4 pmol/l).

Peak values (23.8 pmol/l) were measured for anuric septic patients[5]. In accordance, a 6-fold increase in plasma endothelin occurs in endotoxemic pigs (citation 10 in ref. 5).

Endothelin is among the most potent positive inotropic agents yet described in mammalian heart[275,276] coupling to specific cardiac binding sites,[276,277] that are subject to down-regulation in ischemia.[277]

In isolated rat ventricular CMs, endothelin-1 doubles pulsation amplitude of the cells, at an EC_{50} of 50 pM, a value that approximates the reported K_D of endothelin for its cardiac receptors.[275] This positive inotropic action of endothelin is partly due to a stimulation of the sarcolemmal Na^+-H^+ exchanger via the protein kinase C-mediated pathway, resulting in a rise in pH_i and sensitization of cardiac myofilaments to intracellular Ca^{2+}.[275] In this cascade, a G protein is involved.[278,279] Endothelin action is reduced or abolished by previous exposure of the cells to β-adrenergic agonists.[279]

5-HYDROXYTRYPTAMINE (SEROTONIN)

5-Hydroxytryptamine (5-HT) is released from platelets and from splanchnic visceral organs during the early phase following endotoxin administration, with a rapid return to near control within minutes and a marked decrease thereafter. Its role in the pathogenesis of endotoxin shock appears to be negligible in most species.[261]

5-HT can directly and indirectly modify both the rate and force of contraction in cardiac tissue, including human atria, via an interaction with several 5-HT receptor subtypes.[280-282]

In cultured fetal mouse ventricular myocytes, 5-HT stimulates spontaneous beating via $5-HT_2$ receptors,[281] which are coupled to phospholipase C via a pertussis toxin-insensitive GTP binding protein. Stimulation of $5-HT_2$ receptors results in phospholipase C-mediated hydrolysis of phosphoinositides in these cells, which is counteracted by protein kinase C.[281]

NEUROPEPTIDE Y

Neuropeptide Y (NPY) is colocalized with norepinephrine in many central and peripheral neurons, including the nervous fibers of heart tissue. Plasma concentrations of NPY in 5 patients with septic shock were found to be at least 10-fold increased (47.5 vs ≤ 5 pmol/l).[283] Also, in rats with induced endotoxin shock, plasma NPY levels are raised by 67%, both 30 minutes and 3 hours after toxin administration.[272]

NPY exerts positive chronotropic and inotropic effects in the heart.[284,285]

In adult rat atrial CMs, NPY inhibits β-adrenoceptor-stimulated as well as receptor-independent adenylyl cyclase activity via a pertussis toxin-sensitive pathway, with about half maximal inhibition occurring at 10 nM and maximal inhibition being 40%.[286] In neonatal rat ventricular CMs, chronic exposure of the cells to NPY (10^{-7}M) for 96 hours mimics the onset of sympathetic innervation during ontogeny in switching the α_1-adrenergic chronotropic response from a positive to a negative one.[287]

THROMBIN

Conditions that promote thrombosis and activate coagulation should promote increases in local concentrations of thrombin, although its normal concentration in the blood and extracellular space is unknown.[288]

In isolated frog ventricular cells, thrombin has a positive "inotropic" effect, which has been ascribed to stimulation of the voltage-dependent calcium current.[289] In embryonic chicken CMs, thrombin (1 U/ml) increases both systolic and diastolic $(Ca^{2+})_i$, associated with a rise in force of contraction, beating frequency and action potential duration. Both the increase in $(Ca^{2+})_i$, which is partly due to intracellular Ca^{2+} release, and the thrombin-induced increase in cellular inositol triphosphates are mediated by a pertussis toxin-sensitive G-protein-receptor mechanism.[288]

CONCLUSIONS

The substances discussed in this chapter are, at present, not in the limelight, when septic cardiomyopathy's pathogenesis is discussed. The documented or suspected variations in their plasma and tissue levels might well result in positive or negative cardiac inotropy, either by their own action or by interference with the cardiac effects of other mediators.

With regard to several other candidates potentially affecting myocardial function in sepsis, e.g., histamine,[261] alterations in plasma levels of glucocorticoids, thyroid hormones and vasopressin, the presently available data obtained with CMs are scarce. To the question of histamine release in septic/endotoxic shock there is still a nonconclusive answer.[290]

ACTIVATED BLOOD CELLS

RATIONALE

Critically ill anergic surgical patients with life threatening infections were shown to have increased intravascular activation of polymorphonuclear leukocytes (PMN) which may contribute to oxygen-derived tissue damage in multiple organ failure.[291] Also, in patients with severe trauma, a stimulation of neutrophil oxidative burst (O_2^- production) has been demonstrated.[292] In isolated rat hearts, activated PMN infused into the coronary circulation (about 3×10^5cells/ml) depress cardiac function and increase vascular resistance due to ROS production.[293] These data may suggest a possible involvement of activated leukocytes in myocardial depression in sepsis.

DEPRESSION OF CONTRACTILE FUNCTION IN CARDIOMYOCYTES BY POLYMORPHONUCLEAR LEUKOCYTES

In vitro stimulation of human PMN by 1 nM phorbol-myristate-acetate (PMA) results in an oxidative burst lasting for at least 30 minutes. When coincubated (about 10^6 cells/ml) with spontaneously beating monolayer cultures (ratio 3:1) of neonatal rat CMs, the leukocytes attach to the CMs. Within minutes, arrhythmias occur, and a decrease in contractile function and beating frequency can be observed, with a final standstill of the contractions at about 30 minutes (Fig. 4.33). Separating CMs and PMN by semipermeable membranes during this coincubation allows for a biochemical evaluation of the leucocyte-induced cytotoxicity (e.g. loss in cell potassium) in the heart cells. The detrimental effects of PMN in CMs can be attenuated by catalase, but are enhanced by depleting CMs of GSH by BSO pretreatment prior to the challenge by PMN. These results are in favor of a dominant role of ROS or successor products in the pathogenesis of PMN-induced cell damage of the CMs in this coculture model.[294] The impact of a direct contact of both cell types on PMN-induced injury of CMs in this model warrants further investigation.

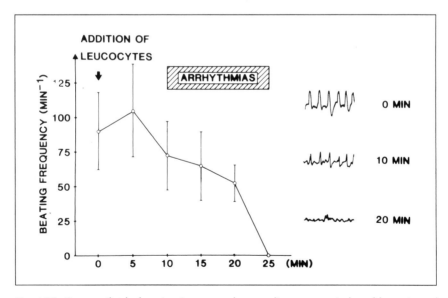

Fig. 4.33. Contractile dysfunction in neonatal rat cardiomyocytes induced by activated polymorphonuclear leukocytes (PMN). Human PMNs, stimulated by phorbol myristate acetate (1 nM), were added to spontaneously beating neonatal rat CMs in culture (ratio 3:1). Thereafter, beating frequency and pulsation amplitude of the CM were monitored by an electrooptical system.[115] For further explanation see ref. 294. (Reproduced with permission from: Werdan K, Müller U, Reithmann C. "Negative inotropic cascades" in cardiomyocytes triggered by substances relevant to sepsis. In: Schlag G, Redl H, eds. Pathophysiology of Shock, Sepsis, and Organ Failure. Berlin, Heidelberg: Springer-Verlag, 1993: 787-832.)

In correspondence to the data described, injury of beating neonatal mouse CMs by PMN was observed during reoxygenation.[295]

INTERACTION OF POLYMORPHONUCLEAR LEUKOCYTES WITH CARDIOMYOCYTES—ROLE OF ADHESION MOLECULES

PMN accumulation, transendothelial migration and adherence to CMs is mediated by several adhesion molecules located on the cell membrane surface of neutrophils and of the target cell (for review see ref. 296). As to the interaction of canine PMN with adult canine ventricular CMs, the course of events has been identified.[296-298] Prerequisite of a strong adhesion is stimulation of both cell types; CMs have to be activated with cytokines like IL-1 and TNF-α, which results in an enhanced protein synthesis, and PMN are stimulated chemotactically. Peak adherence develops within 4 hours after initiation of cytokine treatment. Strong adhesion at a neutrophil/myocyte ratio of 10:1 triggers oxidative burst (H_2O_2 production) at least 20-fold, often associated with contracture of the CMs. An anti-CD 18 monoclonal antibody (R15.7) inhibited stimulated PMN-myocyte adhesion by more than 95% and reduced H_2O_2 production by more than 90%. The adhesion molecule located on the CMs has been identified as ICAM-1, whereas CD18 forms part of the integrins of neutrophils.

These results indicate that sepsis mediators may trigger a strong PMN-CM interaction which can be counteracted by intervention with specific monoclonal antibodies against adhesion molecules.

TOXIC ACTIONS OF EOSINOPHILS IN CARDIOMYOCYTES

Supernatants of zymosan-C3b-stimulated eosinophils obtained from blood of patients with the hypereosinophilic syndrome exert cytotoxicity in adult rat ventricular CMs.[299] This is characterized by an initial increase in the membrane permeability, which may secondarily activate (Na^++K^+)ATPase and increase O_2 uptake. However, toxicity also involves inhibition of pyruvate and oxoglutarate dehydrogenase, but not of lipoamide dehydrogenase, thus entailing a decreased O_2 uptake. The most likely agents accounting for these detrimental effects are the cationic proteins of eosinophils. It is suggested that these mechanisms could contribute to the development of cardiac injury and myocardial disease in clinical situations where many degranulated eosinophils are present.[299]

CARDIOMYOCYTE INJURY AND CONTRACTILE DYSFUNCTION PRODUCED BY CYTOTOXIC T LYMPHOCYTES

Coculture of monolayers of spontaneously beating CMs from fetal mice with sensitized mouse cytotoxic T lymphocytes results in an allospecific cell membrane damage of the CMs, detectable within 1 hour of exposure by ^{51}Cr release, with a maximum by 3-5 hours of coincubation. Myocyte lysis was preceded by an altered myocyte contractile motion (early decrease in amplitude, subsequent development of irregular beating, followed by complete cessation of contraction). This cell injury was calcium dependent; it was prevented by pretreatment of lymphocytes with phorbol ester to deplete protein kinase C, and experiments with antibodies favor involvement of CD8+ cytotoxic T cells.[300]

Lytic granules extracted from cytotoxic T lymphocytes or a purified lytic protein (perforin, 65 kDa) thereof, induces distinct shortening of action potential duration in isolated CMs, probably caused by an attenuation of the L-type Ca^{2+} current and an increase in outward current in the plateau range of membrane potentials. Fura-2 imaging of affected cells shows a doubling of $(Ca^{2+})_i$ prior to significant changes in cell size. Further increase in $(Ca^{2+})_i$ is associated with progressive contracture and destruction of the CMs, suggesting damage to be due to $(Ca^{2+})_i$ overload.[301]

The coincubation models described might be useful to study at the cellular level, the pathogenetic role of cytotoxic T lymphocytes in acute viral myocarditis[301,302] and also in rejection after heart transplantation.[300,301] The data strongly suggest that the expression of MHC class I antigens induced by interferon[127] and killer cells[302] causes the interaction between CMs and T lymphocytes[128,302] and that cytotoxic T lymphocytes in particular may contribute to myocardial damage launched by viral infection.[128]

EFFECT OF PLATELET RELEASE PRODUCTS ON CYTOSOLIC CALCIUM IN CARDIOMYOCYTES

In chick embryonic CMs, cell free filtrate of release products from rabbit platelets activated with thrombin or collagen causes a rapid increase in both systolic and diastolic $(Ca^{2+})_i$ in a dose-dependent manner. This might predispose the cells to arrhythmias. The yet unidentified substance(s) has(have) a low molecular weight (less than 3 kDa) and are thought to represent peptide(s).[303] Though evidence for platelet activation in sepsis has been presented,[304] the relevance of this phenomenon is still unclear.

CONCLUSIONS

With respect to acute septic cardiomyopathy, the activated PMN is the most likely candidate of all blood cell species described which might exert detrimental cardiodepression. The coculture models presented document a direct impairment of contractility and also cytotoxicity in CMs by the PMN action. They build the basis for a further elucidation of the pathogenetic role of mediators secreted and the mechanisms involved. In this context, ROS and successor products, e.g., hydrochloric acid, seem to be of primary importance.[202,305-308] In the target cells, specific metabolic alterations are induced, e.g., inhibition of Ca^{2+}-ATPase activity and of calcium uptake into the sarcoplasmic reticulum.[306] So far, activation of PMN in these experiments is induced by PMA in most cases; with respect to septic cardiomyopathy, it will be of major interest, if various toxins of Gram-negative as well as of Gram-positive bacteria also activate PMN to such an extent that contractile dysfunction of neighboring CMs occurs.

Analyzing the significance of activated PMN, much more is known for myocardial reperfusion injury[202,298] than for acute septic cardiomyopathy; in the postischemic dog heart, a 6-fold rise in neutrophils can be found, amounting to about 6000 neutrophils/mg heart tissue.[202] Depletion of leukocytes by various measures results in a reduction in infarct size of about 50%, which underlines the crucial role of PMN in myocardial ischemia/reperfusion injury.[202] The in vitro experiments presented mimic the clinical setting, as neutrophil concentrations are in the same order of magnitude. Injury of the CMs by activated PMN in vitro demonstrates that the number of PMN accumulated in the postischemic heart in principle suffices for a marked detrimental effect. The abundance of data available for myocardial reperfusion injury does not meet the findings reported about septic cardiomyopathy, thus leaving the relevance of neutrophil-induced injury of CMs in sepsis, at present, an open question.

ENERGY DEPLETION (See also chapter 7)

RATIONALE

^{31}P magnetic resonance spectroscopy reveals a 20% decrease in phosphocreatine/ATP ratios in gastrocnemius muscle of rats in the early phase of sepsis, associated with a quantitatively similar increase in phosphocreatine breakdown. In this early state, ATP concentrations remained constant, and intracellular pH did not change significantly.[309] These data argue for an increased ATP utilization in sepsis to help maintain ionic balance and/or support other metabolic processes, with phosphocreatine stores used to buffer ATP concentrations. In agreement with this finding, increased levels of ATP degradation products can be demonstrated in plasma of patients with sepsis.[310]

With respect to the heart, most data at present argue for a maintenance of normal[311,312] or even elevated[313] ATP levels in sepsis, despite the proven alterations in substrate utilization.[314,315]

IN VITRO MODELS OF ENERGY-DEPLETED CARDIOMYOCYTES

Short-term models (e.g., 1-3 hours)[316] as well as long-term models (e.g., 24 hours)[317] of energy depletion can be established by incubation or cultivation of adult or neonatal/embryonic CMs in the presence of metabolic inhibitors of glycolysis and/or oxidative phosphorylation (e.g. potassium cyanide,[318] iodoacetamide[316,319,320] and iodoacetic acid,[316,319] carbonyl cyanide p-(trifluoromethoxy)phenylhydrazone (FCCP),[320] carbonyl cyanide m-chlorophenylhydrazone (CCCP),[321] dinitrophenol, 2-deoxy-D-glucose (DOG),[317,320] rotenon,[321] oligomycin[321]).

Depending on the experimental conditions chosen, the cellular damage is reversible or irreversible.[316,317,321] The elegant study of van der Laarse et al (1984)[318] proves the applicability of these in vitro models by comparing them with isolated heart preparations.

Short-time exposure of neonatal rat CMs to 30 µM iodoacetic acid results in a fall of cellular ATP contents to 71% (1-hour-exposure), 26% (2-hour-exposure) and 8% (3-hour-exposure) of control. After a 1-hour-exposure, ATP contents fully recovers within 24 hours; after 3-hour-exposure, however, irreversible cell injury is conspicuous by a persistent low ATP level despite the 24-hour-recovery period, by an 11-fold increase in (^{3}H)-arachidonic acid release as an index of membrane phospholipid degradation, and by severe morphological alterations of cell membrane, nucleus, contractile apparatus and mitochondria.[316]

A long-term ATP depletion model[317,321] is accomplished by incubation of neonatal rat CMs with 5 mM DOG for 24 hours resulting in a fall of cellular ATP to about 50-70% of control, of cellular ADP to about 50%, and of ATP/ADP ratio from about 8 to 5. This moderate ATP depletion does not abolish spontaneous beating of the cells, nor does it produce marked morphological alterations, as documented by electron microscopy. However, (^{3}H)leucine incorporation as a measure of protein synthesis is inhibited by about 30%, and the responsiveness of the β-adrenoceptor/adenylyl cyclase is impaired. The cellular ATP pool fully recovers within 24 hours after removal of the inhibitor.

It is worth mentioning that neonatal rat CMs depleted of ATP by use of metabolic inhibitors or low oxygen partial pressure exhibit high mRNA and protein levels of the stress protein HSP70.[322]

EFFECTS OF ENERGY DEPLETION ON β-ADRENOCEPTOR/ADENYLYL CYCLASE COUPLING IN CARDIOMYOCYTES

ATP depletion impairs the β-adrenoceptor/adenylyl cyclase system of the heart resulting in a disturbed catecholamine-induced positive inotropy. However, the data reported hereof are conflicting (for discussion see ref. 317), describing either a decrease or increase in the number of β-adrenoceptors, as well as either an augmentation or an attenuation of isoproterenol-stimulated adenylyl cyclase activity.

In the long-term ATP depletion model with neonatal rat CMs, however, a clear-cut picture emerges:[317]

A fall in cellular ATP by about 40% due to an incubation with 5 mM DOG goes along with a diminution of the number of β$_1$-adrenoceptors by about 23%, leaving receptor affinity unchanged; isoproterenol-stimulated cAMP formation is reduced by 43%, and forskolin-stimulated cAMP production is even cut down by 81%. In contrast to these results obtained with intact cells, isoproterenol-induced adenylyl cyclase activity is not depressed in crude membrane preparations of CMs after ATP-depletion of the very same manner. The discrepancy in results obtained for intact cells and membrane preparations suggests that apart from direct desensitization of the β-adrenoceptor/G protein/adenylyl cyclase by catecholamines alterations in the intracellular environment, e.g., changes in cellular substrate levels like ATP or GTP, induced by ATP depletion have to be taken into account, when interpreting pathological states. Possibly, the intracellular homeostasis is as relevant as catecholamine-desensitization in this system.

CONCLUSIONS

Both short-term and long-term CM culture models are available to study the effect of energy depletion on heart function. Though well established, these in vitro models need further extension, for instance to elucidate the consequences of a partial ATP depletion on the action of positive inotropic agents like digitalis and α-, β₁- and β₂-sympathomimetic substances. Moreover, the question, to what extent an increase in beating frequency[323] can augment the deleterious effects of partial ATP depletion, awaits clarification.

Based on the published data, a significant degree of myocardial ATP depletion in sepsis seems unlikely. As a 30-50% long-term ATP depletion is relatively well tolerated by CMs, severe cytotoxicity by ATP depletion in sepsis seems unlikely. However, if the finding of an increased ATP turnover in sepsis, as documented in skeletal muscle,[309] might also hold true for the heart, then phenomena like impairment of β-adrenoceptor/adenylyl cyclase and inhibition of protein synthesis could also contribute to cardiac depression in sepsis.

HYPOXIA, REOXYGENATION AND "ISCHEMIA"

RATIONALE

Coronary blood flow in patients with septic shock is preserved. In accordance, data of the net myocardial lactate extraction and the increased availability of oxygen in the myocardium of these patients argue against global ischemia as the cause of myocardial depression in human septic shock.[315,324] This is also supported by results of a peritonitis model of sepsis in the rat.[325]

On the other hand, an "oxygen extraction defect" (for citation see ref. 326) and an increased mean skeletal muscle pO_2[326] in patients with sepsis and septic shock have been described, suggesting some kind of intracellular oxygen consumption defect. With respect to the myocardial pO_2 in septic patients, no data are available yet.

IN VITRO MODELS TO STUDY CONTRACTILE DYSFUNCTION IN HYPOXIA, REOXYGENATION AND "ISCHEMIA" IN CARDIOMYOCYTES

A variety of models with adult and neonatal/embryonic CMs has been established to mimic hypoxic and "ischemic" (stasis, substrate deprivation, pH shifts, rise in potassium, and so on) conditions of the heart and to study reperfusion-induced myocardial injury. It is beyond the scope of this article to fully discuss this topic. The interested reader is referred to the articles cited below, dealing preferentially with the pathogenesis,[327,328] the role of acidosis,[329] the ultrastructural damage,[330] the alterations of α-adrenoceptors[331] and β-adrenoceptors,[332] the effects on phospholipid metabolism and prostacyclin synthesis[188,333] and the heterogeneity of contractile dysfunction of individual cells[334] of these conditions.

CONCLUSIONS

Even if coronary blood flow is not suppressed in sepsis, inter- and intracellular myocardial edema[335] could favor cellular hypoxia. The CM models available offer the possibility to reevaluate the effects of bacterial toxins and sepsis mediators on the CM. There might be a different reactivity in the normoxic versus the hypoxic/ischemic state, as has been shown, for instance, for the catecholamine desensitization of the β-adrenoceptor/G protein/adenylyl cyclase system.[336]

REFERENCES

1. Pardini BJ, Jones SB, Filkins JC. Cardiac and splenic norepinephrine turnovers in endotoxic rats. Am J Physiol 1983; 245: H276-H283.
2. Jones SB, Romano FD. Plasma catecholamines in the conscious rat during endotoxicosis. Circ Shock 1984; 14:189-201.
3. Shepherd RE, Lang CH, McDonough KH. Myocardial adrenergic responsiveness after lethal and nonlethal doses of endotoxin. Am J Physiol 1987; 252:H410-H416.
4. Schlag G, Redl H, Hallström S et al. Hyperdynamic sepsis in baboons: I. aspects of hemodynamics. Circ Shock 1991; 34:311-318.
5. Weitzberg E, Lundberg JM, Rudehill A. Elevated plasma levels of endothelin in patients with sepsis syndrome. Circ Shock 1991; 33:222-227.
6. Parratt JR. Myocardial and circulatory effects of *E. coli* endotoxin: modification of responses to catecholamines. Br J Pharmacol 1973; 47:12-25.
7. Romano FD, Jones SB. Beta-adrenergic stimulation of myocardial cyclic AMP in endotoxic rats. Circ Shock 1985; 17:243-252.
8. Smith LW, Winbery SL, Barker LA et al. Cardiac function and chronotropic sensitivity to β-adrenergic stimulation in sepsis. Am J Physiol 1986; 251:H405-H412.
9. Jones SB, Romano FD. Myocardial beta adrenergic receptor coupling to adenylate cyclase during developing septic shock. Circ Shock 1990; 30: 51-61.
10. Bristow MR, Port JD, Sandoval AB et al. β-adrenergic receptor pathways in the failing human heart. Heart Failure 1989; 5:77-90.
11. Romano FD, Jones SB. Characteristics of myocardial β-adrenergic receptors during endotoxicosis in the rat. Am J Physiol 1986; 251: R359-R364.

12. Eisinger MR, Jones SB, Westfall MV et al. Myocardial beta adrenergic receptors in *E. coli* induced septic shock. In: Bond RF, ed. Perspectives in Shock Research. Alan R. Liss, New York, pp 319-324 (Progress in Clinical and Biological Research, vol 264) 1988.

13. Carmona RH, Tsao T, Dae M et al. Myocardial dysfunction in septic shock. Arch Surg 1984; 120:30-35.

14. Reithmann C, Werdan K. Homologous vs. heterologous desensitization of the adenylate cyclase system in chicken heart muscle cells. Eur J Pharmacol 1988; 154:99-104.

15. Werdan K, Reithmann C. Neonatale und embryonale Herzmuskelzellen als Myokardmodell—Regulation kardialer Rezeptoren. Thieme, Stuttgart New York 1987.

16. Marsh JD, Barry WH, Neer EJ et al. Desensitization of chick embryo ventricle to the physiological and biochemical effects of isoproterenol. Circ Res 1980; 47:493-501.

17. Marsh JD, Lachance D, Kim D. Mechanisms of β-adrenergic receptor regulation in cultured chick heart cells—role of cytoskeleton function and protein synthesis. Circ Res 1985; 57:171-181.

18. Bobik A, Campbell JH, Carson V et al. Mechanism of isoprenaline-induced refractoriness of the β-adrenoceptor-adenylate cyclase system in chick embryo cardiac cells. J Cardiovasc Pharmacol 1981; 3:541-553.

19. Bobik A, Little PJ. Role of cyclic AMP in cardiac β-adrenoceptor desensitization: studies using prenalterol and inhibitors of phosphodiesterase. J Cardiovas Pharmacol 1984; 6: 795-801.

20. Karliner JS, Simpson PC, Honbo N et al. Mechanisms and time course of β_1 adrenoceptor desensitization in mammalian cardiac myocytes. Cardiovasc Res 1986; 20:221-228.

21. Limas CJ, Limas C. Rapid recovery of cardiac β-adrenergic receptors after isoproterenol-induced "down-regulation". Circ Res 1984; 55:524-531.

22. Reithmann C, Werdan K. Noradrenaline-induced desensitization in cultured heart cells as a model for the defects of the adenylate cyclase system in severe heart failure. Naunyn-Schmiedeberg's Arch Pharmacol 1989; 339:138-144.

23. Reithmann C, Gierschik P, Sidiropulos D et al. Mechanism of noradrenaline-induced heterologous desensitization of adenylate cyclase stimulation in rat heart muscle cells: increase in the level of inhibitory G-protein α-subunits. Europ J Pharmacol-Mol Pharmacol Section 1989; 172:211-221.

24. Reithmann C, Hallström S, Pilz G et al. Desensitization of rat cardiomyocyte adenylyl cyclase stimulation by plasma of noradrenaline-treated patients with septic shock. Circ Shock 1993; 41:48-59.

25. Jones SM, Kirby MS, Harding SE et al. Adriamycin cardiomyopathy in the rabbit: alterations in contractile proteins and myocyte function. Cardiovasc Res 1991; 24:834-842.

26. Vescovo G, Jones SM, Harding SE et al. Isoproterenol sensitivity of isolated cardiac myocytes from rats with monocrotaline-induced right-sided

hypertrophy and heart failure. J Mol Cell Cardiol 1989; 21:1047-1061.

27. Harding SE, Jones SM, O'Gara P et al. Reduced β-agonist sensitivity in single atrial cells from failing human hearts. Am J Physiol 1990; 259:H1009-H1014.

28. Limas CJ, Goldenberg IF, Limas C. Autoantibodies against β-adrenoceptors in human idiopathic dilated cardiomyopathy. Circ Res 1989; 64:97-103.

29. Limas CJ, Goldenberg IF, Limas C. Effect of antireceptor antibodies in dilated cardiomyopathy on the cycling of cardiac beta receptors. Am Heart J 1991; 122:108-114.

30. Wallukat G, Morwinski R, Kowal K et al. Autoantikörper gegen myokardiale β-Adrenozeptoren im Serum von Patienten mit Myokarditis (MC) und dilativer Kardiomyopathie (DCM): β-adrenerger Agonismus ohne Desensibilisierung. Z Kardiol 1991; 80 (Suppl. 3):141.

31. Wallukat G, Wollenberger A. Circulating autoantibodies from patients with allergic asthma interfering with β₂-adrenoceptor stimulation in cultured neonatal rat heart myocytes. Naunyn-Schmiedeberg's Arch Pharmacol 1991; 344:R99.

32. Suffredini AF, Fromm RE, Parker MM et al. The cardiovascular response of normal humans to the administration of endotoxin. N Engl J Med 1989; 321:280-287.

33. Natanson C, Eichenholz PW, Danner RL et al. Endotoxin and tumor necrosis factor challenges in dogs simulate the cardiovascular profile of human septic shock. J Exp Med 1989; 169:823-832.

34. Cho YW. Direct cardiac action of *E. coli* endotoxin (36856). Proc Soc Exp Biol Med 1972; 141:705-707.

35. Carli A, Auclair MC, Benassayag C et al. Evidence for an early lipid soluble cardiodepressant factor in rat serum after a sublethal dose of endotoxin. Circulatory Shock 1981; 8:301-312.

36. Brenner M, Doerfler ME, Danner RL et al. Determination of direct myocardial contractile effects of eicosanoids, endotoxin, tumor necrosis factor and other mediators using a newly designed quantitative cellular contractile assay. Clin Res 1987; 35:785 A.

37. Hollenberg SM, Cunnion RE, Lawrence M et al. Tumor necrosis factor depresses myocardial cell function: Results using an in vitro assay of myocyte performance. Clin Res 1989; 37:528A.

38. Müller U, Melnitzki SM, Reithmann C et al. Herzmuskelzellkulturen der Ratte: Ein Modell zur Beurteilung kardiotoxischer Effekte von Pseudomonas-aeruginosa-Endotoxin und -Exotoxin A. Intensivmed 1989; 26(Suppl 1):26-31.

39. Werdan K, Melnitzki SM, Pilz G et al. The cultured rat heart cell: a model to study direct cardiotoxic effects of Pseudomonas endo- and exotoxins. In: Schlag G, Redl H, eds. Second Vienna Shock Forum. New York: Alan R Liss, Inc, 1989:247-251 (Progress in Clinical and Biological Research, Vol 308).

40. Melnitzki SM. Direkte Wirkung von Streptokokken- und *Pseudomonas aeruginosa*-Toxinen in kultivierten Ratten-Herzzellen. Medical Thesis, Ludwig-Maximilians-Universität München, Germany 1991.

41. Snell RJ, Parrillo JE. Cardiovascular dysfunction in septic shock. Chest 1991; 99:1000-1009.

42. Werdan K, Müller-Werdan U, Reithmann C et al. Nitric oxide-dependent and nitric-oxide-independent effects of tumor necrosis factor α on cardiomyocyte's beating activity and signal transduction pathways. In: Schlag G, Redl H, eds: 4th Wiggers Bernard Conference. Springer, Berlin Heidelberg, 1995:286-309.

43. Bensard DD, Banerjee A, McIntyre RC et al. Endotoxin disrupts β-adrenergic signal transduction in the heart. Arch Surg 1994; 129:198-205.

44. Balligand J-L, Ungureanu D, Kelly RA et al. Abnormal contractile function due to induction of nitric oxide synthesis in rat cardiac myocytes follows exposure to activated macrophage-conditioned medium. J Clin Invest 1993; 91:2314-2319.

45. Balligand J-L, Kelly RA, Marsden PA et al. Control of cardiac muscle cell function by an endogenous nitric oxide signaling system. Proc Natl Acad Sci USA 1993; 90:347-351.

46. Brady AJB, Poole-Wilson PA, Harding SE et al. Nitric oxide production within cardiac myocytes reduces their contractility in endotoxemia. Am J Physiol 1992; 263:H1963-H1966.

47. Brady AJB, Warren JB, Poole-Wilson PA et al. Nitric oxide attenuates cardiac myocyte contraction. Am J Physiol 1993; 265:H176-182.

48. Hung J, Lew WYW. Cellular mechanisms of endotoxin-induced myocardial depression in rabbits. Circ Res 1993; 73:125-134.

49. Liu M-S. Mechanisms of myocardial membrane alterations in endotoxin shock: roles of phospholipase and phosphorylation. Circ Shock 1990; 30:43-49.

50. Hinshaw LB. Cardiodepressant effects of endotoxin. In: Hinshaw LB, ed. Pathophysiology of Endotoxin. Elsevier Science Publishers, Amsterdam, 1985; pp 16-35 (Handbook of Endotoxin, vol 2).

51. Abel FL. Myocardial function in sepsis and endotoxin shock. Am J Physiol 1989; 257:R1265-R1281.

52. Michie HR, Manogue KR, Spriggs DR et al. Detection of circulating tumor necrosis factor after endotoxin administration. New Engl J Med 1988; 318:1481-1486.

53. Schirmer WJ, Schirmer JM, Fry DE. Recombinant human tumor necrosis factor produces hemodynamic changes characteristic of sepsis and endotoxemia. Arch Surg 1989; 124:445-448.

54. Meyer J, Lentz CW, Stothert JC et al. Effects of nitric oxide synthesis inhibition in hyperdynamic endotoxemia. Crit Care Med 1994; 22:306-312.

55. Smith REA, Palmer RMJ, Moncada S. Coronary vasodilatation induced by endotoxin in the rabbit isolated perfused heart is nitric oxide-dependent and inhibited by dexamethasone. Br J Pharmacol 1991; 104:5-6.

56. Giroir BP, Johnson JH, Brown T et al. The tissue distribution of tumor necrosis factor biosynthesis during endotoxemia. J Clin Invest 1992;

90:693-698.

57. Murad F. Regulation of cytosolic guanylyl cyclase by nitric oxide: the NO-cyclic GMP signal transduction system. Adv Pharmacol 1994; 26:19-33.

58. Schulz R, Nava E, Moncada S. Induction and potential biological relevance of a Ca^{2+}-independent nitric oxide synthase in the myocardium. Br J Pharmacol 1992; 105:575-580.

59. Thiemermann C. The role of the L-arginine: nitric oxide pathway in circulatory shock. Adv Pharmacol 1994; 28:45-79.

60. Ochoa JB, Udekwu AO, Billiar TR et al. Nitrogen oxide levels in patients after trauma and during sepsis. Ann Surg 1991; 214:621-625.

61. Pollack M, Young LS. Protective activity of antibodies to exotoxin A and lipopolysaccharide at the onset of *Pseudomonas aeruginosa* septicemia in man. J Clin Invest 1979; 63:276-286.

62. Cross AS, Sadoff JC, Iglewski BH et al. Evidence for the role of toxin A in the pathogenesis of infection with *Pseudomonas aeruginosa* in humans. J Infect Dis 1980; 142:538-546.

63. Saelinger CB. Use of exotoxin A to inhibit protein synthesis. Methods in Enzymology 1988; 165:226-230.

64. Snell K, Holder IA, Leppla SA et al. Role of exotoxin and protease virulence factors in experimental infections with *Pseudomonas aeruginosa*. Infection and Immunity 1978; 19:839-845.

65. Kwiatkowska-Patzer B, Patzer JA, Heller LJ. *Pseudomonas aeruginosa* exotoxin A enhances automaticity and potentiates hypoxic depression of isolated rat hearts. Proc Soc Exp Biol Med 1993; 202:377-383.

66. Müller-Werdan U, Pfeifer A, Seliger C et al. Partial inhibition of protein synthesis by Pseudomonas exotoxin A deranges catecholamine sensitivity of cultured rat heart myocytes. Submitted for publication.

67. Reithmann C, Gierschik P, Müller U et al. Pseudomonas exotoxin A prevents β-adrenoceptor-induced upregulation of G_i protein α-subunits and adenylyl cyclase desensitization in rat heart muscle cells. Mol Pharmacol 1990; 37:631-638.

68. Reithmann C, Gierschik P, Werdan K et al. Role of inhibitory G protein α-subunits in adenylyl cyclase desensitization. Mol Cell Endocrinol 1991; 82:C215-C221.

69. Rupp H, Berger HJ, Pfeifer A et al. Effect of positive inotropic agents on myosin isoenzyme population and mechanical activity of cultured rat heart myocytes. Circ Res 1991; 68:1164-1173.

70. Vescovo G, Harding SE, Jones SM et al. Comparison between isomyosin pattern and contractility of right ventricular myocytes from rats with right cardiac hypertrophy. Basic Res Cardiol 1989; 84:536-543.

71. Saelinger CB, Morris RE. Intracellular trafficking of Pseudomonas exotoxin A. In: Döring G, Holder IA, Botzenhart K, eds. Basic Research and Clinical Aspects of *Pseudomonas aeruginosa*. Karger, Basel, 1986: 149-159 (Antibiot Chemother, vol 39).

72. Danner RL, Natanson C, Elin RJ et al. *Pseudomonas aeruginosa* compared with *Escherichia coli* produces less endotoxemia but more cardiovascular dysfunction and mortality in a canine model of septic shock. Chest 1990; 98:1480-1487.

73. Pilz G, Class I, Boekstegers P et al. Pseudomonas immunoglobulin therapy in patients with Pseudomonas sepsis and septic shock. Antibiot Chemother 1991; 44:120-135.

74. Pilz G, McGinn P, Boekstegers P et al. Pseudomonas sepsis does not cause more severe cardiovascular dysfunction in patients than Non-Pseudomonas sepsis. Circul Shock 1994; 42:174-182.

75. Thompson A, Halbert SP, Smith U. The toxicity of streptolysin O for beating mammalian heart cells in tissue culture. J Exp Med 1970; 131:745-763.

76. Bombeli T, Bertel O, Vuillioment A. Toxisches Schock-Syndrom bei *Streptokokkus-pyogenes*-Infektionen. Schweiz Med Wschr 1992; 122: 153-157.

77. Bhakdi S, Tranum-Jensen J. Damage to mammalian cells by proteins that form transmembrane pores. Rev Physiol Biochem Pharmacol 1987; 107:147-223.

78. Duncan JL, Buckingham L. Resistance to streptolysin O in mammalian cells treated with oxygenated derivatives of cholesterol—cholesterol content of resistant cells and recovery of streptolysin O sensitivity. Biochim Biophys Acta 1980; 603:278-287.

79. Bhakdi S, Mannhardt U, Muhly M et al. Human hyperimmune globulin protects against the cytotoxic action of staphylococcal alpha-toxin in vitro and in vivo. Infect Immun 1989; 57:3214-3220.

80. Bauriedel G, Bohn I, Werdan K. Direkte Wirkung von Staphylokokken-Toxin (α-Toxin) auf Kontraktions- und Ionenflußverhalten kultivierter Herzmuskelzellen. Z Kardiol 1986; 75(Suppl 1):57.

81. Hildebrand A, Pohl M, Bhakdi S. *Staphylococcus aureus* α-toxin—dual mechanism of binding to target cells. J Biol Chem 1991; 266: 17195-17200.

82. Fisher CJ, Horowitz BZ, Albertson TE. Cardiorespiratory failure in toxic shock syndrome: effect of dobutamine. Crit Care Med 1985; 13:160-165.

83. Natanson C, Danner RL, Elin RJ et al. Role of endotoxemia in cardiovascular dysfunction and mortality. J Clin Invest 1989; 83:243-251.

84. Yarom R, Hasin Y, Raz S et al. T-2 toxin effect on cultured myocardial cells. Toxic Lett 1986; 31:1-8.

85. Marks JD, Marks CB, Luce JM et al. Plasma tumor necrosis factor in patients with septic shock: Mortality rate, incidence of adult respiratory distress syndrome, and effects of methylprednisolone administration. Am Rev Respir Dis 1990; 141:94-97.

86. van der Poll T, Jansen J, van Leenen D et al. Release of soluble receptors for tumor necrosis factor in clinical sepsis and experimental endotoxemia. J Infect Dis 1993; 168:995-960.

87. Levine B, Kalman J, Mayer L et al. Elevated circulating levels of tumor necrosis factor in severe chronic heart failure. N Engl J Med 1990; 323:236-241.

88. McMurray J, Abdhullah I, Dargie HJ et al. Increased concentrations of tumor necrosis factor in "cachectic" patients with severe chronic heart failure. Br Heart J 1991; 66:356-358.

89. Wiedermann CJ, Beimpold H, Herold M et al. Increased levels of serum neopterin and decreased production of neutrophil superoxide anions in chronic heart failure with elevated levels of tumor necrosis factor-alpha. J Am Coll Cardiol 1993; 22:1897-1901.

90. Maury CPJ, Teppo A-M. Circulating tumour necrosis factor-α (cachectin) in myocardial infarction. J Intern Med 1989; 225:333-336.

91. Basaran Y, Basaran MM, Babacan KF et al. Serum tumor necrosis factor levels in acute myocardial infarction and unstable angina pectoris. Angiology 1993; 44:333-337.

92. Latini R, Bianchi M, Correale E et al. Cytokines in acute myocardial infarction: selective increase in circulating tumor necrosis factor, its soluble receptor, and interleukin-1 receptor antagonist. J Cardiovasc Pharmacol 1994; 23:1-6.

93. Squadrito F, Altavilla D, Zingarelli B et al. Tumor necrosis factor involvement in myocardial ischaemia-reperfusion injury. Eur J Pharmacol 1993; 237:223-230.

94. Maury CPJ, Salo E, Pelkonen P. Elevated circulating tumor necrosis factor-α in patients with Kawasaki disease. J Lab Clin Med 1987; 113: 651-654.

95. Smith SC, Allen PM. Neutralization of endogenous tumor necrosis factor ameliorates the severity of myosin-induced myocarditis. Circ Res 1992; 70:856-863.

96. Chollet-Martin S, Depoix JP, Hvass U et al. Raised plasma levels of tumor necrosis factor in heart allograft rejection. Transplant Proc 1990; 22:283-286.

97. Arbustini E, Grasso M, Diegoli M et al. Expression of tumor necrosis factor in human acute cardiac rejection: an immunohistochemical and immunoblotting study. Am J Pathol 1991; 139:709-715.

98. Blick M, Sherwin SA, Rosenblum M et al. Phase I study of recombinant tumor necrosis factor in cancer patients. Cancer Res 1987; 47:2986-2989.

99. Selby P, Hobbs S, Viner C et al. Tumor necrosis factor in man: clinical and biological observations. Br J Cancer 1987; 56:803-808.

100. Spriggs DR, Sherman ML, Michi H et al. Recombinant human tumor necrosis factor administered as a 24-hour intravenous infusion: a phase I and pharmacologic study. J Natl Cancer Inst 1988; 80:1039-1044.

101. Hegewisch S, Weh JH, Hossfeld DK. TNF-induced cardiomyopathy. Lancet 1990; I:294-295.

102. Eichenholz PW, Eichacker PQ, Hoffman WD et al. Tumor necrosis factor challenges in canines: patterns of cardiovascular dysfunction. Am J Physiol 1992; 263:H668-H675.

103. Werdan K, Müller U, Reithmann C. "Negative inotropic cascades" in cardiomyocytes triggered by substances relevant to sepsis. In: Schlag G, Redl H, eds. Pathophysiology of Shock, Sepsis, and Organ Failure. Berlin, Heidelberg: Springer Verlag 1993: 787-832.

104. Odeh M. Tumor necrosis factor-α as a myocardial depressant substance. Int J Cardiol 1993; 42:231-238.

105. Gulick T, Chung MK, Pieper SJ et al. Interleukin 1 and tumor necrosis factor inhibit cardiac myocyte β-adrenergic responsiveness. Proc Natl Acad Sci 1989; 86:6753-6757.

106. Chung MK, Gulick TS, Rotondo RE et al. Mechanism of cytokine inhibition of β-adrenergic agonist stimulation of cyclic AMP in rat cardiac myocytes. Circ Res 1990; 67:753-763.

107. DeMeules JE, Pigula FA, Mueller M et al. Tumor necrosis factor and cardiac function. J Trauma 1992; 32:686-692.

108. Finkel MS, Oddis CV, Jacob TD et al. Negative inotropic effects of cytokines on the heart mediated by nitric oxide. Science 1992; 257:387-389.

109. Reithmann C, Gierschik P, Werdan K et al. Tumor necrosis factor α upregulates $G_{i\alpha}$ and G_β proteins and adenylate cyclase responsiveness in rat cardiomyocytes. Europ J Pharmacol—Mol Pharmacol Section 1991; 206:53-60.

110. Reithmann C, Gierschik P, Jakobs KH et al. Regulation of adenylyl cyclase by noradrenaline and tumor necrosis factor α in rat cardiomyocytes. Europ Heart J 1991; 12(Suppl F):139-142.

111. Yokoyama T, Vaca L, Rossen RD et al. Cellular basis for the negative inotropic effects of tumor necrosis factor-α in the adult mammalian heart. J Clin Invest 1993; 92:2303-2312.

112. Reithmann C, Werdan K. Tumor necrosis factor α decreases inositol phosphate formation and phosphatidiylinositol-bisphosphate (PIP_2) synthesis in rat cardiomyocytes. Naunyn-Schmiedeberg's Arch Pharmacol 1994; 349:175-182.

113. Löw-Friedrich I, Weisensee D, Mitrou P et al. Cytokines induce stress protein formation in cultured cardiac myocytes. Basic Res Cardiol 1992; 87:12-18.

114. Blondel B, Roijen I, Cheneval JP. Heart cells in culture: a simple method for increasing the proportion of myoblasts. Experientia 1971; 27:356-358.

115. Werdan K, Erdmann E. Preparation and culture of embryonic and neonatal heart muscle cells: modification of transport activity. Methods in Enzymology 1989; 173:634-662.

116. Görg A, Postel W, Günther S. The current state of two-dimensional electrophoresis with immobilized pH gradients. Electrophoresis 1988; 9:531-546.

117. Görg A. Two-dimensional electrophoresis with immobilized pH gradients: current state. Biochemical Society Transactions 1993; 21:130-132.

118. Jungblut P, Otto A, Zeindl-Eberhart E et al. Protein composition of the human heart: The construction of a myocardial two-dimensional electro-

phoresis database. Electrophoresis 1994; 15:685-707.

119. Zeindl-Eberhart E, Jungblut PR, Otto A et al. Identification of tumor-associated protein variants during rat hepatocarcinogenesis. J Biol Chem 1994; 269:14589-14594.

120. Chang He, Müller U, Oberthür W et al. Application of high-resolution two-dimensional polyacrylamide gel electrophoresis of polypeptides from cultured neonatal rat cardiomyocytes: Regulation of protein synthesis by catecholamines. Electrophoresis 1992; 13:748-754.

121. Chang He, Müller U, Werdan K. Regulation of protein biosynthesis in neonatal rat cardiomyocytes by adrenoceptor stimulation: Investigations with high-resolution two-dimensional polyacrylamide gel electrophoresis. Electrophoresis 1992; 13:755-756.

122. Girardin E, Roux-Lombard P, Grau GE et al. Imbalance between tumour necrosis factor-alpha and soluble TNF receptor concentrations in severe menigococcaemia. Immunology 1992; 76: 20-23.

123. Isner JM, Dietz WA. Cardiovascular consequences of recombinant DNA technology: interleukin-2. Ann Int Med 1988; 109:933-935.

124. Okusawa S, Gelfand JA, Ikejima T et al. Interleukin 1 induces a shock-like state in rabbits. Synergism with tumor necrosis factor and the effect of cyclooxygenase inhibition. J Clin Invest 1988; 81:1162-1172.

125. Schuchter LM, Hendricks CB, Holland KH et al. Eosinophilic myocarditis associated with high-dose interleukin-2 therapy. Am J Med 1990; 88:439-440.

126. Sonnenblick M, Rosenmann D, Rosin A. Reversible cardiomyopathy induced by interferon. Br Med J 1990; 300:1174-1175.

127. Wang YC, Herskowitz A, Gu LB et al. Influence of cytokines and immunosuppressive drugs in major histocompatibility complex class I/II expression by human cardiac myocytes in vitro. Hum Immunol 1991; 31:123-133.

128. Seko Y, Tsuchimochi H, Nakamura T et al. Expression of major histocompatibility complex class I antigen in murine ventricular myocytes infected with Coxsackievirus B3. Circ Res 1990; 67:360-367.

129. Barthlen W, Stadler J, Lehn NL et al. Serum levels of end products of nitric oxide synthesis correlate positively with tumor necrosis factor α and negatively with body temperature in patients with postoperative abdominal sepsis. Shock 1994; 2:398-401.

130. Parratt JR. Myocardial and circulatory effects of *E. coli* endotoxin; modification of responses to catecholamines. Br J Pharmacol 1973; 47:12-25.

131. Parratt JR, Stoclet JC. Nitric oxide as a mediator of the vascular derangements of sepsis and endotoxemia. In: Lamy M, Thijs LG, eds. Update in Intensive Care and Emergency Medicine 16. Mediators of Sepsis. 1992;174-189.

132. Petros A, Bennett D, Vallance P. Effect of nitric oxide synthase inhibitors on hypotension with septic shock. Lancet 1991; 338:1557-1558.

133. Förstermann U, Pollock JS, Nakane M. Nitric oxide synthases in the cardiovascular system. Trends Cardiovasc Med 1993; 3:104-110.

134. Mery P-F, Lohmann SM, Walter U et al. Ca^{2+} current is regulated by cyclic GMP-dependent protein kinase in mammalian cardiac myocytes. Proc Nat Acad Sci USA 1991; 88:1197-1201.

135. Mery P-F, Pavoine C, Belhassen L et al. Nitric oxide regulates cardiac Ca^{2+} current. J Biol Chem 1993; 35:26286-26295.

136. Kilbourn RG, Cromeens DM, Chelly FD et al. N^G-methyl-L-arginine, an inhibitor of nitric oxide formation, acts synergistically with dobutamine to improve cardiovascular performance in endotoxemic dogs. Crit Care Med 1994; 22:1835-1840.

137. Klabunde RE, Ritger RC. N^G-monomethyl-L-arginine (NMA) restores arterial blood pressure but reduces cardiac output in a canine model of endotoxic shock. Biochem Biophys Res Commun 1991; 178:1135-1140.

138. Statman R, Cheng W, Cunningham JN et al. Nitric oxide inhibition in the treatment of sepsis syndrome is detrimental to tissue oxygenation. J Surg Res 1994; 57:93-98.

139. Petros A, Lamb G, Leone A et al. Effects of a nitric oxide synthase inhibitor in humans with septic shock. Cardiovasc Res 1994; 28:34-39.

140. Benyó Z, Kiss G, Szabó C et al. Importance of basal nitric oxide synthesis in regulation of myocardial blood flow. Cardiovasc Res 1991; 25:700-703.

141. Robertson FM, Ottner PJ, Ciceri DP et al. Detrimental hemodynamic effects of nitric oxide synthase inhibition in septic shock. Arch Surg 1994; 129:149-156.

142. Heideman M, Norder-Hansson B, Bengtson A et al. Terminal complement complexes and anaphylatoxins in septic and ischemic patients. Arch Surg 1988; 123:188-192.

143. Hack CE, Nuijens JH, Felt-Bersma RJF et al. Elevated plasma levels of the anaphylatoxins C3a and C4a are associated with a fatal outcome in sepsis. Am J Med 1989; 86:20-26.

144. Del Balzo UH, Levi R, Polley MJ. Cardiac dysfunction caused by purified human C3a anaphylatoxin. Proc Natl Acad Sci USA 1985; 82:886-890.

145. Del Balzo U, Polley MJ, Levi R. Cardiac anaphylaxis: complement activation as an amplification system. Circ Res 1989; 65:847-857.

146. Hendry PJ, Taichman GC, Biro GP et al. The effects of activated complement on myocardial performance in vitro. J Cardiovasc Surg 1989; 30:351-358.

147. Berger H-J, Taratuska A, Smith TW et al. Activated complement directly modifies the performance of isolated heart muscle cells from guinea pig and rat. Am J Physiol 1993; 265:H267-H272.

148. Braquet P, Touqui L, Shen TY et al. Perspectives in platelet-activating factor research. Pharmacol Rev 1987; 39:97-145.

149. Baum TD, Heard SO, Feldman HS et al. Endotoxin-induced myocardial depression in rats: effect of ibuprofen and SDZ 64-688, a platelet activating factor receptor antagonist. J Surg Res 1990; 48:629-634.

150. Crespo MS, Fernanez-Gallardo S. Pharmacological modulation of PAF: a therapeutic approach to endotoxin shock. J Lipid Mediators 1991; 4:127-144.

151. Moore JM, Earnest MA, DiSimone AG et al. A PAF receptor antagonist, BN 52021, attenuates thromboxane release and improves survival in lethal canine endotoxemia. Circ Shock 1991; 35:53-59.

152. Zhang C, Hsueh W, Caplan MS et al. Platelet activating factor-induced shock and intestinal necrosis in the rat: role of endogenous platelet-activating factor and effect of saline infusion. Crit Care Med 1991; 19:1067-1072.

153. Camussi G, Alloatti G, Montrucchio G et al. Effect of platelet activating factor on guinea-pig papillary muscle. Experientia 1984; 40:697-699.

154. Tamargo J, Tejerina T, Delgado C et al. Electrophysiological effects of platelet-activating factor (PAF-acether) in guinea-pig papillary muscles. Eur J Pharmacol 1985; 109:219-227.

155. Alloatti G, Montrucchio G, Mariano F et al. Effect of platelet-activating factor (PAF) on human cardiac muscle. Int Archs Allergy appl Immun 1986; 79:108-112.

156. Alloatti G, Montrucchio G, Mariano F et al. Protective effect of verapamil on the cardiac and circulatory alterations induced by platelet-activating factor. J Cardiovasc Res 1987; 9:181-186.

157. Robertson DA, Genovese A, Levi R. Negative inotropic effect of platelet-activating factor on human myocardium: a pharmacological study. J Pharmacol Exp Therap 1987; 243:834-839.

158. Robertson DA, Wang D-Y, Ok C et al. Negative inotropic effect of platelet-activating factor: association with a decrease in intracellular sodium activity. J Pharmacol Exp Ther 1988; 245:124-128.

159. Felix SB, Baumann G, Raschke P et al. Cardiovascular reactions and respiratory events during platelet activating factor-induced shock. Basic Res Cardiol 1990; 85:217-226.

160. Felix SB, Steger A, Baumann G et al. Platelet-activating factor-induced coronary constriction in the isolated perfused guinea pig heart and antagonistic effects of the PAF antagonist WEB 2086. J Lipid Med 1990; 2:9-20.

161. Koltai M, Hosford D, Guinot P et al. Platelet activating factor (PAF)—A review of its effects, antagonists and possible future clinical implications (part I). Drugs 1991; 42:9-29.

162. Pugsley MK, Salari H, Walker MJA. Actions of platelet-activating factor on isolated rat hearts. Circ Shock 1991; 35:207-214.

163. Massey CV, Kohout TA, Gaa St et al. Molecular and cellular actions of platelet-activating factor in rat heart cells. J Clin Invest 1991; 88: 2106-2116.

164. Wahler GM, Coyle DE, Sperelakis N. Effects of platelet-activating factor on single potassium channel currents in guinea pig ventricular myocytes. Mol Cell Biochem 1990; 93:69-76.

165. Schwinger RHG, Böhm M, Rosee KL et al. Existence of PAF-receptors in human platelets and human lung tissue but not in the human myocardium. Am Heart J 1992; 124:320-330.

166. Ball HA, Cook JA, Wise WC et al. Role of thromboxane, prostaglandins and leukotrienes in endotoxic and septic shock. Intensive Care Med 1986; 12:116-126.

167. Oettinger W, Berger D, Beger HG. The clinical significance of prostaglandins and thromboxane as mediators of septic shock. Klin Wochenschr 1987; 65:61-68.

168. Klosterhalfen B, Hörstmann-Jungemann K, Vogel P et al. Hemodynamic variables and plasma levels of PGI_2, TxA_2 and IL-6 in a porcine model of recurrent endotoxemia. Circ Shock 1991; 35:237-244.

169. Mozes T, Zijlstra FJ, Heiligers JPC et al. Sequential release of tumour necrosis factor, platelet activating factor and eicosanoids during endotoxin shock in anaesthetized pigs: protective effects of indomethacin. Br J Pharmacol 1991; 104:691-699.

170. Haupt MT, Jastremski MS, Clemmer TP et al. Effect of ibuprofen in patients with severe sepsis: A randomized, double-blind, multicenter study. Crit Care Med 1991; 19:1339-1347.

171. Morinelli TA, Haluska PV. Thromboxane-A_2/prostaglandin/H_2-receptors—characterization and antagonism. Trends Cardiovasc Med 1991; 1:157-161.

172. Smith EF, Slivjak MJ, Bartus JO et al. SK&F 86002 inhibits tumor necrosis factor formation and improves survival in endotoxemic rats. J Cardiovasc Pharmacol 1991; 18:721-728.

173. Michelassi F, Castorena G, Hill RD et al. Effects of leukotrienes B_4 and C_4 on coronary circulation and myocardial contractility. Surgery 1983; 94:267-275.

174. Burke JA, Levi R, Guo Z-G et al. Leukotrienes C_4, D_4 and E_4: Effects on human and guinea pig cardiac preparations in vitro. J Pharmacol Exp Ther 1982; 221:235-241.

175. Roth DM, Lefer DJ, Hock CE et al. Effects of peptide leukotrienes on cardiac dynamics in rat, cat, and guinea pig hearts. Am J Physiol 1985; 249:H477-H484.

176. Fauler J, Frölich JC. Cardiovascular effects of leukotrienes. Cardiovas Drugs Ther 1989; 3:499-505.

177. Semb AG, Vaage J, Mjos OD. Oxygen free radical producing leukocytes cause functional depression of isolated rat hearts: role of leukotrienes. J Mol Cell Cardiol 1990; 22:555-563.

178. Sterin-Borda L, Canga L, Borda ES et al. Inotropic effect of prostacyclin (PGI_2) on isolated rat atria at different contraction frequencies. Naunyn-Schmiedeberg's Arch Pharmacol 1980; 313:95-100.

179. Soulsby ME, Jacobs ER, Perlmutter BH et al. Protection of myocardial function during endotoxin shock by ibuprofen. Prostaglandins, Leukotrienes and Medicine 1984; 13:295-305.

180. Heard SO, Baum TD, Feldman HS et al. Lipopolysaccharide-induced myocardial depression is not mediated by cyclooxygenase products. Crit Care Med 1991; 19:723-727.

181. Schneider J. Beneficial effects of the prostacyclin analogue taprostene on cardiovascular, pulmonary and renal disturbances in endotoxin-shocked rabbits. Eicosanoids 1991; 4:99-105.

182. Clapham DE. Arachidonic acid and its metabolites in the regulation of G-protein gated K^+ channels in atrial myocytes. Biochem Pharmacol 1990; 39:813-815.

183. Hallaq H, Sellmayer A, Smith TW et al. Protective effect of eicosapentaenoic acid on ouabain toxicity in neonatal rat cardiac myocytes. Proc Natl Acad Sci USA 1990; 87:7834-7838.

184. Kim D, Duff RA. Regulation of K^+ channels in cardiac myocytes by free fatty acids. Circ Res 1990; 67:1040-1046.

185. Schmilinsky Fluri G, Rüdisüli A, Willi M et al. Effects of arachidonic acid on the gap junctions of neonatal rat heart cells. Pflügers Arch 1990; 417:149-156.

186. Freyss-Beguin M, Millanvoye-Van Brussel E, Simon J et al. Effect of isoproterenol on lipid metabolism and prostaglandin production in cultures of newborn rat heart cells, under normoxic and hypoxic conditions. Prostaglandins, Leukotrienes and Essential Fatty Acids 1990; 41:235-242.

187. Härtel B, Morwinski R, Heydeck D et al. Arachidonic acid metabolism in cultured adult myocardial cells under short-term hypoxic conditions. Mol Cell Biochem 1991; 106:67-74.

188. Kawaguchi H, Shoki M, Iizuka K et al. Phospholipid metabolism and prostacyclin synthesis in hypoxic myocytes. Biochim Biophys Acta 1991; 1094:161-167.

189. Wallukat G, Kuehn H, Wollenberger A. Supersensitivity to isoprenaline induced in cultured neonatal rat heart cells by certain eicosatetraenoic acids. Europ Heart J 1991; 12(Supplement F)145-148.

190. Wallukat G, Nemecz G, Farkas T et al. Modulation of the beta-adrenergic response in cultured rat heart cells—I. Beta-adrenergic supersensitivity is induced by lactate via a phospholipase A_2 and 15-lipoxygenase involving pathway. Mol Cell Biochem 1991; 102:35-47.

191. Wallukat G, Boehmer F-D, Engstroem U et al. Modulation of the beta-adrenergic-response in cultured rat heart cells—II. Mammary-derived growth inhibitor (MDGI) blocks induction of beta-adrenergic supersensitivity. Dissociation from lipid-binding activity of MDGI. Mol Cell Biochem 1991; 102:49-60.

192. Lefer AM. Pharmacologic and surgical modulation of myocardial depressant formation and action during shock. In: Molecular and Cellular Aspects of Shock and Trauma. New York: Alan R Liss Inc, 1983:111-123.

193. Sagher U, Rosen H, Sarel O et al. Studies on a pancreatic cardiodepressant factor. Circ Shock 1986; 19:319-327.

194. Carli A, Auclair M-C. Role of humoral cardiodepressant factors in septic shock—A brief review. In: Lewis DH, Haglund U, eds. Shock Research. Amsterdam: Elsevier Science Publishers BV, 1983:203 -214.

195. Parrillo JE, Burch C, Shelhamer JH et al. A circulating myocardial depressant substance in humans with septic shock. J Clin Invest 1985; 76:1539-1553.

196. Hallström S, Koidl B, Müller U et al. A cardiodepressant factor isolated from blood blocks Ca²⁺ current in cardiomyocytes. Am J Physiol 1991; 260:H869-H876.

197. Werdan K, Müller U, Reithmann C et al. Mechanisms in acute septic cardiomyopathy: evidence from isolated myocytes. Basic Res Cardiol 1991; 86:411-421.

198. Hallström S, Koidl B, Müller U et al. Cardiodepressant factors. In: G Schlag, H Redl, eds. Pathophysiology of Shock, Sepsis, and Organ Failure. Berlin, Heidelberg: Springer-Verlag, 1993: 200-214.

199. Parrillo JE. Pathogenetic mechanisms of septic shock. N Engl J Med 1993; 328:1471-1477.

200. Hallström S, Bernhart E, Müller U et al. A cardiodepressant factor (CDF) isolated from hemofiltrates of patients in septic and/or cardiogenic shock blocks calcium inward current in cardiomyocytes. Shock 1994; Suppl to Vol 2: abstract 1.

201. Hearse DJ, Bolli R. Reperfusion-induced injury—manifestations, mechanisms, and clinical relevance. Trends Cardiovasc Med 1991; 1:233-240.

202. Mullane K. Neutrophil and endothelial changes in reperfusion injury. Trends Cardiovasc Med 1991; 1:282-289.

203. Parrillo JE. The cardiovascular pathophysiology of sepsis. Ann Rev Med 1989; 40:469-485.

204. Schoenberg MH. The participation of oxygen free radicals in septic shock. In: Vincent JL, Thijs LG, eds. Update in Intensive Care and Emergency Medicine 4. Septic Shock. Berlin, Heidelberg: Springer-Verlag, 1987:51-73.

205. Wagenknecht B, Hug M, Hübner G et al. Myokardiale Wirkungen von Mediatoren. Intensivmed 1989; 26(Suppl 1):32-40.

206. Rao PS, Rujikarn N, Weinstein GS et al. Effect of oxygen free radicals and lipid peroxides on cardiac isoenzymes. Biomed Biochim Acta 1990; 49:439-443.

207. Mickle DAG, Li R-K, Weisel RD et al. Water-soluble antioxidant specificity against free radical injury using cultured human ventricular myocytes and fibroblasts and saphenous vein endothelial cells. J Mol Cell Cardiol 1990; 22:1297-1304.

208. Xie Z, Wang Y, Askari A et al. Studies on the specificity of the effects of oxygen metabolites on cardiac sodium pump. J Mol Cell Cardiol 1990; 22:911-920.

209. Burton KP, Morris AC, Massey KD et al. Free radicals alter ionic calcium levels and membrane phospholipids in cultured rat ventricular myocytes. J Mol Cell Cardiol 1990; 22:1035-1047.

210. Josephson RA, Silverman HS, Lakatta EG et al. Study of the mechanisms of hydrogen peroxide and hydroxyl free radical-induced cellular injury and calcium overload in cardiac myocytes. J Biol Chem 1991; 266:2354-2361.

211. Barrington PL. Effects of free radicals on the electrophysiological function of cardiac membranes. Free Radical Biology & Medicine 1990; 9:355-365.

212. Cerbai E, Ambrosio G, Porciatti F et al. Cellular electrophysiological ba-

sis for oxygen radical-induced arrhythmias—a patch-clamp study in guinea pig ventricular myocytes. Circulation 1991; 84:1773-1782.

213. Mak IT, Kramer JH, Freedman AM et al. Oxygen radical-mediated injury of myocytes—protection by propranolol. J Mol Cell Cardiol 1990; 22:687-695.

214. Scott JA, Fischman AJ, Khaw B-A et al. Free radical-mediated membrane depolarization in renal and cardiac cells. Biochim Biophys Acta 1987; 899:76-82.

215. Fliss H. Oxidation of proteins in rat heart and lungs by polymorphonuclear leukocyte oxidants. Mol Cell Biochem 1988; 84:177-188.

216. Beresewicz A, Horackova M. Alterations in electrical and contractile behavior of isolated cardiomyocytes by hydrogen peroxide: possible ionic mechanisms. J Mol Cell Cardiol 1991; 23:899-918.

217. Janero DR, Hreniuk D, Sharif HM. Hydrogen peroxide-induced oxidative stress to the mammalian heart-muscle cell (cardiomyocyte): lethal peroxidative membrane injury. J Cell Physiol 1991; 149:347-364.

218. Konno N, Kako KJ. Effects of hydrogen peroxide and hypochlorite on membrane potential of mitochondria in situ in rat heart cells. Can J Physiol Pharmacol 1991; 69:1705-1712.

219. Bhatnagar A, Srivastava SK, Szabo G. Oxidative stress alters specific membrane currents in isolated cardiac myocytes. Circ Res 1990; 67:535-549.

220. Timerman AP, Altschuld RA, Hohl CM et al. Cellular glutathione and the response of adult rat heart myocytes to oxidant stress. J Mol Cell Cardiol 1990; 22:565-575.

221. Vlessis AA, Muller P, Bartos D et al. Mechanism of peroxide-induced cellular injury in cultured adult cardiac myocytes. FASEB J 1991; 5:2600-2605.

222. Eley DW, Eley JM, Korecky B et al. Impairment of cardiac contractility and sarcoplasmic reticulum Ca^{2+} ATPase activity by hypochlorous acid: reversal by dithiothreitol. Can J Physiol Pharmacol 1991; 69:1677-1685.

223. Turner JJO, Rice-Evans CA, Davies MJ et al. The formation of free radicals by cardiac myocytes under oxidative stress and the effects of electron-donating drugs. Biochem J 1991; 277:833-837.

224. VerDonck L, Van Reempts J, Vandeplassche G et al. A new method to study activated oxygen species induced damage in cardiomyocytes and protection by Ca^{2+}-antagonists. J Mol Cell Cardiol 1988; 20:811-823.

225. Vandeplassche G, Bernier M, Thone F et al. Singlet oxygen and myocardial injury: ultrastructural, cytochemical and electrocardiographic consequences of photoactivation of rose bengal. J Mol Cell Cardiol 1990; 22:287-301.

226. Matsuura H, Shattock MJ. Effects of oxidant stress on steady-state background currents in isolated ventricular myocytes. Am J Physiol 1991; 261:H1358-H1365.

227. Wagenknecht B, Hug M, Freudenrich C et al. Oxygen free radical-induced cell injury in rat heart muscle cells. Circ Shock 1991; 34:abstracts 153-154.

228. Hug M. Wirkung von Sauerstoffradikalen auf kultivierte neonatale Rattenherzmuskelzellen—Untersuchungen zu Kardiodepression, Kardiotoxizität sowie zum protektiven Effekt von Schutzsubstanzen. Medical thesis, Ludwig-Maximilians-Universität München, Germany, 1993.

229. Tate RM, Vanbenthuysen KM, Shasby M et al. Oxygen-radical-mediated permeability edema and vasoconstriction in isolated perfused rabbit lungs. Am Rev Respir Dis 1982; 126:802-806.

230. Massey KD, Burton KP. Free radical damage in neonatal rat cardiac myocyte cultures: effects of α-tocopherol, trolox and phytol. Free Radical Biology & Medicine 1990; 8:449-458.

231. Löw-Friedrich I, Schoeppe W. Effects of calcium channel blockers on stress protein synthesis in cardiac myocytes. J Cardiovasc Pharmacol 1991; 17:800-806.

232. McDonough KH, Henry JJ, Spitzer JJ. Effects of oxygen radicals on substrate oxidation by cardiac myocytes. Biochim Biophys Acta 1987; 926:127-131.

233. Barrington PL, Meier CF, Weglicki WB. Abnormal electrical activity induced by free radical generating systems in isolated cardiocytes. J Mol Cell Cardiol 1988; 20:1163-1178.

234. Kaneko M, Lee S-L, Wolf CM et al. Reduction of calcium channel antagonist binding sites by oxygen free radicals in rat heart. J Mol Cell Cardiol 1989; 21:935-943.

235. Kaneko M, Chapman DC, Ganguly PK et al. Modification of cardiac adrenergic receptors by oxygen free radicals. Am J Physiol 1991; 260:H821-H826.

236. Burton KP, Morris AC, Massey KD et al. Cellular ionic calcium increases in cultured neonatal rat ventricular myocytes exposed to a free radical generating system. J Mol Cell Cardiol 1988; 20(Suppl V):38.

237. Eley DW, Korecky B, Fliss H et al. Calcium homeostasis in rabbit ventriuclar myocytes—Disruption by hypochlorous acid and restoration by dithiothreitol. Circ Res 1991; 69:1132-1138.

238. Müller U, Greger C, Hallström S et al. Sensitisation of spontaneously beating neonatal rat cardiomyocytes to oxygen free radicals by depletion of glutathione. Circ Shock 1991; 34:abstract 409.

239. Unterberg C, Buchwald A, Grüning B et al. Protektion von Rattenherzmyozyten gegen freie Radikale durch Radikalfänger, Verapamil und deren Kombination. Z Kardiol 1989; 78 Suppl I:84.

240. Sedlis SP, Sequeira JM, Altszuler HM. Potentiation of the depressant effects of lysophosphatidylcholine on contractile properties of cultured cardiac myocytes by acidosis and superoxide radical. J Lab Clin Med 1990; 115:203-216.

241. Samuni A, Winkelsberg D, Pinson A et al. Nitroxide stable radicals protect beating cardiomyocytes against oxidative damage. J Clin Invest 1991; 87:1526-1530.

242. Jornot L, Petersen H, Junod AF. Differential protective effects of o-phenantroline and catalase on H_2O_2-induced DNA damage and inhibi-

tion of protein synthesis in endothelial cells. J Cell Physiol 1991; 149:408-413.

243. Kirkland JB. Lipid peroxidation, protein thiol oxidation and DNA damage in hydrogen peroxide-induced injury to endothelial cells: role of activation of poly(ADP-ribose)polymerase. Biochim Biophys Acta 1991; 1092:319-325.

244. Burton KP, McCord JM, Ghai G. Myocardial alterations due to free-radical generation. Am J Physiol 1984; 246:H776-H783.

245. Jackson CV, Mickelson JK, Pope TK et al. O_2 free radical-mediated myocardial and vascular dysfunction. Am J Physiol 1986; 251:H1225-H1231.

246. Schrier GM, Hess ML. Quantitative identification of superoxide anion as a negative inotropic species. Am J Physiol 1988; 255:H138-H143.

247. Brigham KL. Oxygen radicals—an important mediator of sepsis and septic shock. Klin Wochenschr 1991; 69:1004-1008.

248. Ogilvie AC, Groeneveld ABJ, Straub JP et al. Plasma lipid peroxides and antioxidants in human septic shock. Intensive Care Med 1991; 17:40-44.

249. Gurll NJ, Reynolds DG, Holaday JW. Evidence for a role of endorphins in the cardiovascular pathophysiology of primate shock. Crit Care Med 1988; 16:521-530.

250. Parker JL, Keller RS, Behm LL et al. Left ventricular dysfunction in early *E. coli* endotoxemia: effects of naloxone. Am J Physiol 1990; 28:H504-H511.

251. Safani M, Blair J, Ross D et al. Prospective, controlled, randomized trial of naloxone infusion in early hyperdynamic septic shock. Crit Care Med 1989; 17:1004-1009.

252. Laurent S, Marsh JD, Smith TW. Enkephalins have a direct positive inotropic effect on cultured cardiac myocytes. Proc Natl Acad Sci USA 1985; 82:5930-5934.

253. Ela C, Hasin Y, Eilam Y. Dual effects of opioids on contractility and cytosolic Ca^{2+} transients in cultured rat-cardiomyocytes. Circulation 1990; 82 Suppl III:III-141.

254. Ventura C, Spurgeon HA, Lakatta EG et al. Specific opioid receptor agonists alter the twitch and cytosolic Ca^{2+} transient of rat myocytes. Circulation 1989; Suppl II:II-196.

255. Ventura C, Guarnieri C, Lakatta EG et al. An increase in inositol-1,4,5-triphosphate accompanies K opioid alterations in Ca^{2+} homeostasis in cardiac myocytes. Circulation 1990; Suppl III:III-141.

256. Ventura C, Guarnieri C, Stefanelli C et al. Comparison between alpha-adrenergic- and K-opiodergic-mediated inositol(1,4,5)P_3/inositol(1,3,4,5)P_4 formation in adult cultured rat ventricular cardiomyocytes. Biochem Biophys Res Commun 1991; 179:972-979.

257. Ventura C, Muscari C, Spampinato S et al. Inhibitory action of opioid peptides on ouabain-sensitive Na^+-K^+ and Ca^{2+}-dependent ATPase activities in bovine cardiac sarcolemma. Peptides 1987; 8:709-713.

258. Ventura C, Guarnieri C, Bastagli L et al. Opioids stimulate sarcolemmal NAD(P)H-vanadate dehydrogenase activity. Bas Res Cardiol 1988; 83:376-383.

259. Gu H, Gaugl JF, Barron BA et al. Naloxone enhances cardiac contractile responses to epinephrine without altering epinephrine uptake from plasma. Circ Shock 1990; 32:257-271.

260. Schaller MD, Waeber B, Nussberger J et al. Angiotensin II, vasopressin, and sympathetic activity in conscious rats with endotoxemia. Am J Physiol 1985; 249:H1086-H1092.

261. Emerson Jr TE. Release and vascular effects of histamine, serotonin, angiotensin II and renin following endotoxin. In: Hinshaw LB, ed. Pathophysiology of Endotoxin. Handbook of Endotoxin, vol 2. Amsterdam: Elsevier Science Publishers, 1985:173-202.

262. Thomas VL, Nielsen MS. Administration of angiotensin II in refractory septic shock. Crit Care Med 1991; 19:1084-1086.

263. Baker KM, Singer HA, Aceto JF. Angiotensin II receptor-mediated stimulation of cytosolic-free calcium and inositol phosphates in chick myocytes. J Pharmacol Exp Therap 1989; 251:578-585.

264. Rogers TB, Gaa ST, Allen IS. Identification and characterization of functional angiotensin II receptors on cultured heart myocytes. J Pharmacol Exp Therap 1986; 236:438-444.

265. Allen IS, Cohen NM, Dhallan RS et al. Angiotensin II increases spontaneous contractile frequency and stimulates calcium current in cultured neonatal rat heart myocytes: insights into the underlying biochemical mechanisms. Circ Res 1988; 62:524-534.

266. Dösemeci A, Dhallan RS, Cohen NM et al. Phorbol ester increases calcium current and simulates the effects of angiotensin II on cultured neonatal rat heart myocytes. Circ Res 1988; 62:347-357.

267. Moorman JR, Kirsch GE, Lacerda AE et al. Angiotensin II modulates cardiac Na+ channels in neonatal rat. Circ Res 1989; 65:1804-1809.

268. Anand-Srivastava MB. Angiotensin II receptors negatively coupled to adenylate cyclase in rat myocardial sarcolemma—involvement of inhibitory guanine nucleotide regulatory protein. Biochem Pharmacol 1989; 38:489-496.

269. Robalino BD, Petrella RW, Jubran FY et al. Atrial natriuretic factor in patients with right ventricular infarction. J Am Coll Cardiol 1990; 15:546-553.

270. McCall D, Fried TA. Effect of atriopeptin II on Ca influx, contractile behavior and cyclic nucleotide content of cultured neonatal rat myocardial cells. J Mol Cell Cardiol 1990; 22:201-212.

271. Anand-Srivastava MB, Cantin M. Atrial natriuretic factor receptors are negatively coupled to adenylate cyclase in cultured atrial and ventricular cardiocytes. Biochem Biopyhs Res Commun 1986; 138:427-436.

272. Wang X, Jones SB, Zhou Z et al. Calcitonin gene-related peptide (CGRP) and neuropeptide Y (NPY) levels are elevated in plasma and decreased in vena cava during endotoxin shock in the rat. Circ Shock 1992; 36:21-30.

273. Wang X, Fiscus RR. Calcitonin gene-related peptide increases cAMP, tension, and rate in rat atria. Am J Physiol 1989; 256:R421-R428.

274. Joyce CD, Prinz RA, Thomas JX et al. Calcitonin gene-related peptide increases coronary flow and decreases coronary resistance. J Surg Res 1990;

49:435-440.

275. Krämer BK, Smith TW, Kelly RA. Endothelin and increased contractility in adult rat ventricular myocytes—role of intracellular alkalosis induced by activation of the protein kinase C-dependent Na^+-H^+ exchanger. Circ Res 1991; 68:269-279.

276. Takanashi M, Endoh M. Characterization of positive inotropic effect of endothelin on mammalian ventricular myocardium. Am J Physiol 1991; 261:H611-H619.

277. Nambi P, Pullen M, Egan JW et al. Identification of cardiac endothelin binding sites in rats: downregulation of left atrial endothelin binding sites in response to myocardial infarction. Pharmacology 1991; 43:84-89.

278. Galron R, Bdolah A, Kloog Y et al. Endothelin/sarafotoxin receptor induced phosphoinositide turnover: effects of pertussis and cholera toxins and of phorbol ester. Biochem Biophys Res Commun 1990; 171:949-954.

279. Kelly RA, Eid H, Krämer BK et al. Endothelin enhances the contractile responsiveness of adult rat ventricular myocytes to calcium by a pertussis toxin-sensitive pathway. J Clin Invest 1990; 86:1164-1171.

280. Connor HE, Humphrey PA, Feniuk W. Serotonin receptors—therapeutic prospects in cardiovascular disease. Trends Cardiovasc Med 1991; 1:205-210.

281. Hamamori Y, Yokoyama M, Yamada M et al. 5-Hydroxytryptamine induces phospholipase C-mediated hydrolysis of phosphoinositides through 5-hydroxytryptamine-2 receptors in cultured fetal mouse ventricular myocytes. Circ Res 1991; 66:1474-1483.

282. Saxena PR, Villalon CM. 5-Hydroxytryptamine: a chameleon in the heart. Trends Pharmacol Science 1991; 12:223-227.

283. Watson JD, Sury MRJ, Corder R et al. Plasma levels of neuropeptide tyrosine (NPY) are increased in human sepsis but are unchanged during canine endotoxin shock despite raised catecholamine concentrations. J Endocrinol 1988; 116:421-426.

284. Lundberg JM, Hua X-Y, Franco-Cereceda A. Effects of neuropeptide Y (NPY) on mechanical activity and neurotransmission in the heart, vas deferens and urinary bladder of the guinea-pig. Acta Physiol Scand 1984; 121:325-332.

285. Walker P, Grouzmann E, Burnier M et al. The role of neuropeptide Y in cardiovascular regulation. Trends Pharmacol Science 1991; 12:111-115.

286. Kassis S, Olasmaa M, Terenius L et al. Neuropeptide Y inhibits cardiac adenylate cyclase through a pertussis toxin-sensitive G protein. J Biol Chem 1987; 262:3429-3431.

287. Sun LS, Ursell PC, Robinson RB. Chronic exposure to neuropeptide Y determines cardiac α_1-adrenergic responsiveness. Am J Physiol 1991; 261:H969-H973.

288. Chien WW, Mohabir R, Clusin WT. Effect of thrombin on calcium homeostasis in chick embryonic heart cells—receptor-operated calcium entry with inositol triphosphate and a pertussis toxin-sensitive G protein as second messenger. J Clin Invest 1990; 85:1436-1443.

289. Markwardt F, Albitz R, Franke T et al. Thrombin stimulates Ca-channel currents in isolated frog ventricular cells. Pflüger's Arch Eur J Physiol 1988; 412:668-670.

290. Neugebauer E, Rixen D, Lorenz W. Histamine in septic/endotoxic shock. In: Neugebauer EA, Holaday JW, eds. Handbook of Mediators in Septic Shock. Boca Raton: CRC Press, Inc. 1993:51-126.

291. Tellado JM, Christou NV. Critically ill anergic patients demonstrate polymorphonuclear neutrophil activation in the intravascular compartment with decreased cell delivery to inflammatory foci. J Leukocyte Biol 1991; 50:547-553.

292. Tanaka H, Ogura H, Yokota J et al. Acceleration of superoxide production from leukocytes in trauma patients. Ann Surg 1991; 214:187-192.

293. Semb AG, Ytrehus K, Vaage J et al. Functional impairment in isolated rat hearts induced by activated leukocytes: protective effect of oxygen free radical scavengers. J Mol Cell Cardiol 1989; 21:877-887.

294. Müller U, Greger C, Finkenzeller C et al. In vitro interactions of PMN-leukocytes with heart muscle cells. Abstract: Workshop "Cellular Aspects of Impaired Heart Function: Sepsis Versus Ischemia"; organized by Werdan K, Eckert P, Groß R; Bayer AG, Wuppertal 1991.

295. Fuji H, Kuzuya T, Hoshida S et al. Free radicals derived from neutrophils mediate reoxygenation-induced myocardial injury. Circulation 1988; 78 Suppl II: II-56.

296. Smith CW, Anderson DC, Taylor AA et al. Leukocyte adhesion molecules and myocardial ischemia. Trends Cardiovasc Med 1991; 1:167-170.

297. Entman ML, Youker K, Shappell SB et al. Neutrophil adherence to isolated adult canine myocytes—evidence for a CD18-dependent mechanism. J Clin Invest 1990; 85:1497-1506.

298. Entman ML, Michael L, Rossen RD et al. Inflammation in the course of early myocardial ischemia. FASEB J 1991; 5:2529-2537.

299. Tai P-C, Hayes DJ, Clark JB et al. Toxic effects of human eosinophil secretion products on isolated rat heart cells in vitro. Biochem J 1982; 204:75-80.

300. Woodley SL, McMillan M, Shelby J et al. Myocyte injury and contraction abnormalitites produced by cytotoxic T lymphocytes. Circulation 1991; 83:1410-1418.

301. Berke G. How cytolytic T-lymphocytes(CTL) damage myocardial tissues in heart transplant rejection and in acute myocarditis. Abstract: Workshop "Cellular Aspects of Impaired Heart Function: Sepsis versus Ischemia"; organized by Werdan K, Eckert P, Groß R; Bayer AG Wuppertal 1991.

302. Seko Y, Shinkai Y, Kawasaki A et al. Expression of perforin in infiltrating cells in murine hearts with acute myocarditis caused by Coxsackievirus B3. Circ Res 1991; 84:788-795.

303. Chien WW, Mohabir R, Newman D et al. Effect of platelet release products on cytosolic calcium in cardiac myocytes. Biochem Biopyhs Res Commun 1990; 170:1121-1127.

304. Taniguchi T, Takagi D, Takeyama N et al. Platelet size and function in septic rats: changes in the adenylate pool. J Surg Res 1990; 49:400-407.

305. Capodici C, Muthukumaran G, Amoruso MA et al. Activation of neutrophil collagenase by cathepsin G. Inflammation 1989; 13:245-258.

306. Kukreja RC, Weaver AB, Hess ML. Stimulated human neutrophils damage cardiac sarcoplasmic reticulum function by generation of oxidants. Biochim Biophys Acta 1989; 990:198-205.

307. Chung Y, Kercsmar CM, Davis PB. Ferret tracheal epithelial cells grown in vitro are resistant to lethal injury by activated neutrophils. Am J Respir Cell Mol Biol 1991; 5:125-132.

308. Ricevuti G, Mazzone A, Pasotti D et al. Role of granulocytes in endothelial injury in coronary heart disease in humans. Atherosclerosis 1991, 91:1-14.

309. Jacobs DO, Kobayashi T, Imagire J et al. Sepsis alters skeletal muscle energetics and membrane function. Surgery 1991; 110:318-326.

310. Grum CM, Simon RH, Dantzker DR et al. Evidence for adenosine triphosphate degradation in critically-ill patients. Chest 1985; 88:763-767.

311. Chaudry IH, Wichterman KA, Baue AE. Effect of sepsis on tissue adenine nucleotide levels. Surgery 1979; 85:205-211.

312. McDonough KH, Lang CH, Spitzer JJ. The effect of hyperdynamic sepsis on myocardial performance. Circ Shock 1985; 15:247-259.

313. Pasque MK, Murphy CE, Van Trigt P et al. Myocardial adenosine triphosphate levels during early sepsis. Arch Surg 1983; 118:1437-1440.

314. D'Orio V, El Allaf D, Vaira S et al. Lack of defective cardiac oxidative metabolism in intact dogs subjected to a prolonged low-dose infusion of *Escherichia coli* endotoxin. Circ Shock 1986; 18:43-52.

315. Dhainaut J-F, Huyghebaert M-F, Monsallier JF et al. Coronary hemodynamics and myocardial metabolism of lactate, free fatty acids, glucose, and ketones in patients with septic shock. Circulation 1987; 75:533-541.

316. Buja LM, Fattor RA, Miller JC et al. Effects of calcium loading and impaired energy production on metabolic and ultrastructural features of cell injury in cultured neonatal rat cardiac myocytes. Lab Invest 1990; 63:320-331.

317. Wagenknecht B, Beuttler C. Alterations of β-receptor-adenylyl cyclase coupling by long-term ATP depletion in cultured rat cardiomyocytes. Eur J Pharmacol—Mol Pharmacol Section 1991; 208:261-264.

318. van der Laarse A, Altona IC, van Dijkman RM et al. Metabolic blocker-induced damage in rat cardiac tissue—comparison of three models currently used: the isolated heart, heart cell cultures and isolated myocytes. Res Commun Chem Path Pharmacol 1984; 43:43-54.

319. Miyazaki Y, Gross RW, Sobel BE et al. Selective turnover of sarcolemmal phospholipids with lethal cardiac myocyte injury. Am J Physiol 1990; 259:C325-C331.

320. Goldhaber JI, Parker JM, Weiss JN. Mechanisms of excitation-contraction coupling failure during metabolic inhibition in guinea-pig ventricular myocytes. J Physiol 1991; 443:371-386.

321. Beuttler C. Das β-Adrenozeptor-Adenylatzyklasesystem kultivierter Rattenherzmuskelzellen—Effekte chronischer Energieverarmung und erhöhter Katecholaminkonzentrationenals Teilkomponenten der chronischen Myokardischämie. Medical Thesis, Ludwig-Maximilians-Universität München, Germany, 1993.

322. Mestril R, Dillmann WH. Heat shock and adaptive response to ischemia. Trends Cardiovasc Med 1991; 1:241-244.

323. Montgomery C, Hamilton N, Ianuzzo CD. Effects of different rates of cardiac pacing on rat myocardial energy status. Mol Cell Biochem 1991; 102:95-100.

324. Cunnion RE, Schaer GL, Parker MM et al. The coronary circulation in human septic shock. Circulation 1986; 73:637-644.

325. Hotchkiss RS, Rust RS, Dence CS et al. Evaluation of the role of cellular hypoxia in sepsis by the hypoxic marker (^{18}F)fluoromisonidazole. Am J Physiol 1991; 261:R965-R972.

326. Boekstegers P, Weidenhöfer S, Pilz G et al. Peripheral oxygen availability within skeletal muscle in sepsis and septic shock: comparison to limited infection and cardiogenic shock. Infection 1991; 19:317-323.

327. Barry WH. Calcium and ischemic injury. Trends Cardiovasc Med 1991; 1:162-166.

328. Quaife RA, Kohmoto O, Barry WH. Mechanisms of reoxygenation injury in cultured ventricular myocytes. Circulation 1991; 83:566-577.

329. Bond JM, Herman B, Lemasters JJ. Protection by acidotic pH against anoxia/reoxygenation injury to rat neonatal cardiac myocytes. Biochem Biophys Res Commun 1991; 179:798-803.

330. Musters RJP, Post JA, Verkleij AJ. The isolated neonatal rat—cardiomyocyte used in an invitro model for "ischemia". I. A morphological study. Biochim Biopyhs Acta 1991; 1091:270-277.

331. Heathers GP, Evers AS, Corr PB. Enhanced inositol triphosphate response to α_1-adrenergic stimulation in cardiac myocytes exposed to hypoxia. J Clin Invest 1989; 83:1409-1413.

332. Marsh JD, Sweeney KA. β-adrenergic receptor regulation during hypoxia in intact cultured heart cells. Am J Physiol 1989; 256:H275-H281.

333. Hagve T-A, Sprecher H, Hohl CM. The effect of anoxia on lipid metabolism in isolated adult rat cardiac myocytes. J Mol Cell Cardiol 1990; 22:1467-1475.

334. Boekstegers P, Pfeifer A, Peter W et al. Contractile dysfunction of "reperfused" neonatal rat heart cells: a model for studying "myocardial stunning" at the cellular level? Adv Exp Med Biol 1992; 14:573-582.

335. Gotloib L, Shostak A, Galdi P et al. Loss of microvascular negative charges accompanied by interstitial edema in septic rats' heart. Circ Shock 1992; 36:45-56.

336. Strasser RH, Marquetant R. Sensitization of the β-adrenergic system in acute myocardial ischemia by a protein kinase C-dependent mechanism. Eur Heart J 1991; 12(Supplement F):48-53.

337. Reithmann C, Wieland F, Jakobs KH et al. Intrinsic sympathomimetic activity of β-adrenoceptor antagonists: downregulation of cardiac β_1- and

β_2-adrenoceptors. Eur J Pharmacol 1989; 170:243-255.

338. Reithmann C, Gierschik P, Werdan K et al. Einfluß von Pseudomonas Exotoxin A auf die Regulation der Adenylatzyklase des Herzens—Blockkade der Noradrenalin-induzierten heterologen Desensibilisierung in Rattenherzmuskelzellen. Intensivmed 1989; 26 (Suppl 1):50-54.

339. Marsh JD, Roberts DJ. Adenylate cyclase regulation in intact cultured myocardial cells. Am J Physiol 1987; 252:C47-C54.

340. Reithmann C, Thomschke A, Werdan K. The role of endogenous noradrenaline in the beta-blocker withdrawal phenomenon—studies with cultured heart cells. Klin Wochenschr 1987; 65:308-316.

341. Porzig H, Becker C, Reuter H. Competitive and non-competitive interactions between specific ligands and β-adrenoceptors in living cardiac cells. Naunyn-Schmiedeberg's Arch Pharmacol 1982; 321:89-99.

342. Wallukat G, Wollenberger A. Modulation of β_2-adrenergic receptor function in cultured rat heart cells by L(+) lactate and pyruvate. In: Tucek S, Stipek S, Stastny F, Krivanek J, eds. Molecular basis of nerval function. Abstracts of the Sixth General Meeting of the European Society for Neurochemistry, 1986:165.

343. Kupfer LE, Bilezikian JP, Robinson RB. Regulation of alpha and beta adrenergic receptors by triiodothyronine in cultured rat myocardial cells. Naunyn-Schmiedeberg's Arch Pharmacol 1986; 334:275-281.

344. Lau YH, Robinson RB, Rosen MR et al. Subclassification of β-adrenergic receptors in cultured rat cardiac myoblasts and fibroblasts. Circ Res 1980; 47:41-48.

345. Kaumann AJ. Cultured heart cells as a model for β-adrenoceptors in a heart pacemaker—chronotropic spare β-adrenoceptors and spare adenylyl cyclase for (-)-isoprenaline but not for (-)-dichloroisoprenaline in rat cardiocytes. Naunyn-Schmiedeberg's Arch Pharmacol 1982; 320:119-129.

346. Hazeki O, Ui M. Beta$_1$- and beta$_2$-adrenergic receptors responsible for cyclic AMP accumulation in isolated heart and lung cells. Mol Pharmacol 1980; 17:8-13.

347. Freissmuth M, Hausleithner V, Nees S et al. Cardiac ventricular β_2-adrenoceptors in guinea-pigs and rats are localized on the coronary endothelium. Naunyn-Schmiedeberg's Arch Pharmacol 1986; 334:56-62.

348. Mauz ABM, Pelzer H. β-Adrenoceptor-binding studies of the cardioselective β-blockers bisoprolol, H-I 42 BS, and HX-CH 44 BS to heart membranes and intact ventricular myocytes of adult rats: two β_1-binding sites for bisoprolol. J Cardiovasc Pharmacol 1990; 15:421-427.

349. Muntz KH, Calianos TA, Vandermolen DT et al. Differences in affinity of cardiac β-adrenergic receptors for (^{3}H)dihydroalprenolol. Am J Physiol 1986; 250:H490-H497.

350. Buxton ILO, Brunton LL. Compartments of cyclic AMP and protein kinase in mammalian cardiomyocytes. J Biol Chem 1982; 258:10233-10239.

351. Reithmann C, Panzner B, Werdan K. Distinct pathways for β-adrenoceptor-induced up-regulation of muscarinic acetylcholine receptors and inhibitory G-protein α-subunits in chicken cardiomyocytes. Naunyn-Schmiedeberg's Arch Pharmacol 1992; 345:530-540.

352. Liang BT. Characterization of the adenosine receptor in cultured embryonic chick atrial myocytes: coupling to modulation of contractility and adenylate cyclase activity and identification by direct radioligand binding. J Pharmacol Exp Ther 1989; 249:775-784.

353. Foster KA, McDermott PJ, Robishax JD. Expression of G proteins in rat cardiac myocytes: effects of KCl depolarization. Am J Physiol 1990; 259:H432-H441.

354. Foster KA, Robishaw JD. Effect of calcium and cAMP on $G_{o\alpha}$ expression in neonatal rat cardiac myocytes. Am J Physiol Suppl 1991; 261:15-20.

355. Liang BT, Galper JB. Differential sensitivity of α_o and α_i to ADP-ribosylation by pertussis toxin in the intact cultured embryonic chick ventricular myocyte. Biochem Pharmacol 1988; 37:4549-4555.

356. Reuter H, Porzig H. Regulation by 8-Br-cAMP of β-adrenoceptors in cultured myocardial cells. J Mol Cell Cardiol 1985; 17: 307-316.

357. Weisensee D, Bereiter-Hahn J, Schoeppe W et al. Effects of cytokines on the contractility of cultured cardiac myocytes. Int J Immunopharmac 1993; 15:581-587.

358. Kumar A, Dimou C, Hollenberg SM et al. Tumor necrosis factor produces a concentration-dependent depression of myocardial cell contraction in vitro. Circ Res 1991; 39:321A.

CHAPTER 5

DERANGEMENT
OF CARDIAC STRUCTURE

FINDINGS IN THE PREANTIBIOTIC ERA

Romberg[1] described the morphological changes seen in septic myocarditis: "Septic myocarditis is mostly due to an invasion of septic material into the coronary arteries. In the surroundings of the occluded vessel, inflammation arises, often resulting in a liquefaction of the tissue, an abscess. These abscesses are often miliar in nature and usually intersperse the heart muscle in a large number. Rarely, direct invading of the septic process from the valves or from the mural endocardium into the heart muscle results in larger abscesses. The suppurations thus originating occasionally perforate the walls and pour into the lumen of the heart. Blood flows into the abscess cavern. Cardiac rupture can result, and also an abnormal communication between two cavities of the heart." (Free translation of the authors.)

PATHOMORPHOLOGICAL CORRELATES
OF SEPTIC CARDIOMYOPATHY IN PATIENTS

To the surprise of the clinicians often fighting unsuccessfully against heart failure in sepsis, pathomorphological correlates of septic cardiomyopathy are scarce.[2] In recent textbooks of cardiovascular pathology,[3] sepsis of the heart is not specifically delineated as it was 75 years ago.[1] In a recent review, Müller-Höcker and Haerty[4] state, "Specific pathomorphological alterations of the heart in sepsis have not been described, however, and the question remains whether they exist." The authors have nicely summarized the available information. Their review forms the basis of the following short synopsis:

PRIMARY INFECTIVE HEART DISEASE AS A CAUSE OF SEPSIS

Endocarditis—predominantly of the aortic and/or mitral valves—is the putative source. It results either from primary bacterial attacks on the valves, or from nonbacterial thrombotic endocarditis caused by endothelial injury with secondary bacterial infection. Vegetations are composed of platelets admixed with fibrin, red blood cells, and especially polymorphonuclear leukocytes and bacteria. In immunocompromised patients, not only bacteria, but also fungi like *Candida albicans* and *Aspergillus fumigatus* can destroy the valves. Besides the resulting valvular incompetence, vegetations of the aortic valve can also occlude orifices of the coronary arteries, resulting in myocardial ischemia or embolic heart disease.

MYOCARDIAL ABSCESS FORMATION

Two routes of abscess formation can be discerned: continuous spread of the infectious organisms from an infected valve into the paravalvular myocardium and in case of bacteremia, dissemination and proliferation of bacteria and fungi in the heart via the vascular route. Besides the abscess type of myocarditis in sepsis, diffuse infiltration by neutrophils, granulocytic myocarditis can also be observed. Though transient bacteremias are common events in infections, with the microorganisms entering the blood through lymphatics or by crossing the vessel walls, in most of the cases the human body has efficient defense mechanisms to prevent infectious endocarditis. In immunocompromised patients, however, abscess formation in the heart can be severe, especially by fungi. The hyphae not only escape from the vessels into the tissue, but also invade the parenchymal vessels and thus lead to additional ischemic muscle necrosis.

However, these pathomorphological changes are even less frequently encountered in sepsis and septic shock than are positive blood cultures nowadays. If anything is seen at all, then these changes are usually nonspecific.

NONSPECIFIC PATHOMORPHOLOGICAL CHANGES OF THE HEART SEEN IN SEPSIS

Gross Morphology

Enlargement of the left ventricle due to dilatation with rounding of the apex, increased heart weight because of interstitial fluid overload, and small thrombotic, noninfectious vegetations on the heart valves in the course of accelerated coagulation are macroscopic alterations of the heart which can be seen in sepsis.

Histological Findings

While fragmentation of the heart muscle with separation of the cardiomyocytes from each other at the intercalated discs is a typical feature of the nonseptic heart at autopsy, elongated and undulated wavy fibers lacking fragmentation can be seen in sepsis. The latter phenomenon is due to an impairment of contractility caused by loss of adenosine triphosphate. It indicates a prenecrotic but probably fully reversible state of cardiomyocyte damage which is especially common in ischemic heart disease. The wavy appearance is induced by the regularly contracting and relaxing muscle cells in the vicinity of the damaged region.

Hypercontraction bands with clumping of filaments are attributed to increased endogenous or pharmacologically applied catecholamine levels, representing a reversible injury, with the potential of irreversible cell necrosis. An increase in cytoplasmic calcium level is probably the causative mechanism.

Ultrastructure

Severe calcium overload can occasionally be detected by the typical staining aspect of a blueish appearance of the cardiomyocyte. Electron microscopy reveals mitochondria as stores of excess calcium. On the other hand, calcium overload is also the consequence of cell death.

Mitochondria may often present with swelling of their matrices, with nonspecific damage of their cristae and also with an accumulation of lipid droplets, the latter seen preferentially in regions with lower oxygen tissue tension, like the subendocardial area of papillary muscle.

However, as Müller-Höcker and Haerty[4] state, "all these changes are by no means specific. They merely indicate disturbance of energy production. Similar changes therefore may be present during ischemia and probably also after therapeutic administration of catecholamines."

PATHOMORPHOLOGICAL CORRELATES IN ANIMAL SEPSIS MODELS

A BRIEF OVERVIEW

Myocardial edema and hemorrhage represent two prominent morphological signs of endotoxin shock in animals:[2] accumulation of edema between and within myocardial myofibrils and in mitochondria is found during endotoxin shock in the dog,[5,6] with the edema severe enough in some cases to cause mitochondrial rupture. Also in baboons subjected to *E. coli* endotoxin[7] and live *E. coli*,[8,9] the morphological picture is dominated by myofibrils and mitochondria separated by edema (intra- and interfiber edema) by high amplitude swelling of mitochondria and by an increased number of contraction bands. Discrete hemorrhages of epicardium are observed in LD_{100} *E. coli*-shocked baboons.[10] In endotoxin-shocked dogs, myocardial hemorrhage can be detected five hours post-endotoxin, it increases in severity from five to twelve hours post-endotoxin, but thereafter, only a minimum of new cardiac lesions appears.[11]

As a third important finding, morphological correlates of a microcirculatory dysfunction seem to exist in the septic heart:[12] myocardial biopsies of hyperdynamic septic sheep demonstrated patchy cell necroses,[13] as typically seen when cardiac vessels are damaged on the microcirculatory level.[14]

LOSS OF MICROVASCULAR NEGATIVE CHARGES ACCOMPANIED BY INTERSTITIAL EDEMA

With myocardial edema being a prominent feature of experimental septic cardiomyopathy, we must look for its etiology. Very elegant experimental work from Gotloib and coworkers[15] point to a loss of microvascular negative charges as the underlying cause:

All microvascular basement membranes show anionic fixed charges, whose main role is to prevent the escape of anionic plasma proteins from the blood compartment. The negative charges of heart capillaries and of cardiomyocytes can be documented by transmission electron microscopy with the cationic binding tracers ruthenium red and poly-ethylene imine. Twenty-four hours after intraperitoneal injection of live *E. coli* in rats ($LD_{68/24 h}$) negative charges decrease in glycocalyx and basement membrane of myocardial capillary endothelial cells. There is a substantial amount of edema. The density of anionic charges in the sarcolemmal glycocalyx and basement membrane of cardiomyocytes is also markedly reduced. Myocardial cells' mitochondria consistently show morphological changes, their severity ranging between stages II and IV C of Trump.[16] Thirteen days after induction of sepsis, capillary endothelial and myocardial cells will recover almost completely, lacking intracellular edema.

The data of Gotloib and his group[15] argue for a significant reduction in negative charges during Gram-negative sepsis, which are normally present in the microvascular wall as well as on cardiomyocytes. As a consequence, several membranes limiting the various compartments of the heart tissue lose their structural integrity. The authors conclude, "This morphometric data could explain the development of protein-rich interstitial edema and defective cell volume regulation observed in cardiac muscle of endotoxin-shocked animals. This myocardial edema may be at the origin of the cardiac dysfunction observed in both experimental and human septic shock."

The heart is not the only organ where a loss of microvascular negative charges can be found in sepsis. A significant decrease in anionic sites also takes place in skeletal muscle microvasculature of septic rats.[17] Therefore, this loss of negative charges of cell membranes seems to represent a more general phenomenon in sepsis, being responsible for the leakage of protein-rich fluid into the interstitium and for cell volume dysregulation. Preventing this loss of charges by therapeutic measures could be a potent approach to reduce the functional impairment of septic multiple organ dysfunction syndrome including that of the heart.

WHAT REMAINS TO BE DONE ?
—A NONPATHOLOGIST'S VIEW

Looking for molecular mechanisms of septic cardiomyopathy, the pathomorphological findings available today do not seem to be very helpful. In patients, only scarce, if any, and mostly nonspecific observations have been reported. To make the story even more puzzling, these nonspecific pathological findings are similar to those being present during myocardial ischemia, while pathophysiological data strongly argue against myocardial ischemia as the main cause of heart failure in sepsis.

In animal models, edema, hemorrhage as well as signs of microcirculatory dysfunction and their consequences dominate the morphological alterations in septic hearts. The documented loss of negative charges of the vessels and cardiomyocytes[15] is a first, important step from a purely descriptive to a more pathophysiologically oriented pathology of septic cardiomyopathy. With great interest, we will await future results regarding the expression of cytokines, adhesion molecules and other mediators in the course of the development of heart failure in sepsis. We are convinced that those data might contribute a considerable part to the understanding of the mechanisms underlying septic cardiomyopathy.

REFERENCES

1. Romberg E. Die septische akute Myokarditis. In: Romberg E, ed. Krankheiten des Herzens und der Blutgefäße. 3rd edition. Stuttgart: Ferdinand Enke, 1921:494.

2. Archer LT. Pathological manifestations of septic shock. In: Proctor R.A., ed. Clinical Aspects of Endotoxin Shock (Handbook of Endotoxin 4, Proctor RA, series editor). Amsterdam, New York, Oxford: Elsevier, 1986:18-54.

3. Silver MD, ed. Cardiovascular Pathology. 2nd edition. Edinburgh: Churchill Livingstone, 1991.

4. Müller-Höcker J, Haerty W. Pathomorphological aspects of the heart in septic patients. In: Schlag G, Redl H, eds. Pathophysiology of Shock, Sepsis, and Organ Failure. Berlin, Heidelberg, New York: Springer-Verlag, 1993:853-858.

5. Coalson JJ, Woodruff HK, Greenfield LJ et al. Effects of digoxin on myocardial ultrastructure in endotoxin shock. Surg Gynec Obstet 1972; 135:908-912.

6. Mela L, Hinshaw LB, Coalson JJ. Correlation of cardiac performance, ultrastructural morphology and mitochondrial function in endotoxemia in the dog. Circ Shock 1974; 1:265- 272.

7. Coalson JJ, Benjamin B, Archer LT et al. Prolonged shock in the baboon subjected to infusion of E. coli endotoxin. Circ Shock 1978; 5:423-437.

8. Coalson JJ, Hinshaw LB, Guenter CA et al. Pathophysiologic responses of the subhuman primate in experimental septic shock. Lab Invest 1975; 32:561-569.

9. Coalson JJ, Archer LT, Benjamin BA et al. A morphologic study of live Escherichia coli organism shock in baboons. Exp Mol Pathol 1979; 31:10-22.

10. Archer LT, Kosanke SD, Beller BK et al. Prevention or amelioration of morphologic lesions in LD_{100} *E. coli*-shocked baboons with steroid/antibiotic therapy. In: Reichard SM, Reynolds DG, Adams HR, eds. Advances in Shock Research 10. New York: Alan R Liss, 1983:195-215.

11. Brunson JG, Schulz DM, Angevine DM et al. Evaluation of therapeutic agents: morphologic changes and survival data in dogs subjected to endotoxin during the shock tour. J Oklahoma State Med Assoc 1966; 59:479-484.

12. Bloos F, Sibbald WJ. Cardiocirculation in sepsis. In: Reinhart K, Eyrich K, Sprung C, eds. Sepsis—Current Perspectives in Pathophysiology and Therapy (Update in Intensive Care and Emergency Medicine 18). Berlin, Heidelberg: Springer; 1994:139-149.

13. Hersch M, Gnidec AA, Bersten AD et al. Histologic and ultrastructural changes in nonpulmonary organs during early hyperdynamic sepsis. Surgery 1990;107:397-410.

14. Ince C, Ashruf JF, Avontuur JAM et al. Heterogeneity of the hypoxic state in rat heart is determined at capillary level. Am J Physiol 1993;264:H294-301.

15. Gotloib L, Shostak A, Galdi P et al. Loss of microvascular negative charges accompanied by interstitial edema in septic rats' heart. Circ Shock 1992; 36:45-56.

16. Trump BF, Berezesky IK, Cowley RA. The cellular and subcellular characteristics of acute and chronic injury with emphasis on the role of calcium. In: Cowley RA, Trump BF, eds. Pathophysiology of Shock, Anoxia and Ischemia. Baltimore: Williams and Wilkins, 1982:6-60.

17. Gotloib L, Shostak, Jaichenko J et al. Decreased density distribution of mesenteric and diaphragmatic microvascular anionic charges during murine abdominal sepsis. Resuscitation 1988; 16:179-182.

CHAPTER 6

DERANGEMENT OF CORONARY CIRCULATION AND MYOCARDIAL OXYGEN SUPPLY

In coronary artery disease, myocardial impairment is due to a reduced supply of the heart with blood, resulting in a deficit in O_2 supply in relation to O_2 demand. In septic cardiomyopathy, not an inadequate O_2 supply by the coronary macrocirculation, but the impaired coronary reserve based on disturbances in coronary microcirculation seems to be a problem.

CORONARY CIRCULATION

Coronary circulation in patients with septic shock was studied by measuring coronary sinus blood flow and major cardiac vein blood flow.[1]

Cunnion et al[2] compared coronary blood flow in seven patients with septic shock with measurements in subjects with normal coronary arteries at rest and during pacing. No significant differences were noted in coronary blood flow at heart rates below 100 beats/min. At heart rates above 100 beats/min, septic patients had higher coronary sinus blood flow and major cardiac vein blood flow than paced normal subjects. Despite elevated arterial lactate levels, net myocardial lactate production was never observed. Coronary perfusion was characterized by a high coronary sinus oxygen saturation at low arterial oxygen extraction, abnormalities typical of the peripheral vasculature in septic shock. Similar findings were obtained by Dhainaut et al[3] in 40 patients with septic shock in comparison to 13 control patients. Coronary sinus blood flow was higher in septic patients than in the control group due to marked coronary vasodilatation, particularly in the subgroup of nonsurvivors. Myocardial oxygen consumption, myocardial work loads and myocardial efficiency were not significantly different in the control and septic patients.

In contrast to the uniform findings in patients with septic shock documenting a high coronary blood flow, experimental data in animal models of septic shock are more heterogenous, both an increase[4] and a decrease[5-7] of coronary perfusion having been reported (for review see Dhainaut et al[1] and Bloos and Sibbald[8]). In detail, the following observations have been published:

- In isolated hearts from endotoxemic dogs, Cho[9] noticed that endotoxin constricts coronary arteries.
- From data obtained with endotoxemic dogs, Bohs et al[5] concluded that myocardial dysfunction may be associated with cardiac ischemia.
- Kleinman et al[7] found in endotoxemic dogs a nonuniform coronary perfusion and histological damage of the heart.
- In endotoxemic pigs, myocardial dysfunction was attributed to a relative hypoperfusion of the subendocardium.[4]
- A coronary blood flow high enough to maintain myocardial O_2 need was noticed by D'Orio et al[6] in endotoxemic dogs. He argued that endotoxemia reduces heart work because of a decrease in afterload, with the consequence of a diminished myocardial O_2 need and an autoregulatory fall in coronary blood flow. This hypothesis, however, is inconsistent with the finding of an improved coronary blood flow in a canine model of endotoxemic shock after infusion of glucose-insulin-potassium, accompanied by a restoration of myocardial performance.[10]
- Based on their findings in endotoxemic dogs, Groeneveld et al[11] postulated an increased heterogeneity of coronary blood flow causing focal myocardial ischemia.

While the animal septic shock models described above probably mimic human septic shock of a relatively late phase, animal normotensive sepsis models with adequate fluid resuscitation better represent the early phase of human sepsis. After inducing an intraperitoneal inflammatory focus and avoiding hypotension by adequate fluid resuscitation, in all the studies describing normotensive experimental sepsis uniformly an increased coronary blood flow was shown, due to coronary vasodilatation.[12-16]

CORONARY RESERVE

The heart, unlike skeletal muscle, cannot accept an O_2 debt. Therefore, O_2 supply to the myocardium must always match the O_2 need of the heart, and any failure to do so will cause myocardial dysfunction, even if no necrosis occurs.[17] Coronary autoregulation and coronary metabolic regulation are aimed at providing O_2 also under critical conditions, and thereby mismatch of supply and demand is avoided (for review see Bloos and Sibbald[8]). In coronary vasculature, the autoregulatory range, i.e., the ability to maintain blood flow independent of arterial perfusion pressure, lies between 70 to 130 mm Hg, with the site of autoregulation located mainly in arterioles with a diameter < 100 μm. If myocardial O_2 demand rises, coronary blood flow will increase by vasodilatation, which results in a narrowing of the autoregulatory range up to a complete loss in case of maximal vasodilatation.

The coronary metabolic regulation relies on the release of substances (adenosine, prostacyclins) which are apt to dilate coronary arteries and thereby increase coronary blood flow within 20 seconds, with the prize of shifting blood from "nonvital" organs, which have a higher O_2 extraction reserve than the myocardium. In addition to the "flow" reserve, some increase in myocardial O_2 extraction, which even at rest is relatively high (about 70%), can provide the heart with more O_2.

In sepsis with its enhanced coronary blood flow, coronary autoregulation is limited, making the septic heart more susceptible to low perfusion pressures.[18,19] Coronary metabolic regulation remains intact in sepsis, an increase in heart work being accompanied by an increase in coronary blood flow,[14,16] yet its reserve still is significantly depressed;[8] coronary flow reserve during a severe hypoxic stress is three times larger in control sheep than in septic sheep ($419 \pm 126\%$ vs $143 \pm 48\%$). Only in control but not in septic sheep, myocardial O_2 extraction reserve could be mobilized ($11 \pm 5\%$ vs $1 \pm 4\%$). Moreover, splanchnic organs did not contribute to the redistribution of cardiac output to the heart as encountered in healthy animals. The hearts of septic sheep could not maintain their O_2 need when arterial oxygen dropped below about 80 ml O_2/ml compared to about 55 ml O_2/ml in healthy sheep. These experimental findings in sheep[16] confirm similar results in rhesus monkeys,[20] documenting that the septic heart is more sensitive to even brief hypoxia than healthy ones.

MICROCIRCULATION AND MYOCARDIAL O_2 SUPPLY/DEMAND RATIO

In the balance of tissue O_2 supply and demand, the microcirculation plays a prominent role. In many organs, microcirculatory dysfunction has been shown to occur during sepsis (for review see Bloos and Sibbald,[8] Menger et al[21]), with the number of nonperfused capillaries being higher in sepsis than under normal conditions. The multifactorial pathogenesis of microcirculatory dysfunction[8,21] may include endothelial cell damage, adhesion of leukocytes to endothelial cells, plugging of capillaries by stiff erythrocytes, as well as a left-shift in the O_2 dissociation curve.[22]

With regard to the microcirculation of the septic heart, however, only a few findings are available. Biopsies from hearts of hyperdynamic septic sheep demonstrate patchy cell necrosis,[23] which strongly suggests that myocardial vessels are damaged on the microcirculatory level.[24] More data are necessary to unequivocally document the suggested dysfunction of coronary microcirculation in sepsis.

In sepsis, disturbances in microcirculation are usually accompanied by a diminished O_2 extraction capacity. Also in humans, myocardial O_2 extraction is depressed in sepsis;[1-3] patients with septic shock extract less O_2 from the coronary circulation than controls. In agreement, an O_2 extraction defect has also been demonstrated in the hearts of septic sheep during hypoxic stress (see above).

With the finding of a reduced O_2 extraction capacity of the heart in sepsis, the role of a pathological oxygen supply dependency also comes into play, i.e., the fact that the O_2 uptake in septic organs depends on a wider concentration range of O_2 delivery than under physiological conditions, and thus higher O_2 delivery levels are necessary to optimize and plateau the O_2 uptake. It is beyond the scope of this article to fully elaborate on the topic of a pathological oxygen supply dependency in sepsis, its relevance presently being under vivid discussion,[25] but two aspects will be viewed. First, the concept of a pathological oxygen supply in sepsis demands a supranormal O_2 delivery to the organs, which can only be achieved by a high cardiac output. Taking into account the severely stressed heart in sepsis, an additional stress by catecholamines to raise cardiac output might eventually harm the organ even more. With this respect it is worthwhile mentioning that, in contrast to earlier findings, in a very well conducted recent trial[26] supranormal O_2 delivery achieved by dobutamine treatment could not improve the outcome of septic patients.

Second, the question arises if the heart itself benefits from supranormal oxygen delivery. At present, no clear-cut answer to this question is yet available. However, it is the opinion of the authors that it might not. The argument for this assumption is indirect, inferred from our group's measurements of skeletal muscle pO_2 in septic patients: by means of needle electrodes it is possible to measure partial oxygen pressure in skeletal muscle. By doing this in patients with well-defined sepsis, surprisingly not a decreased, but even an increased oxygen partial pressure is found, while pO_2 in patients with cardiogenic shock is, as expected, low (Fig. 6.1). Fever alone is not the cause of this elevated pO_2 (Fig. 6.1).[27,28] During patients' recovery, skeletal muscle pO_2 normalizes by going down (Fig. 6.2).[28] Of the septic patients treated with anti-TNF-α-antibody, only those who respond exhibit a fall of the increased skeletal muscle pO_2.[29] The data of Reinhart et al[30] as well are in agreement with the concept of an increased but not decreased skeletal muscle O_2 partial pressure in sepsis. Rising O_2 delivery from 692 to 830 ml x min^{-1} m^{-2} in patients with hyperdynamic septic shock did not further enhance the skeletal muscle pO_2 slightly elevated from the start. As these skeletal muscle pO_2 measurements are representative of both extracellular (interstitial) and intracellular pO_2 in skeletal muscle tissue, the muscle cell apparently is not deprived of O_2. And even if a pathological O_2 supply/O_2 demand ratio would prevail, then pharmacological interventions to increase oxygen

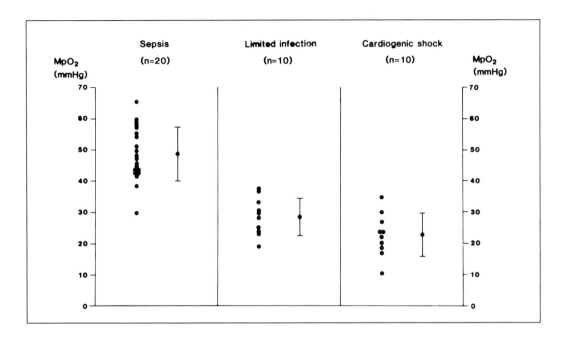

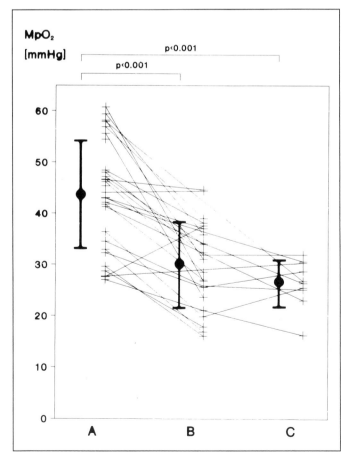

Fig. 6.1. Above: Comparison of individual mean skeletal muscle pO_2 in septic patients, patients with limited infection without sepsis and patients with cardiogenic shock. MpO_2 = mean skeletal muscle pO_2. In addition to the individual values (points) means ± SDs are given.
(Reproduced with permission from: Boekstegers P, Weidenhöfer S, Pilz G et al. Peripheral oxygen availability within skeletal muscle in sepsis and septic shock: Comparison to limited infection and cardiogenic shock. Infection 1991; 19:317-323.)

Fig. 6.2. Left: Serial intermittent determinations of skeletal muscle pO_2 in 28 patients with sepsis during seven consecutive days. A) days of septic state; B) days of intermediate state; C) days of nonseptic state. Values of each patient and the mean ± SD of each state are given. To convert torr to kPa, multiply the torr value by 0.1333. (Reproduced with permission from: Boekstegers P, Weidenhöfer S, Kapsner T et al. Skeletal muscle partial pressure of oxygen in patients with sepsis. Crit Care Med 1994; 22:640-650.)

supply (delivery) would be without success. These data, in our opinion, strongly argue for a reduced O_2 extraction not only due to disturbed microcirculation, but also to an additional defect in intracellular O_2 utilization, at least in skeletal muscle. If this holds true for the heart muscle, too, then an increase in O_2 delivery to the myocardium should not be helpful, but septic cardiomyopathy might rather improve by a therapeutic approach aiming at the reactivation of the impaired cellular metabolism (see chapter 7) and recovery of the deranged inotropic cascades of the cardiomyocyte (see chapter 8).

CONCLUSIONS
1. Coronary blood flow in the early phases of normotensive human sepsis is not diminished, but probably even increased; and in the later phase, during septic shock, global coronary blood flow neither is decreased but increased, however regional myocardial ischemia may occur.
2. The metabolic reserve of the heart is significantly depressed in sepsis, due to its inability to sufficiently raise coronary blood flow and myocardial O_2 extraction. Therefore, the septic myocardium becomes more sensitive to hypoxia and hypotension. The O_2 availability of the healthy heart is unaffected by anemia over a large range of hematocrits due to the large cardiac metabolic reserve. However, with the metabolic reserve being depressed in sepsis a normal hemoglobin might be necessary to maintain myocardial O_2 need in a hyperdynamic state.

REFERENCES
1. Dhainaut J-F, Dall'Ava J, Mira JP. Coronary hemodynamics and myocardial metabolism in sepsis and septic shock. In: Schlag G, Redl H, eds. Pathophysiology of Shock, Sepsis, and Organ Failure. Berlin, Heidelberg, New York: Springer-Verlag, 1993:882-892.
2. Cunnion RE, Schaer GL, Parker MM et al. The coronary circulation in human septic shock. Circulation 1986; 73:637-644.
3. Dhainaut JF, Hughebaert M-F, Monsallier JF et al. Coronary hemodynamics and myocardial metabolism of lactate, free fatty acids, glucose, and ketones in patients with septic shock. Circulation 1987; 75:533-541.
4. Goldfarb RD, Nightingale LM, Kish P et al. Left ventricular function during lethal and sublethal endotoxemia in swine. Am J Physiol 1986; 251:H364-H373.
5. Bohs CT, Turbow ME, Kolmen SN et al. Coronary blood flow alterations in endotoxin shock and response to dipyridamole. Circ Shock 1976; 3:281-286.
6. D'Orio V, El Allaf D, Vaira S et al. Lack of defective cardiac oxidative metabolism in intact dogs subjected to a prolonged low-dose infusion of *Escherichia coli* endotoxin. Circ Shock 1986; 18:43-52.

7. Kleinman WM, Krause SM, Hess ML. Differential subendocardial perfusion and injury during the course of gram-negative endotoxemia. Adv Shock Res 1980; 4:139-152.

8. Bloos F, Sibbald WJ. Cardiocirculation in sepsis. In: Reinhart K, Eyrich K, Sprung C, eds. Sepsis—Current Perspectives in Pathophysiology and Therapy (Update in Intensive Care and Emergency Medicine 18). Berlin, Heidelberg: Springer-Verlag, 1994:139-149.

9. Cho YW. Direct cardiac action of *E. coli* endotoxin (36856). Proc Soc Exp Biol Med 1972;141:705-707.

10. Bronsveld W, van Lambalgen AA, van Velzen D et al. Myocardial metabolic and morphometric changes during canine endotoxin shock before and after glucose-insulin-potassium. Cardiovasc Res 1985; 19:455-464.

11. Groeneveld ABJ, van Lambalgen AA, van den Bos GC et al. Maldistribution of heterogenous coronary blood flow during canine endotoxin shock. Cardiovasc Res 1991; 25:80-88.

12. Lang CH, Bagby GJ, Ferguson JL et al. Cardiac output and redistribution of organ blood flow in hypermetabolic sepsis. Am J Physiol 1984; 246:R331-R337.

13. Fish RE, Burns AH, Lang CH et al. Myocardial dysfunction in a nonlethal, nonshock model of chronic endotoxemia. Circ Shock 1985; 16:241-252.

14. Fish RE, Lang CH, Spitzer JA. Regional blood flow during continuous low-dose endotoxin infusion. Circ Shock 1986; 18:267-275.

15. Lee KJ, Dziuban SW Jr, van der Zee H et al. Cardiac function and coronary flow in chronic endotoxemic pigs (42805). Proc Soc Exp Biol Med 1988; 189:245-252.

16. Bloos F, Morisaki H, Neal A et al. Is the circulatory "reserve" supporting tissue O_2 availability depressed in normotensive hyperdynamic sepsis? Crit Care Med 1992; 20:S55.

17. Laxson DD, Homans DC, Dai X-Z et al. Oxygen consumption and coronary flow in chronic endotoxemic pigs (42805). Proc Soc Exp Biol Med 1989; 189:245-252.

18. Elkins RC, McCurdy JR, Brown PP et al. Effects of coronary perfusion on myocardial performance during endotoxin shock. Surg Gynecol Obstet 1973; 137:991-996.

19. Hinshaw LB, Archer LT, Spitzer JJ et al. Effects of coronary hypotension and endotoxin on myocardial performance. Am J Physiol 1974; 227:1051-1057.

20. Snow TR, Dickey DT, Hinshaw LB et al. Early myocardial dysfunction induced with endotoxin in rhesus monkeys. Can J Cardiol 1990; 6:130-136.

21. Menger MD, Vollmar B, Messmer K. Sepsis and nutritional blood flow. In: Reinhart K, Eyrich K, Sprung, eds. Sepsis - Current Perspectives in Pathophysiology and Therapy (Update in Intensive Care and Emergency Medicine 18). Berlin, Heidelberg: Springer-Verlag, 1994:163-173.

22. Bloos F, Neal A, Pitt M et al. A left-shifted O_2 dissociation curve contributes to the depressed O_2 extraction in hyperdynamic septic sheep. Chest 1993; 104:152S.

23. Hersch M, Gnidec AA, Bersten AD et al. Histologic and ultrastructural changes in non pulmonary organs during early hyperdynamic sepsis. Surgery 1990; 107:397-410.

24. Ince C, Ashruf JF, Avontuur JAM et al. Heterogeneity of the hypoxic state in rat heart is determined at capillary level. Am J Physiol 1993; 264:H294-H301

25. Cain SM. A Current view of oxygen supply dependency. In: Reinhart K, Eyrich K, Sprung C, eds. Sepsis - Current Perspectives in Pathophysiology and Therapy (Update in Intensive Care and Emergency Medicine 18). Berlin, Heidelberg: Springer-Verlag, 1994:150-162.

26. Hayes MA, Timmins AC, Yau EHS et al. Elevation of systemic oxygen delivery in the treatment of critically ill patients. N Engl J Med 1994; 330:1717-1722.

27. Boekstegers P, Weidenhöfer S, Pilz G et al. Peripheral oxygen availability within skeletal muscle in sepsis and septic shock: Comparison to limited infection and cardiogenic shock. Infection 1991; 19:317-323.

28. Boekstegers P, Weidenhöfer S, Kapsner T et al. Skeletal muscle partial pressure of oxygen in patients with sepsis. Crit Care Med 1994; 22:640-650.

29. Boekstegers P, Weidenhöfer S, Zell R et al. Changes in skeletal muscle pO_2 after administration of anti-TNF-α-antibody in patients with severe sepsis: comparison to interleukin-6 serum levels, APACHE II, and Elebute scores. Shock 1994;1:246-253.

30. Reinhart K, Hannemann L, Meier-Hellmann A et al. Monitoring of O_2 transport and tissue oxygenation in septic shock. In: Reinhart K, Eyrich K, Sprung C, eds. Sepsis—Current Perspectives in Pathophysiology and Therapy (Update in Intensive Care and Emergency Medicine 18). Berlin, Heidelberg: Springer-Verlag, 1994:193-213.

CHAPTER 7

DERANGEMENT OF MYOCARDIAL METABOLISM

OVERVIEW ON MYOCARDIAL METABOLISM

The mechanical work carried out by the heart can vary tremendously during a 24-hour-period, with a relatively low cardiac energy demand during sleep (oxygen consumption about 8 ml/100 g tissue/min) and a several fold increase during strenuous exercise (oxygen consumption about 80 ml/100g tissue/min). Consequently the heart is not only an organ with a high energy production and consumption, but also one with a high degree of regulation.

This brief overview consists of a short description of the varying energy demands of the heart, the substrates used for ATP synthesis, the different ways of aerobic and anaerobic energy production, as well as its different modes of regulation; finally, some pathophysiological aspects will be discussed concerning the impaired myocardial energy metabolism in patients with various nonseptic heart diseases.

ENERGY DEMAND OF THE HEART

The Energy-Rich Molecules

Adenosine triphosphate (ATP) is the energy source for contraction (Table 7.1): the myosin ATPase splits ATP in adenosine diphosphate (ADP) and inorganic phosphate (P_i), with the release of free energy. Lost ATP is rapidly restored by the energy-rich creatine phosphate (CP): the creatine phosphokinases (CP-kinases) transfer the energy of CP to ADP, yielding ATP and creatine (C), with the equilibrium favoring formation of ATP by 50 times. In the heart, several CP-kinase isoenzymes exist; the larger proportion is present in the cytosol as the MB isoenzyme, consisting of one subunit of the muscle (M) type and one subunit of the brain (B) type isoenzyme. Small amounts of the MM isoenzyme are located in the myofibrils and possibly also in the microsomes.

At the outer side of the inner mitochondrial membrane, probably in close vicinity to the adenine nucleotide translocator (see below), a mitochondrial CP-kinase isoenzyme is located. It is supposed that this isoenzyme converts the newly synthesized and exported mitochondrial ATP into cytosolic CP. This CP is then reconverted to ATP by other CP-kinase isoenzymes at the cytosolic site of its use.

Table 7.1. The energy-rich molecules

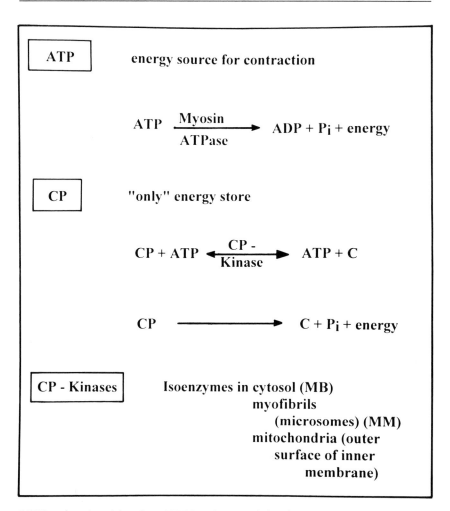

"ATP" = adenosine triphosphate; "ADP" = adenosine diphosphate; "P$_i$" = inorganic phosphate; "CP" = creatine phosphate; "C" = creatine; "CP-Kinases" = creatine phosphokinases; "MB" = muscle/brain isoenzyme; "MM" = muscle/muscle isoenzyme

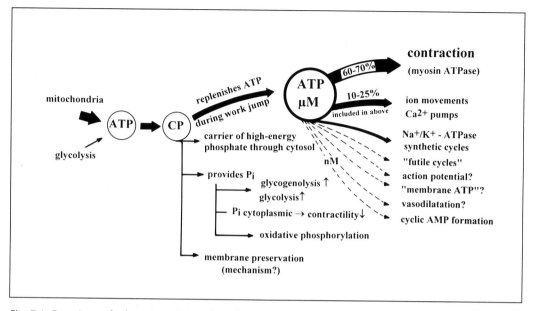

Fig. 7.1. Functions of adenosine triphosphate (ATP) and creatine phosphate (CP) in the heart. For further explanation see text. (Modified from Opie LH. The Heart–Physiology and Metabolism. New York: Raven Press, 1991.)

Consumption of Adenosine Triphosphate and Creatine Phosphate in the Heart

The functions of ATP and CP in the heart (Fig. 7.1) are nicely summarized by Opie[1] (pp. 259-266):

Rough estimates of myocardial energy expenditure suggest that about 60-70% of ATP use is for contractile purposes, including the associated obligatory phenomena like calcium uptake by the sarcoplasmic reticulum and active transport of Na^+ and K^+ across the cell membrane, mediated by the Na^+/K^+-ATPase (about 10-15%). Only very little (less than 5%) ATP is used for the actual generation of the action potential and the conduction of the cardiac impulse, and even less for the protein kinase-mediated phosphorylation of proteins and cyclic AMP formation, the latter mediating important regulatory key functions of the cardiomyocyte. Small amounts of ATP are required to maintain normal mitochondrial volume and structure, for synthetic purposes (synthesis of glycogen, triglycerides and protein), to function as membrane-associated superficially located ATP and to run futile cycles like glycogen turnover, synthesis and breakdown of triglycerides in the triglyceride-fatty acid cycle, and the constant uptake and release of Ca^{2+} by the mitochondria. Since myocardial protein turns over at a relatively high rate, there must be a constant requirement of ATP for protein synthesis; in neonatal rat cardiomyocytes in culture, ATP depletion by 42% results in an inhibition of global protein synthesis by

34%.[2] Overall, the efficiency of conversion of chemical energy (ATP) into mechanical work in the heart is about 20-25%.

Replenishment of ATP stores and carrying high-energy phosphate through the cytosol are the main, but not the only functions of CP; it also works as a store of inorganic phosphate (P_i), which is liberated in the formation of ATP. The rapid increase of P_i in the cytosol is a striking feature of increased heart work or anoxia; it stimulates glycolysis by increasing the activity of the key glycolytic enzyme phosphofructokinase; it acts as a substrate for phosphorylase b to stimulate glycogenolysis, and it also stimulates oxidative phosphorylation by a yet unproven mechanism (alteration of the extramitochondrial phosphorylation potential (ATP)/(ADP)(P_i); increased uptake of P_i by mitochondria ?). Excess accumulation of P_i during ischemia can paradoxically inhibit contractility and thereby diminish oxygen demand.

Compartmentation and Transfer of Energy Rich Phosphates in Cardiomyocytes

Compartmentation of ATP (Fig. 7.2) between its site of production in mitochondria and its sites of use in the cytosol is a well-known phenomenon, with at least 90% of ATP prevalent in the cytosol. During

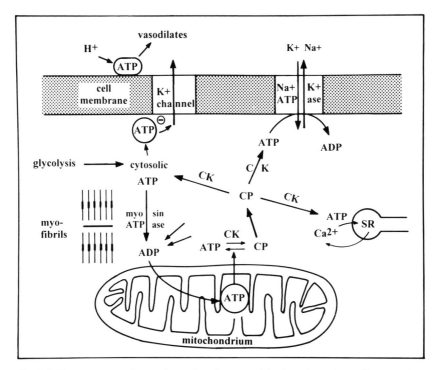

Fig. 7.2. Compartmentation and transfer of energy-rich phosphates in cardiomyocytes. CP = creatine phosphate; CK = creatine phosphokinase; ATP = adenosine triphopshate; ADP = adenosine diphosphate; SR = sarcoplasmic reticulum. For further explanation see text. (Modified from Opie LH. The Heart–Physiology and Metabolism. New York: Raven Press, 1991.)

heart work, cytosolic ATP breaks down and results in a doubling of the very small amount of cytosolic ADP, the rise in which then can stimulate mitochondrial respiration (see below).

The concept of subcompartments of ATP within the cytoplasm (Fig. 7.2) is increasingly accepted, though still discussed controversially (Opie,[1] pp. 264-265); minor localized cytoplasmic pools are associated with the potassium channel (ATP blocks K^+-flux through the channel) and the external surface ATP, which may function as a vasodilator. Uneven CP-kinase isoenzyme distribution within the cytosol (see above) argues for local ATP gradients around myofibrils and the sarcoplasmic reticulum (energy-dependent uptake of Ca^{2+}). The mitochondrial CP-kinase isoenzyme is located on the outer site of the inner mitochondrial membrane; it uses the ATP synthesized in the mitochondria and transported into the intermembrane space by the adenine nucleotide translocator to form CP from C. As the outer mitochondrial membrane is freely permeable for CP, it can diffuse into the cytoplasm where cytoplasmic CP-kinase isoenzymes can rebuild ATP from ADP with the energy of CP.

Nuclear Magnetic Resonance (NMR) Spectroscopy to Study Myocardial Energy Metabolism in the Intact Heart

Most information about energy-rich phosphates in the heart has been obtained from animal experiments by rapidly freezing myocardial tissue and analyzing the content of energy-rich phosphates by, for instance, high pressure liquid chromatography (HPLC). [31]P nuclear magnetic resonance (NMR) spectroscopy allows measurement, among others, of CP and ATP, even in intact hearts of animals and also in humans,[3,4] with a relatively good correlation of both methods as studied in myocardial ischemia[5] (also see below).

NMR spectroscopy renders the study of pathological states of the myocardium[6] possible (Fig. 7.3); in comparison to control hearts (Fig. 7.3A), inhibition of glycolysis in hearts perfused with pyruvate led to decreased levels of CP and ATP (Fig. 7.3B). However, contractile activity fell only slightly. During ischemia (Fig. 7.3C), there is a marked decrease in high-energy phosphates, particularly in CP. During reperfusion (Fig. 7.3D) resynthesis of CP precedes that of ATP. Left ventricular pressure generation is somewhat limited (stunning), but adequate despite the low ATP levels. In addition to CP and ATP, inorganic phosphate can also be monitored adequately by this method, while the low cytosolic level of ADP, a crucial regulator of mitochondrial activity, is not. The decline of myocardial contractility during a lack of oxygen can be linked not so much to decreased high-energy phosphate levels, but rather to decreased rates of production of ATP and CP.[7]

Also in humans, myocardial energy metabolism has been studied with ^{31}P NMR-spectroscopy under various physiological (exercise) and pathological states, as well as after heart transplantation (see below).

^{31}P NMR spectroscopy also allows measurement of the rate constant for phosphoryl transfer from CP to (γ-P)ATP catalyzed by creatine phosphokinase.[3,4] By this method it was demonstrated that the velocity of the creatine phosphokinase reaction in vivo is about one order of magnitude faster than ATP synthesis rates by oxidative phosphorylation. It also established the surprising finding that during hypoxia and ischemia, not only myocardial ATP synthesis and ATP utilization are decelerated, but also the ATP turnover via phosphoryl transfer between ATP and CP; the creatine phosphokinase reaction velocity in the hypoxic rat heart is reduced to one fourth.[7]

NMR spectroscopy also provides the opportunity to compare unidirectional ATP synthesis rates from different substrates (glucose, pyruvate

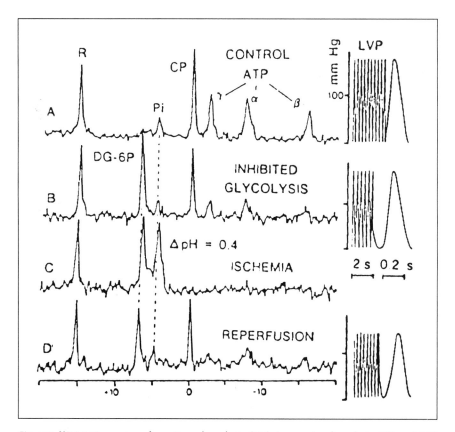

Fig. 7.3. [31]*P NMR spectra of creatine phosphate (CP), inorganic phosphate (Pi) and ATP (the three spectra reflecting the three phosphate groups) in rat heart, during control conditions (A), inhibition of glycolysis by deoxyglucose (B), inhibited glycolysis plus ischemia (C) and the same plus perfusion (D). LV = left ventricular pressure; R = reference; DG-6P = 2-deoxyglucose 6-phosphate. (Reproduced with permission from: Kupriyanov W, Lakomkin VL, Steinschneider AYa et al. Relationships between preischemic ATP and glycogen content and postischemic recovery of rat heart. J Mol Cell Cardiol 1988; 20:1151-1162.)*

Table 7.2. Respiratory quotients and comparative energy yields of various fuels per molecule fully oxidized in the heart

Molecule	Respiratory quotient (RQ)	ATP yield per molecule	ATP yield per carbon atom	ATP yield per oxygen atom taken up (P/O ratio)
Glucose	1.0	38	6.3	3.17
Lactate	1.0	18	6.0	3.00
Pyruvate	0.83	15	5.0	3.00
Palmitrate	0.70	130	8.1	2.83

For further explanation see text. (Modified from Opie LH. The Heart—Physiology and Metabolism. New York: Raven Press, 1991.)

and acetate); using ^{13}C NMR spectroscopy and ^{13}C-labeled substrates, one can investigate the metabolism of glycogen, glucose and Krebs cycle intermediates in the heart and obtain an indirect measure of flux through the citric acid cycle.[8,9]

FUELS FOR MYOCARDIAL ENERGY SUPPLY

Knowledge of the fuels of the human heart can be achieved by measuring the chemical composition of arterial blood entering the heart and that of coronary sinus blood leaving the heart. By this method, glucose, lactate and fatty acids were established as the heart's major sources of energy.[10] By calculation of the respiratory quotient (Table 7.2; ratio of the number of molecules of oxygen taken up and carbon dioxide produced), the type of fuel used by the heart can be estimated. The energy yield per molecule fully oxidized in the heart is highest for fatty acids (Table 7.2), in terms of the highest yield per carbon atom. On the other hand, fatty acids require about 12% more oxygen to produce the same amount of ATP than when using only glucose (Table 7.2; "ATP yield per oxygen atom taken up"). The explanation for this oxygen-wasting is that during fatty acid degradation by β-oxidation not only NADH+H$^+$, but also FADH$_2$ are built as substrates for the respiratory chain, with FADH$_2$ entering the respiratory chain at a later stage than NADH+H$^+$ and thereby yielding less ATP than NADH+H$^+$.

Principles of Fuel Oxidation in the Heart

The common final pathway of fuel oxidation (Fig. 7.4) is represented by the Krebs cycle (citrate cycle, tricarboxylic acid cycle) and the respiratory chain, both located in the mitochondrion. From all fuels metabolized under aerobic conditions in the heart, acetyl-CoA is built in the mitochondrion, in the case of carbohydrates by the pyruvate dehydrogenase from pyruvate, in the case of lipids by the β-oxidation from activated fatty acids (acyl-CoA), and in the case of ketone bodies by activation with CoA. Acetyl-CoA is then put into the Krebs cycle (Fig. 7.5), where the acetyl backbone is converted to hydrogen (H^+ and electron), carried by $NADH+H^+$ and $FADH_2$, and carbon dioxide. For one molecule of acetyl-CoA, a total of three molecules of $NADH+H^+$, one molecule of $FADH_2$ and one molecule of GTP are created. Hydrogen finally is channeled to the electron chain (Fig. 7.6);

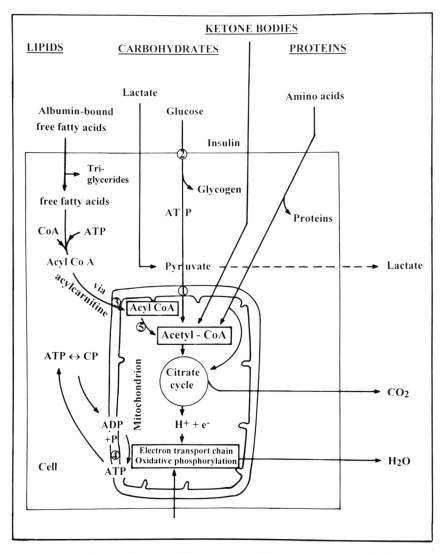

Fig. 7.4. Fuel pathways of myocardial oxygen metabolism. 1 = pyruvate dehydrogenase complex; 2 = glucose carrier; 3 = carnitine-acyl carnitine translocase; 4 = adenine nucleotide translocator; 5 = fatty acid β-oxidation. For further explanation see text.

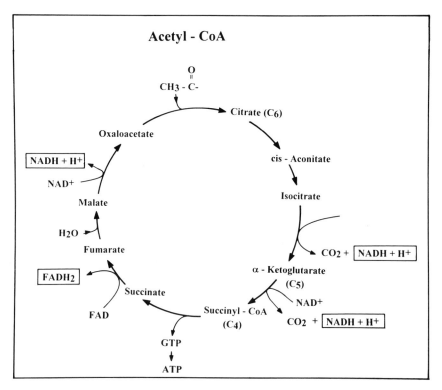

Fig. 7.5. The Krebs cycle of cardiomyocytes. For further explanation see text.

By the electron transfer along the NADH-Q reductase (NADH-dehydrogenase; site 1), where NADH is starting, followed by the ubichinol-cytochrome c reductase complex (cytochrome-reductase, b-c_1 complex; site 2) where $FADH_2$ is included, and the cytochrome c oxidase complex (cytochrome a,a_3; site 3) with final transfer to oxygen, a proton gradient is built across the inner mitochondrial membrane. The electrochemical energy of this proton gradient is converted into chemical energy in the form of ATP via the ATP synthetase also located at the inner face of the inner mitochondrial membrane. Each proton translocation yields the generation of one molecule of ATP, with NADH+H^+ forming six ATP molecules and $FADH_2$ forming four ATP molecules. So, in summary, from one molecule of acetyl-CoA fully metabolized and oxidized via Krebs cycle, one molecule of energy-rich GTP, one molecule $FADH_2$ and three molecules NADH+H^+ are built, resulting in a total of 11 ATP molecules in the subsequent respiratory chain electron transfer, with a total of 12 energy-rich molecules per acetyl-CoA molecule.

In the case of hypoxia/anoxia/ischemia, fuel oxidation is impaired. In this case, ATP production is warranted only via glycolysis, with glucose metabolized to lactate (Fig. 7.4), yielding only a very limited energy production of two molecules of ATP per molecule glucose, in comparison to 38 molecules of ATP produced by fully oxidizing one molecule of glucose (see below).

Substrate Metabolism of Human Heart

In humans, the major myocardial substrates are carbohydrates and lipids (Table 7.3; Opie[1] [pp. 212-216]). The proportion of fuels oxidized depends on the nutritional state and exercise, and is determined by a competition and mutual inhibition of the metabolic pathways; in the fasted state, blood free fatty acids (FFAs) are high. The high rate of FFA uptake by the heart inhibits oxidation of glucose, so that fatty acids become the major source of energy, while the glucose taken up is converted to glycogen. After a carbohydrate(CHO)-rich meal or after a glucose-insulin infusion, circulating FFAs fall, their uptake into the heart is suppressed, the inhibition of glycolysis by FFA is derepressed and glucose oxidation increases. After a lipid-rich meal, there is a marked rise in blood triglycerides during postprandial lipemia. Triglycerides, which then become the major myocardial fuel, are converted to FFA by the lipoprotein lipase located in the vascular endothelium; FFAs then enter the pathway of fatty acid oxidation (see below). During acute exercise, blood lactate rises, and lactate becomes the major fuel. In this circumstance, lactate inhibits oxidation of glucose and uptake of FFAs, each of which now makes up for only 15-20% of the energy need of the heart during exercise. Ketone bodies are not a major substrate of the normal human heart (Table 7.3), with the exception of severe diabetic ketoacidosis.

Aerobic and Anaerobic Glycolysis

Glucose is taken up into the cardiomyocyte in an energy-independent manner by the insulin-sensitive glucose carrier. Inside the cell, it is phosphorylated and channeled into the glycolytic pathway (Fig. 7.4), the end product of which is pyruvate. In the case of aerobic conditions, pyruvate is then transported from the cytosol into mitochondria, where pyruvate dehydrogenase splits the molecule into acetyl-CoA and carbon dioxide by oxidative decarboxylation. The NADH+H$^+$ formed during glycolysis (Fig. 7.7) is transported into mitochondria by the malate aspartate shuttle located in the inner mitochondrial membrane. Under anaerobic conditions, pyruvate is reduced to lactate and transported outside the cell.

Energy gain of glycolysis up to pyruvate is poor: per each molecule of pyruvate, a net production of only one molecule of ATP (two molecules of ATP per molecule of glucose) is accomplished, which, in the case of anaerobic glycolysis, is the final balance. Under aerobic conditions, however, full oxidation accounts for a total of 19 molecules of ATP per pyruvate: one ATP as net production during glycolysis; 12 ATP by oxidative phosphorylation from acetyl-CoA (see above), three ATP from the NADH+H$^+$ produced by the formation of 1,

Table 7.3. Effect of nutritional state or exercise on fuel oxidative metabolism of the human heart: percentage of oxygen uptake accounted for, if various substrates taken up are fully oxidized

Nutritional state or exercise	Substrates oxidized (OER%)								Respiratory quotient
	Glucose	Pyruvate	Lactate	Total CHO	FFA	TG	Ketones	Amino acids	
Postprandial, CHO meal	68	4	28	100	—	—	—	—	0.94
Postprandial, lipid meal	10	—	10	20	30	50	5	—	—
Fasting, few hours	31	2	28	61	34	—	5	0	—
Same during exercise	16	0	61	77	21	—	2	0	—
Fasting overnight resting	27	1	11	38	62	14	7	0	0.74

"OER" = oxygen extraction ratio; "CHO" = carbohydrate; "FFA" = free fatty acids; "TG" = triglycerides; "—" = absence of data. (Modified from Opie LH. The Heart–Physiology and Metabolism. New York: Raven Press, 1991.)

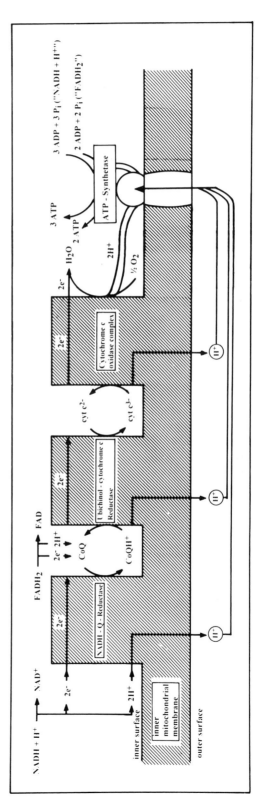

Fig. 7.6. The mitochondrial respiratory chain of cardiomyocytes. For further explanation see text.

3-diphosphoglycerate from glyceraldehyde 3-phosphate (Fig. 7.7), and three ATP from the NADH+H[+] of the pyruvate dehydrogenase reaction. In total, 2 x 19 = 38 molecules of ATP are provided for one molecule of glucose oxidized.

Comparison of aerobic with anaerobic energy production clearly demonstrates that the, at best modest, stimulation of anaerobic glycolysis during anoxia is much too less to fulfill the energy demand of the heart; this could only be achieved if glycolytic flux would be accelerated 20-fold (Opie,[1] p. 233). While the working rat heart requires about 80 μmoles ATP/g wet weight/min, only 10 μmoles are produced during anoxia and even less during severe ischemia, which would only meet the energy demand of the heart in cardioplegia and hypothermia (Opie,[1] p. 233).

Besides its function as an essential pathway for general energy supply, glycolysis may have additional importance: during acute strenuous exercise, it is probably the fastest mode of energy supply, as documented by an activation within 5 seconds,[11] while the pathway of fatty acid oxidation is unlikely to be accelerated so quickly, especially because there may be a transient lack of oxygen available to the heart at the beginning of exercise. Glycolytic ATP also seems important for the maintenance of normal membrane function, at least in the case of ATP-sensitive potassium channels, both under normoxic as well as under ischemic conditions.[12] This beneficial effect might be mediated by glycolytic enzymes located near the sarcolemma. Finally, although currently discussed controversially, glycolysis is probably operative to sustain maximal heart work and to promote diastolic function (Opie,[1] pp. 222 and 234; Owen et al[13]).

Glycogen

The physiological function of cardiac glycogen at present is poorly understood. The glycogen pool is supposed to be reserved for hypoxic emergencies with an abrupt onset of suddenly increased heart work. Glycogen synthesis proceeds at a high rate in the fed state under the influence of insulin, after intense heart work and after ischemia has depleted the glycogen stores. Glycogenolysis is stimulated by hypoxia and ischemia.

Free Fatty Acids

Free fatty acids (FFAs; nonesterified free fatty acids) circulate in the blood in the albumin-bound form. Uptake into the heart probably occurs after binding of this complex to the albumin receptor of the sarcolemma, thus FFAs rapidly cross the membrane. The higher the FFA level and the FFA/albumin molar ratio, the greater the uptake of FFAs by the myocardium.[14]

In humans, the chief fatty acid taken up is oleic acid (C18:1), which consists of about 30-45% of total plasma FFAs and whose up-take

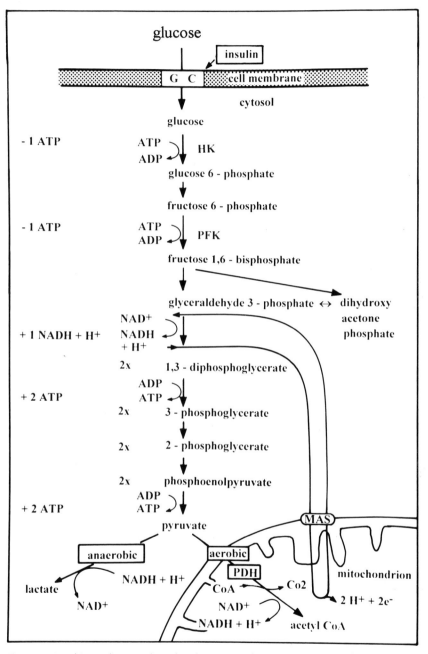

Fig. 7.7. Aerobic and anaerobic glycolysis in cardiomyocytes. GC = glucose carrier; HK = hexokinase; PFK = phosphofructokinase; PDH = pyruvate dehydrogenase; MAS = malate aspartate shuttle. The enzyme glyceraldehyde 3-phosphate dehydrogenase catalyzes the oxidative phosphorylation of glyceraldehyde 3-phosphate to 1,3-diphosphoglycerate. Under anaerobic conditions, the enzyme lactate dehydrogenase converts pyruvate and NADH+H⁺ to lactate and NAD⁺. For further explanation see text.

amounts to about 50% of total FFA uptake in the fasting state (Opie,[1] pp. 235-236). The uptake of palmitic acid (C:16:0) makes up for 16% and of stearic acid (C:18:0) and of linoleic acid (C18:2) for 7% of FFA each (Opie,[1] p. 236). Within the cytosol, FFAs are activated by the energy-consuming thiokinase reaction to yield acyl CoA (Fig. 7.8). The activated fatty acids can either form triglycerides and structural lipids, or they can be transferred as acyl carnitine into mitochondria for β-oxidation (see below). Acyl carnitine is formed in the cytosol from acyl CoA and carnitine; it is transported by the mitochondrial carnitine-acyl carnitine translocase, located in the inner mitochondrial membrane, into the mitochondrial space. Catalyzed by the mitochondrial carnitine acyltransferase, intramitochondrial acyl carnitine reacts with CoA, to yield carnitine and acyl CoA. The carnitine released is exported into the cytosol by the carnitine-acyl carnitine transferase system, and the acyl CoA is channeled into the β-oxidation spiral (Fig. 7.8).

The multienzyme complex of β-oxidation continuously removes acetyl CoA from the carboxyl-end of the fatty acid. By this breakdown, one molecule of $FADH_2$ and one molecule of $NADH+H^+$ is formed per one molecule of acetyl-CoA released. Acetyl CoA is finally channeled into the Krebs cycle.

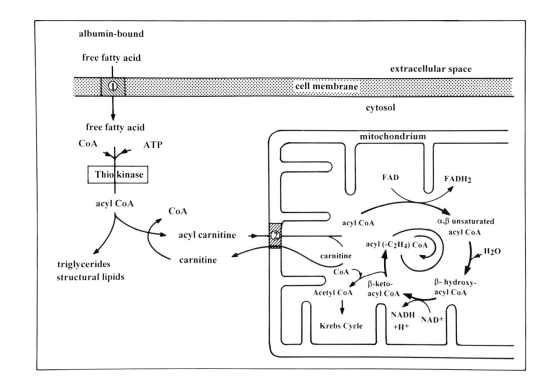

Fig. 7.8. The fatty acid pathway in cardiomyocytes. 1 = albumin receptor; 2 = carnitine-acyl carnitine translocase. For further explanation see text.

In the case of palmitoyl CoA, 130 molecules of ATP are formed during breakdown: 96 ATP from the 8 acetyl-CoA channeled into the Krebs cycle; from the 7 runs of the β-oxidation spiral, 14 ATP result from the 7 $FADH_2$ formed, and 21 ATP from the 7 NADH+H⁺. Taking into account one ATP necessary for fatty acid activation by thiokinase (see above), a net production of 130 ATP molecules per one molecule of palmitic acid results.

Metabolic Imaging of Myocardial Fuels in Humans by Positron Emission Tomography

The technique of positron emission tomography (PET) allows noninvasive monitoring of myocardial metabolic pathways in humans. Suitable markers are ^{18}F-2-deoxy-D-glucose, ^{11}C-acetate and $^{13}NH_3$, the latter for measurement of coronary blood flow. 2-deoxy-D-glucose is an inhibitor of glycolysis, which is taken up into the cell via the glucose carrier and phosphorylated in the cytosol to 2-deoxy-D-glucose 6-phosphate; as further metabolism is blocked, it accumulates and inhibits glycolysis. When ^{18}F-2-deoxy-D-glucose is given in tracer amounts, it can be monitored by PET, and in combination with $^{13}NH_3$, uptake of glucose into the heart can be estimated.[15]

Uptake of ^{11}C-acetate is directly related to the rate of acetate oxidation and thereby to myocardial oxygen uptake, representing a mode of noninvasive determination of oxygen uptake of the intact human heart.[16] Applications of this method in clinical medicine are given below.

REGULATION OF MYOCARDIAL ENERGY METABOLISM

In the heart oxidative phosphorylation in mitochondria is the dominant way of energy production, with glycolysis being quantitatively a much less important source, due to the relatively low activities of the enzymes constituting the pathway. In consequence, substrates that yield energy only by mitochondrial metabolism, such as free fatty acids and lactate, are preferred to glucose, which can support additional energy by glycolysis. In conditions with an adequate coronary blood flow and unrestricted fuel delivery to the heart, the various substrates compete for oxygen, with the suppression of glucose oxidation by free fatty acids being a representative example (Opie,[1] p. 210).

Due to the extremely variable demand of energy-rich substrates in the heart, the traits of energy metabolism are subject to strict regulation. Accumulated and/or depleted substrates and products of the energy pathway have been identified as main regulators, with a number of carriers and key enzymes involved (Fig. 7.4). Understanding of these steps may help to get insight into the adaptive changes of energy metabolism, seen not only in myocardial hypoxia and ischemia,[17] but also in septic cardiomyopathy.

Glycolysis—Regulatory Steps and Control of Anaerobic Glycolysis

Concerning regulatory carriers and key enzymes, the activity of the glucose carrier (Fig. 7.7) is a rate-limiting step in glycolysis (Table 7.4). Insulin raises the number of active carrier molecules, probably by translocating them from internal sites unavailable for transport purposes to external available sites. Glucose uptake is stimulated during hypoxia, increased heart work and in the fed state; in contrast, the fasted state, a low workload, severe ischemia and uncontrolled diabetes mellitus all reduce glucose uptake.

Another key enzyme of glycolysis—phosphofructokinase—phosphorylates fructose 6-phosphate to fructose 1,6-bisphosphate in an unidirectional, irreversible way, as the enzyme fructose 1,6-bisphosphatase, which catalyzes the reverse process, apparently is absent from the heart. Stimulation of phosphofructokinase by the substances and states listed in Table 7.4 lowers the level of glucose 6-phosphate, hence derepressing the activity of hexokinase (Table 7.4). Consequently, stimulation of phosphofructokinase enhances glucose phosphorylation, glucose uptake, and thereby the global glycolytic flux, and vice versa. Fructose 2,6-bisphosphate, a byproduct of glycolysis, whose enzymatic synthesis is enhanced by a rise in inorganic phosphate and adenosine monophosphate, is a potent stimulator of phosphofructokinase, which may override the inhibitory effects of ATP and citrate. Thereby the accelerating effects of insulin and of increased heart work on glycolysis might at least in part be explained.[18] Accumulation of H^+ inhibits the phosphofructokinase, a mechanism responsible for the rapid inhibition of glycolysis during severe ischemia (Table 7.4).

Another major regulator of glycolysis is the enzyme glyceraldehyde 3-phosphate dehydrogenase (Table 7.4). It is inhibited by the products of glycolysis, $NADH+H^+$, H^+ and lactate, which accumulate during severe ischemia.

Under anaerobic conditions, pyruvate is converted to lactate by the lactate dehydrogenase (LDH). The activities of the five LDH isoenzymes in the heart are high enough to make a controlling role of this enzyme in lactate metabolism unlikely (Opie,[1] p. 225).

Phosphofructokinase and glyceraldehyde 3-phosphate dehydrogenase mainly determine the flux of glucose through the glycolytic pathway (Table 7.4, Fig. 7.7). Under normoxia, glycolytic flux is inhibited by high levels of citrate and ATP, formed by oxidative metabolism (Table 7.4). During hypoxia, oxidative phosphorylation is depressed, with a subsequent fall in citrate and ATP and a rise in inorganic phosphate. Consequently, inhibition of glycolysis is turned off, and glucose metabolism to lactate is stimulated by the fall in ATP and the rise in inorganic phosphate. In the presence of not only hypoxia but also severe ischemia with poor blood flow, products of anaerobic glycolysis—protons and lactate—accumulate and inhibit both key enzymes (Table 7.4). By this inhibition, further worsening of myocardial energy supply occurs during severe ischemia, with potentially very harmful consequences.

Table 7.4. Regulation of myocardial energy metabolism by carriers and key enzymes

Pathway	Carrier/Enzyme	Mode of regulation	Relevance
Glycolysis	Global	citrate and ATP inhibit aTP ↓, P_i ↑ stimulate H+ ↑, lactate ↑ inhibit, overcoming stimulation by persistent ATP ↓ and P_i ↑	normoxemia hypoxia, mild ischemia severe ischemia
	Glucose carrier	insulin: increase in the number of carriers	insulin ↑ in fed state
		glucose uptake increased by	→ hypoxia, increased heart work, fed state, mild ischemia
		(signal: lowering of high energy phosphates?) glucose uptake depressed by	→ fasted state, low workload, severe ischemia, uncontrolled diabetes mellitus
	Hexokinase Phosphofructokinase	inhibition by glucose 6-phosphate ↑ inhibition by ATP, citrate, CP stimulation by AMP ↑, P_i ↑, α-adrenergic stimulation (?) fructose 2, 6-biphosphate: potent stimulator	starvation, fatty acids, ketones, severe ischemia increased heart work, inotropic agents fed state, insulin, hypoxia, mild ischemia overrides the inhibitory effects of ATP and citrate; mediates the accelerating effects of insulin and of increased heart work on glycolysis
		inhibition by H+	severe ischemia
	Glyceraldehyde 3-Phosphate Dehydrogenase	inhibition by NADH + H+, lactate H+	severe ischemia
Linkage Glycolysis - Krebs Cycle	Pyruvate Dehydrogenase phosphorylated: inactive dephosphorylated: active	stimulation by Ca^{2+} mitochondrial ↑ inhibition by NADH + H+ ≠	catecholamines, inotropic agents ischemia, hypoxia, fatty acid oxidation

Table 7.4. *Regulation of myocardial energy metabolism by carriers and key enzymes (continued)*

Pathway	Carrier/Enzyme	Mode of regulation	Relevance
Krebs Cycle	Isocitrate Dehydrogenase α-Ketoglutarate Dehydrogenase Malate Dehydrogenase	stimulation by a rise of mitochondrial $NAD^+/NADH + H^+$ ratio inhibition by a fall of mitochondrial $NAD^+/NADH + H^+$ ratio	increased work hypoxia, ischemia
	Citrate Synthase	increased activity by substrate supply: Oxaloacetate ↑ by $NAD^+/NADH + H^+$ ↑ Acetyl CoA ↑ by glycolysis ↑ and fatty acid β oxidation ↑	increased heart work
	Isocitrate Dehydrogenase α-Ketoglutarate Dehydrogenase	stimulation by mitochondrial Ca^{2+}	inotropic stimuli
	Bypassing the slow part of the Krebs Cycle	?	sudden increase of heart work
Fatty Acid Metabolism	Fatty acid uptake	inhibition by low tissue CoA	avoidance of harmful excess of fatty acid uptake
	Thiokinase	lowering of activity by CoA ↓ increased activity by low Acyl CoA and high CoA levels due to high mitochondrial Acyl CoA oxidation rate	avoidance of harmful excess of fatty acid uptake increased heart work
	β-Oxidation Spiral	stimulation by higher oxidized state of mitochondrial $NAD^+/NADH + H^+$ and $FAD/FADH_2$ inhibition by lower oxidized of $NAD^+/NADH + H^+$ and $FAD/FADH_2$	increased heart work anaerobiosis

Table 7.4. Regulation of myocardial energy metabolism by carriers and key enzymes (continued)

Pathway	Carrier/Enzyme	Mode of regulation	Relevance
Fatty Acid Metabolism	Acyl Carnitine and Carnitine-Acyl Carnitine Translocase	high transport turnover increases fatty acid entry into the cell & activation in the cytosol; high acyl carnitine: potentially arrhythmogenic	high energy demand; ischemia
Mitochondrial Respiratory Chain/Oxidative Phosphorylation	Adenine Nucleotide Transporter	transport activity depends on ADP supply	respiratory control (hypoxia, mild ischemia)
	via: fatty acid β-oxidation, Krebs Cycle, Pyruvate Dehydrogenase	stimulation by a rise in mitochondrial $NAD^+/NADH + H^+$ ratio	respiratory control (normoxia)
	via: Isocitrate Dehydrogenase, α-Ketoglutarate Dehydrogenase, Pyruvate Dehydrogenase	stimulation by a rise in mitochondrial Ca^{2+}	respiratory control
	Cytochrome C Oxidase Complex	supply of oxygen	respiratory control (severe ischemia, coronary occlusion)
Glycogen Synthesis Breakdown	Glycogen Synthase	stimulation by a complex mechanism; stimulation by glycogen depletion; high glucose 6-phosphate levels due to inhibition of glycolysis by free fatty acids	fed state under the influence of insulin; ischemia, after intense heart work; fasted state
	Phosphorylase Phosphorylase b (inactive) Phosphorylase a (active)	stimulation of conversion b→a by cAMP; fall of high energy phosphates	catecholamines; work, ischemia, hypoxia

For abbreviations and further explanation see text.

Pyruvate Dehydrogenase

Pyruvate dehydrogenase, located in the inner mitochondrial membrane, links glycolysis to the Krebs cycle; it decarboxylates pyruvate with the aid of coenzyme A to acetyl-CoA, releasing carbon dioxide and NADH+H[+]. Acetyl-CoA can be channeled into the Krebs cycle, and NADH+H[+] into the respiratory chain to eventually form ATP (Fig. 7.4). Normally, only about 20% of the enzyme is present in the active, phosphorylated form. When glycolytic flux is stimulated, as during increased heart work, 60-90% can be active, possibly due to the increased cell calcium or changes in the levels of the various energy-rich phosphate compounds; an increase in mitochondrial Ca^{2+} is thought to convert the inactive form of the enzyme to the active form during stimulation by catecholamines and other inotropic agents;[19] on the other hand, ischemia, hypoxia and fatty acid oxidation form NADH+H[+] which inhibits pyruvate dehydrogenase. The inactivation of the enzyme is a key factor in the inhibition of glycolysis during concurrent provision of the heart with fatty acids.[20]

Stimulation of the enzyme can be achieved by dichloroacetate, with the consequence of an increased aerobic and a decreased anaerobic glycolytic flux. This pharmacological approach has been applied for the treatment of patients with lactic acidosis.[21]

The Citrate Cycle of Krebs

The rate of turnover of the Krebs cycle is tightly coupled to the mitochondrial redox state, which is balanced by the production of NADH+H[+]—among others via the Krebs cycle itself (isocitrate dehydrogenase and α-ketoglutarate dehydrogenase)—and its consumption via the respiratory chain; key enzymes of the cycle (Table 7.4) respond to the redox state of the mitochondrial NAD[+]/NADH+H[+]-system; a rise of this ratio (up to 4-fold) during increased heart work stimulates and a fall in this ratio in hypoxia inhibits the activity of these key enzymes of the Krebs cycle, with an up to 4-fold increase in turnover.

Activity of another key enzyme—citrate synthase—is accelerated by the availability of its substrates; the supply of oxaloacetate is increased when the ratio of NAD[+]/NADH+H[+] rises and thereby stimulates malate dehydrogenase activity, and accumulation of acetyl-CoA can result from an increased flux through glycolysis and fatty acid β-oxidation.

Two of the Krebs cycle enzymes are Ca^{2+}-sensitive; the activities of isocitrate dehydrogenase and α-ketoglutarate dehydrogenase are increased when the mitochondrial Ca^{2+} rises, as it is thought to occur by a rise in cytosolic Ca^{2+} during inotropic stimulation. Besides these regulatory steps of the Krebs cycle, mainly by the mitochondrial NAD[+]/NADH+H[+]-ratio, it is suggested that the rate of part of the Krebs cycle is just too slow for certain extreme situations, as during a sudden increase in heart work, when the cycle must spin very rapidly. The slow part of the cycle can then be bypassed (Opie,[1] p. 248).

Fatty Acid Metabolism

Free fatty acid (FFA) uptake, thiokinase, acyl carnitine transport and the enzymes of the β-oxidation spiral represent the regulatory cornerstones of myocardial fatty acid metabolism (Table 7.4, Fig. 7.8). Low tissue CoA is suggested to limit free fatty acid uptake and avoid harmful intracellular accumulation. The same mechanism lowers fatty acid activation in the cytosol by inhibition of thiokinase. During increased heart work, stimulation of mitochondrial acyl CoA oxidation lowers acyl CoA and increases CoA levels, with the consequence of a stimulation of thiokinase activity.

The redox state of mitochondrial $NAD^+/NADH+H^+$ and $FAD/FADH_2$ determines the rate of β-oxidation of the activated fatty acids, with a more oxidized redox state stimulating and a more reduced redox state inhibiting β-oxidation activity. This explains the higher rates of β-oxidation during increased work and the suppression during anaerobiosis.

At low rates of mitochondrial oxidation, long-chain acyl CoA may accumulate in both the mitochondria and the cytosol. In sub-mitochondrial particles, long-chain fatty acyl CoA can inhibit the adenine nucleotide translocase. However, in ischemia, acyl CoA levels are no higher than under normoxic conditions.[22] Therefore it remains questionable, whether acyl CoA contributes to the impairment of energy metabolism and mitochondrial energy transport seen in ischemia. With this respect, acyl carnitine might represent a more likely candidate; it rises dramatically during ischemia, it can inhibit Na^+/K^+-ATPase and it is potentially arrhythmogenic.[23]

Respiratory Chain and Oxidative Phosphorylation

A loss in cellular ATP stimulates mitochondrial energy production to replenish the energy-rich compounds consumed, with the breakdown products ADP and inorganic phosphate belonging to the trigger substances.

The energy status of the cardiomyocyte (Opie,[1] p. 258; Kammermeier[24]) can be characterized either by the energy charge or, more simply, by the phosphorylation potential $(ATP)/(ADP)(P_i)$. There is a good correlation between the phosphorylation potential and the oxygen uptake of the isolated rat heart.[25] A reciprocal relationship exists between the phosphorylation potential and the rate of mitochondrial oxidative metabolism,[26] with a proportional stimulation of oxidative phosphorylation by the ATP breakdown products ADP and inorganic phosphate. However, recent data have given convincing evidence that the ADP and P_i alterations in the living heart are too small to account for all the marked changes in the rate of oxidative phosphorylation seen under all the different conditions.[27]

The current view of the different mechanisms involved in the control of mitochondrial respiratory chain is the following (Table 7.4): Stimulation of the respiratory chain and thereby energy production is achieved by an increased transport of ADP into the mitochondrium via the adenine nucleotide translocator, by a rise in the mitochondrial $NAD^+/NADH+H^+$-ratio stimulating $NADH+H^+$-generating enzymes, by elevation of mitochondrial Ca^{2+} concentration which also stimulates some of the $NADH+H^+$-generating enzymes[17] and finally also by the mitochondrial supply with oxygen. The response of mitochondria to oxygen is steep, needing only minute amounts of O_2 (Michaelis constant less than 1 μM) for full operation. Under all but the most extreme conditions of hypoxia, the high oxygen affinity of the mitochondria warrants a normal rate of oxidative phosphorylation; thus oxygen seems unlikely to be a physiological regulator of oxidative phosphorylation (Katz,[28] p.122).

Taking all data together, the following picture of respiratory control emerges (Table 7.4; Katz,[28] p. 122-123). In the well oxygenated heart, oxygen and ATP levels are high and ADP levels are low but stable. Under this condition, the availability of $NADH+H^+$ is probably rate-limiting for the mitochondrial energy production, as the $NAD^+/NADH+H^+$-ratio is relatively high. Under hypoxia or mildly ischemic conditions, ADP accumulates and $NADH+H^+$ rises. When this occurs, the elevated ADP levels may become important for the respiratory control. In severe ischemia or coronary occlusion, $NADH+H^+$ and $FADH_2$ accumulate and so cease to control the rate of oxidation. Although ADP also accumulates, it does not play a regulatory role, because the suppression in oxygen supply becomes rate-limiting. However, as the mitochondrial oxygen stores are very small, respiration soon ceases, and the cardiomyocyte will die.

Glycogen

Glycogen synthase (Table 7.4) is the key enzyme of glycogen synthesis. It is stimulated by a complex mechanism in the fed state under the influence of insulin and by glycogen depletion, as it occurs after intense heart work or during ischemia.[15,29] In the fasted state, free fatty acids inhibit glycolysis, with a subsequent rise in glucose 6-phosphate (Fig. 7.7). After conversion to glucose 1-phosphate, glycogen synthase activity rises as a consequence of this increased substrate concentration, though to a lesser degree than in the fed state. However, despite the lack of insulin, glycogen synthesis also runs in the fasted state, albeit at a lower rate, due to the raised glucose 6-phophate levels.

Conversion of the inactive phosphorylase b into the active phosphorylase a stimulates glycogen breakdown, with the rise of cyclic AMP and the fall in energy rich phosphates being the main trigger mechanisms (Table 7.4). The former is initiated by catecholamines via β-adrenoceptor binding and activation of the adenylyl cyclase; the latter signals the energy deficit during intense work, ischemia and hypoxia. While phosphorylase activation is the enzyme controlling the initial burst of glycogenolysis during ischemia and hypoxia, the activity of the debranching enzyme determines the rate of glycogen breakdown thereafter (Opie,[1] p. 227).

IMPAIRMENT OF MYOCARDIAL ENERGY METABOLISM IN PATIENTS WITH NON-SEPTIC HEART DISEASE

It is of course far beyond the scope of this article to discuss this topic in full detail. With this respect, the reader is referred to comprehensive reviews.[1,3,17,28,30,31] This article is focused on in vivo data obtained in patients with nonseptic heart disease, which could be also of relevance for septic cardiomyopathy.

Recent advances in nuclear magnetic resonance (NMR) spectroscopy have allowed the transition to be made from using animal models for the studies of myocardial energy metabolism to direct measurements in human myocardium.[32] ^{31}P NMR spectroscopy is now being used to define changes in the relative concentrations of creatine phosphate and ATP in normal, ischemic, hypertrophied and failing human hearts, as well as after cardiac transplantation.[3]

ENERGY METABOLISM OF HUMAN HEART AT REST AND DURING EXERCISE

Recent estimates by ^{31}P NMR spectroscopy for CP and ATP in normal human myocardium are 11 ± 2.7 and 6.9 ± 1.6 µmol/g wet weight, respectively, values close to those obtained for isolated animal hearts.[33] These data confirm a CP/ATP ratio of about 2:1.

During exercise, myocardial CP/ATP ratios did not differ from the ratio at rest.[34,35] This suggests that neither ATP or ADP levels nor their ratio regulate the rise in cardiac oxygen consumption that accompanies an increase in cardiac work.

MYOCARDIAL ISCHEMIA

In animal hearts, severe myocardial ischemia causes depletion of CP and ATP, with a concomitant increase in inorganic phosphate (P_i). Measured by ^{31}P NMR spectroscopy in patients with ischemic heart disease, the CP/P_i- and CP/ATP ratios show the same patterns; after anterior myocardial infarction, the CP/P_i ratios are reduced at rest.[36] During exercise, the CP/ATP ratio falls, as it has been documented in impressive findings by ^{31}P NMR spectrocopy in patients with critical coronary artery stenoses.[35] The mean CP/ATP ratio at rest was 1.45 ± 0.31, slightly lower than in normal subjects; it fell significantly during exercise in almost all individuals to a mean of 0.91 ± 0.24, associated with ischemic symptoms in only three patients, and it increased to pre-exercise levels during immediate postexercise recovery. In 11 control subjects without coronary artery disease, no decrease in CP/ATP ratio during exercise was observed.

The impaired energy production in coronary artery disease is accompanied by a change in fuel utilization, as can be measured by positron emission tomography (see also above); in patients with unstable angina, the myocardial uptake of (^{18}F)deoxy-D-glucose is increased 4-fold.[15] This finding allows discrimination of ischemic but viable (increased uptake of glucose) from nonviable (decreased glucose uptake) segments of the heart, and can be helpful in selecting patients which might benefit from coronary artery surgery. The uptake of ^{11}C-acetate can be taken as a method for noninvasive determination of the oxygen uptake into the intact heart, since ^{11}C-acetate uptake is related directly to the acetate oxidation via Krebs cycle.[16]

CARDIOMYOPATHIES AND HEART FAILURE

In patients with cardiomyopathies ^{31}P NMR spectroscopy yielded conflicting results as to myocardial CP/ATP ratio, which was reported to be significantly lowered in patients with dilated cardiomyopathy, whereas others found it to be unaltered;[3] in a patient with left ventricular hypertrophy and heart failure, a reduced CP/ATP ratio at rest was described.[37] By critically analyzing the data it becomes obvious that the severely impaired heart function and not the dilated or hypertrophic form of the cardiomyopathy per se seems to represent the determining factor of a disturbed energy metabolism. This conclusion would be in agreement with the finding of a reduced total creatine pool measured by classic techniques in biopsy samples from failing hearts (class IV).[38]

CARDIAC TRANSPLANT REJECTION

Myocardial energy levels and CP/ATP ratios as measured noninvasively by ^{31}P-NMR spectroscopy are reduced in patients with histologically proven cardiac transplant rejection.[3,39] However, in agreement with animal experiments,[40,41] this method does not reliably differentiate mild from more severe rejection in patients.[39] This limits the applicability of this method, since clinical decisions on immunosuppressive therapy are typically based on the severity rather than just the presence of rejection.[3]

METABOLICALLY DERANGED CARDIOMYOPATHY OF SEPSIS AND SIRS—A PRELIMINARY DRAFT

WHAT ARGUES FOR A METABOLIC DERANGEMENT IN SEPTIC CARDIOMYOPATHY?

It remains an intriguing clinical finding that the function of the cardiovascular system becomes rapidly impaired during systemic inflammatory response syndrome (SIRS)[42] and sepsis. Of major pathogenetic importance is the peripheral vasodilatation that results in a reduction of peripheral resistance down to 30% (Fig. 7.9; see also chapters 1 and 2). The vasodilatation cannot be attributed to fever (Fig. 7.9), but arises from vascular degeneration and interstitial edema. Vascular responsiveness to α-adrenergic agonists, angiotensin and calcium entry blockers is depressed, rendering pharmacologic vasoconstrictive interventions inefficient.[43] In an adaptive response, the cardiac output of the intact heart should increase by a factor of 2 to 3. However, this is not the case in septic cardiomyopathy, owing to myocardial depression. Accompanying impaired myocardial functions are reduced ejection fraction and an increased left ventricular diastolic pressure (chapter 2). Although the peripheral oxygen supply is increased at least in some organs, as can be deduced from the tissue oxygen partial pressure of skeletal muscle (Fig. 7.9), a cellular energy imbalance might exist in various organs owing to disturbances in oxygen diffusion and utilization. Thus, the impaired cardiac performance associated with inadequate rise in cardiac output might have detrimental consequences for the oxidative metabolism of peripheral organs. Although the causes of septic cardiomyopathy are multifactorial, coronary hypoperfusion does not play a relevant role (chapter 6). It appears, however, that alterations in cardiac metabolism are of great relevance.

OVERVIEW ON CELLULAR METABOLISM IN SEPSIS AND SIRS

Among the numerous actions of bacterial toxins, cytokines and other mediators, the present discussion will focus on their metabolic effects.[44] When reflecting these substances, also the increased concentrations of

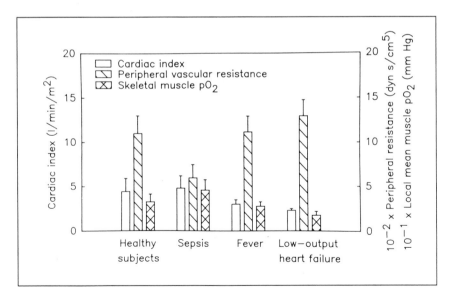

Fig. 7.9. Cardiovascular parameters and skeletal muscle partial oxygen pressure (pO₂) in intensive care patients with sepsis, with fever without sepsis, or with low-output failure. Healthy subjects = non-smoking volunteers (Reproduced with permission from: Rupp H, Müller U, Werdan K. Metabolically deranged cardiomyopathy of the trauma-sepsis syndrome. In: Nagano M, Takeda N, Dhalla NS, eds. The Cardiomyopathic Heart. New York, Raven Press, 1994:257-267.)

blood catecholamines, glucagon and cortisol must be taken into account.[44] This neuroendocrine imbalance results in various metabolic disturbances. Thus, interleukin-1 (IL-1) stimulates proteolysis,[45] which is further potentiated by the effect of the increased glucagon and cortisol levels.[44] The ensuing protein catabolism does not only affect skeletal muscle, particularly endangering the respiratory system, but would be expected to influence heart muscle as well. The thus mobilized amino acids are used for protein synthesis of acute phase proteins and also for gluconeogenesis.[44] The increased blood glucose level provides the fuel for glucose-dependent cells. Yet glucose uptake by the major glucose-utilizing organ of the body, the skeletal muscle, becomes gradually depressed during sepsis. One of the main causes is the reduced activity of the pyruvate dehydrogenase (PDH) complex,[44] which has a key role in the regulation of the glycolytic flux.[46] Noteworthy is the fact that skeletal muscle PDH is affected already during mild sepsis, whereas hepatic PDH is depressed maximally only during severe sepsis.[47] Although data on cardiac PDH are currently not available, it seems most likely that, as in skeletal muscle, it is reduced. As the blood insulin levels are normal (or even increased) and the insulin receptor does not appear to be impaired,[44] the hyperglycemia has to be caused by postreceptor defects. The reduced pyruvate oxidation of skeletal muscle results in an increased release of pyruvate and lactate, which are primarily used in the liver for gluconeogenesis.[44] The increased lipolysis during sepsis and SIRS arises most probably from high blood levels of catecholamines, cortisol and glucagon.[48] Tumor necrosis factor alpha (TNF-α) contributes to the increased triglyceride levels via inhibition of endothelial lipoprotein lipase.[49]

Taken together, the metabolic status of the body during sepsis and SIRS mimics in various aspects a state typically observed during severe starvation or insulin-dependent diabetes mellitus; it is aggravated, however, by the specific actions of various cytokines.

But what are the cellular and molecular mechanisms underlying these metabolic changes in sepsis and SIRS? Recently, Gutierrez[50] gave an excellent survey of the general aspects of the disturbances of cellular metabolism in sepsis. He sees an overwhelming evidence of blood flow redistribution among the different organs including kidneys, liver, intestines, cerebrum, spleen, skeletal muscle and also the heart. Evidence is accumulating pointing towards nitric oxide (NO)-induced guanylyl cyclase activation as the mediator of the vascular manifestations of sepsis.[43] Without questioning this finding, Gutierrez[50] states, "In my opinion, NO probably plays a very important role in mediating the systemic vasodilation of sepsis; however, these vascular abnormalities may be the manifestation, not the cause, of cellular metabolic damage set in motion by sepsis-related cytokines. In other words, the initial result is directed to the tissue cells which, in turn, signal the endothelium to produce NO and perhaps other vasodilator substances."

Are these initial cellular manifestations of sepsis the result of hypoxia? The answer is probably no, at least for the initial stages of the disease. When achieving similar hemodynamic and metabolic impairment in rabbits, either by endotoxin infusion or by inflating a balloon placed in the right ventricle, a similar decrease in O_2 transport, O_2 consumption and skeletal muscle pO_2 results, but the septic animals have greater increases in arterial lactate concentration.[51] This suggests that lactate production in sepsis may be unrelated to changes in systemic O_2 transport. Also Hotchkiss et al,[52] using [18F]fluoromisonidazole as a marker of tissue hypoxia, found no evidence of tissue hypoxia in various organs including skeletal muscle and heart in rats made septic by cecal ligation and perforation. Neither seen were changes in creatine phosphate content in muscle biopsies obtained from 31 patients with sepsis, letting Tresadern et al[53] conclude that tissue hypoxia was not present in these patients.

Are these initial manifestations of sepsis the result of an imbalance of cellular energetics? Again, the answer appears to be no, as the majority of studies in septic animals does not show decreases in ATP levels, with the exception of the late phase in liver and kidney,[54] despite increased arterial lactate concentrations.[54-59] So, even if aerobic metabolism should be impaired in sepsis, increases in oxygen extraction ratio, which is large in skeletal muscle and lesser in extent in the heart, and anaerobic energy production seem sufficiently compensatory. Anaerobic ATP production can be achieved by the enzymes lactate dehydrogenase, adenylate kinase and creatine phosphokinase. The byproducts of these enzymatic reactions—lactate, adenosine monophophate (AMP), xanthine, uric acid, fall in creatine phosphate—provide markers which allow grading the severity of tissue hypoxia.

Profound alterations in glucose homeostasis are foremost among the metabolic derangements that occur in sepsis,[44,60] an early state of hyperglycemia[61,62] with increased glucose turnover and elevated lactic acid levels,[63-65] later on progressing to life-threatening hypoglycemia and lactatacidemia.[66] Specific metabolic consequences of sepsis include enhanced peripheral glucose utilization, acceleration of glycogenolysis, decreased glycogen synthesis and depressed hepatic gluconeogenesis.[60] Increased glucose utilization may lead to hypoglycemia[67] and a decrease in muscle glycogen.[55] As arterial glucose concentration falls and skeletal muscle glucose rises, despite normal levels of plasma insulin, an "insulin-like" effect or an increased sensitivity of tissues to insulin has been postulated for endotoxemia.[64] Further insight into the complex pattern of the disturbed glucose homeostasis in sepsis comes from a more detailed consideration of cellular glucose uptake mechanisms;[60] glucose disposal in peripheral tissues occurs by two complementary processes, by an insulin-mediated glucose uptake (IMGU) and by a noninsulin-mediated glucose uptake (NIMGU).[68,69] In the fasted state, NIMGU is the predominant pathway, while in the fed state IMGU prevails. The molecular basis of cellular glucose uptake is represented by five glucose transporter isoforms (GLUT1-GLUT5), whose abundance, regulation and expression is variable in different tissues, thereby allowing adaptation of glucose uptake to the unique requirement of individual cells.[60] With respect to the heart, GLUT4 is of special relevance; this isoform is only expressed in tissues, in which glucose uptake is regulated by insulin, i.e., fat, skeletal muscle and heart.[70,71] In rats with Gram-negative infection, this insulinopenic, either eu- or hypoglycemic condition is characterized by an enhanced NIMGU in macrophage rich and barrier tissues (liver, spleen, lung, intestine, skin), resulting in an elevated rate of total body glucose utilization.[69,72] On the other hand, both septic patients[73] and infected animals[74] exhibit a whole body insulin resistance, for which the decreased IMGU rate in muscle is primarily responsible.[68] From a quantitative point of view, skeletal IMGU depression can override the rise in NIMGU in other tissues.[68]

Such opposite effects of the septic condition, decreasing glucose uptake in muscle while increasing glucose uptake in other tissues, seem paradoxical, but are well explained by the differential regulation of glucose transporter isoforms in sepsis.[75] Six to eight hours after treatment of rats with endotoxin, bringing about a decompensated, hypoglycemic and lactacidemic phase of shock, messenger RNA transcripts encoding glucose transporter isoforms show specific changes; GLUT1 mRNA abundance is increased in liver (871%), muscle (314%) and fat (660%); at the same time, GLUT2 mRNA levels are markedly decreased (-58%), thus clearly indicating differential regulation of transporter isoform expression in endotoxemic rats. While it is not possible to determine whether such changes in transporter isoform expression reflect or cause changes in glucose transport itself, it is logical to speculate that such changes may be linked with increased peripheral glucose utilization and decreased liver glucose output.[60] Cytokines were supposed[65] and finally confirmed to be the mediators of endotoxin induction of GLUT mRNA; both supernatants from endotoxin-treated macrophages and tumor necrosis factor α (TNF-α) stimulate glucose uptake and glycogen breakdown in L6 skeletal muscle cells; stimulation requires an induction period of about 15 hours and is dependent on synthesis and insertion of glucose transporters,[76] with GLUT1 being the predominant form in L6 cells. Also in fibroblasts, an increase in GLUT1 mRNA and glucose transporter isoforms can be induced by prolonged exposure of the cells either to TNF-α[77] or to interleukin-1 (IL-1).[78]

However, a number of questions remain open today regarding the molecular mechanisms that underlie endotoxin-mediated alterations of glucose transport. One of these questions, the mechanism of sepsis-mediated insulin resistance, may be clarified in the future by full investigation of the sepsis-induced changes in GLUT4 mRNA and protein levels in red, white and mixed muscle subtypes.[60]

Also key enzymes of glucose metabolism—phosphofructokinase (PFK) and pyruvate dehydrogenase (PDH)[46]—might make targets for toxins and cytokines. In the case of PFK, activation of the enzyme was postulated,[79] but inhibition was found[80] in sepsis and endotoxin exposure. Under these conditions, also a higher proportion of the inactive form of PDH was described.[81,82] Dichloroacetate (DCA) promotes formation of the active form of PDH and decreases lactic acidosis, however, with no beneficial effects on O_2 consumption, hemodynamics and survival.[21,83-86] These and other experimental findings[87] support the hypothesis that the lactic acidosis of sepsis may also reflect a decreased enzyme activity of PDH, but may not always be related to an anaerobic state or tissue hypoxia.

Is the mitochondrion the primarily impaired organelle of the cell in sepsis?[88] At least distinct effects of various cytokines on mitochondrial function can be demonstrated in animal and cell culture models (Table 7.5). However, the current opinion disfavors that notion, though there are arguments pro and con; a defective O_2 consumption of skeletal muscle mitochondria in patients with septic shock was described,[89] and it was hypothesized that endotoxin inhibits mitochondrial respiration.[88,90] On the other hand, enhanced respiration in rat liver mitochondria following lethal doses of *E. coli* endotoxin was seen, as well.[91] Also in the case of the mitochondrial tricarboxylic acid (TCA) cycle,

Table 7.5. Evidence for cytokine-induced impairment of energy metabolism (animal and cell models)

Model	Cytokine(s)	Effect(s)	Ref.
Rabbit	TNF-α, IL-1	Reduced oxygen consumption	144
Mouse fibroblasts	TNF-α	Inhibition of mitochondrial respiration	145
Human fibroblasts	TNF-α, γ-interferon	Reduced glucose oxidation	146
Rat aortic smooth muscle cells	TNF-α, γ-interferon	Inhibition of mitochondrial respiration mediated by NO	147
L929 cells	TNF-α, γ-interferon	Inhibition of mitochondrial respiration	148
Neonatal rat cardiomyocytes	TNF-α	Lowering of cellular ATP	149
Neonatal rat cardiomyocytes	TNF-α, IL-1	Inhibition of mitochondrial respiration and of pyruvate dehydrogenase activity	150
Rat hepatocytes	Nitric oxide	Inhibition of mitochondrial respiration	151
Rat hepatocytes	TNF-α	Inhibition of mitochondrial respiration	152

the findings are equivocal; a slower turnover rate has been suspected as the cause of decreased O_2 consumption in sepsis.[92] Yet, no differences in TCA cycle intermediates or high energy phosphates were found in vivo in septic rat brain.[93]

Finally, also the cell membrane with its resting and action potential could be a primary target of bacterial toxins and sepsis mediators. The available findings include a relatively early lowering of resting membrane potential in skeletal muscle of rabbits[59] and in diaphragm of rats[94] given I.V. endotoxin, while an increase in resting membrane potential was observed in endotoxin-exposed mouse neuroblastoma cells.[82] Also, a circulating shock protein with a molecular mass of 200 kDa depolarizes cells in hemorrhage and sepsis.[95] The corresponding effects in cardiomyocytes will be discussed in chapters 4 and 8.

In his overview, Gutierrez[50] concludes that sepsis results in a fairly predictable pattern of metabolic alterations consisting of increased glucose utilization and increased lactate production in most organs in the absence of tissue hypoxia.[96] Gutierrez hypothesizes: "it is possible that selected organs with a low injury threshold to hypoxia, such as the gut and the kidney, may be responsible for initiating a cascade of events leading to these abnormalities. However, another possibility is that the cytokines associated with endotoxemia—TNF-α, IL-1 etc.—set in motion a series of intracellular events leading to a preprogrammed cellular reaction to stress...as part of a misdirected effort of the organism. Perhaps cellular reaction to stress represents a uniform pattern of physiological and biochemical actions aimed at increasing the activity of organs involved in locomotion as part of the "fight or flight" reaction. Thus, the systemic manifestations to the stress imposed by sepsis may be a misdirected effort of the organism to flee from danger. This concept may be useful as a point of departure in our efforts to unravel the more puzzling aspects of the septic response."

CARDIAC METABOLISM IN SEPSIS AND SIRS

The general catabolic effects of sepsis and SIRS can also be expected to affect heart muscle in an unfavorable manner. The function of heart mitochondria was found to be impaired 18 hours after intraperitoneal injection of an LD_{50} dose of *E. coli* endotoxin in rats: the respiratory capacities of these mitochondria in state 3, and thus their ATP synthetic rates, were significantly below normal when α-ketoglutarate was used as substrate.[97-99] Mela et al,[100] however, found no significant deterioration in cardiac mitochondrial function 4.5-6.5 hours after an intravenous injection of an LD_{60-80} dose of *E.coli* endotoxin in dogs. In spite of the onset of myocardial performance failure, myocardial blood flow and oxygen consumption remained normal, and the mitochondria showed regular morphology without swelling. The mitochondrial state 3 respiratory capacity, respiratory control ratios, efficiency of oxidative phosphorylation and ATPase activities were all normal. In a further study with E. coli endotoxemia in the rat, even an increased rate of mitochondrial state 3 respiratory capacity of heart and skeletal muscle was found.[101] Thus, these data in endotoxemia suggest that the lethal in vivo effects of endotoxin on mitochondrial function may not be direct but are most likely a result of changes in tissue perfusion and the resulting tissue ischemia.[88] However, the question of a direct mitochondrial dysfunction in sepsis is anew, highly topical by recent findings of nitric oxide and cytokine effects on mitochondrial function (Table 7.5).[86]

In case it should occur in sepsis, a reduction in myocardial PDH activity would be of particular importance, reducing glucose oxidation and resulting in an increased fatty acid oxidation. Additional citrate would be formed, which should be transformed into malonyl-coenzyme A (CoA) in the cytoplasm. By this mechanism, the carnitine palmitoyl transferase-1 activity is reduced, and the mitochondrial long chain fatty acid uptake is adjusted to the functional demands (Fig. 7.10). The metabolic regulation of the heart in sepsis appears, however, to be more complex, because the uptake of fatty acids and glucose was found to be markedly diminished, whereas the lactate uptake is increased (Fig. 7.11).[102] Furthermore, about 35% to 55% of oxygen uptake could not be accounted for by identifiable exogenous substrates (Fig. 7.11).[102,103] As the relationship between myocardial oxygen consumption and myocardial work was not altered, a normal myocardial oxidative phosphorylation was inferred. One could assume, then, that in septic shock the heart depends to a great extent on endogenous energy sources and that perhaps the depletion of energy reserves might underlie the evidenced progressive cardiac depression.[102,103] However, the currently available data suggest normal[96,104] or even elevated[105] adenosine triphosphate (ATP) levels in the septic heart, demonstrating that energy depletion represents a late process. With regard to the endogenous substrate reserves that could be utilized by the heart, one has to take into account the fact that glycogen stores are depleted much earlier than lipid stores, and the heart would thus be expected to depend primarily on fatty acid oxidation. Thus, the energy status of the heart muscle would be altered in a manner similar to that observed in severe diabetes mellitus. As there is increasing evidence that glucose oxidation and the formation of glycolytic ATP are essential for the maintenance of various subcellular processes (see also above),[106] the metabolic status of heart muscle during sepsis is unfavorable. Little is known about the mechanisms that result in the deranged cardiac metabolism (Fig. 7.10). Thus, the question arises why fatty acid uptake and glucose uptake are reduced in septic shock. The finding that TNF-α inhibits endothelial lipoprotein lipase[107] only partially accounts for the reduced fatty acid uptake. With respect to glucose utilization, various inconsistencies remain. One of the missing links is the activity of glucose transporters (see above) which relates to the PDH activity. Particularly intriguing is the finding of an increased lactate utilization in conjunction with a possibly reduced PDH activity.

Taken together, it appears that a major unsolved issue of heart muscle in sepsis and SIRS is the imbalance of substrate utilization. Currently, the importance of substrate utilization is best documented for diabetic cardiomyopathy,[108] in which glucose oxidation is greatly depressed and mechanical performance is impaired.[109] Although it is not clear to what extent glucose utilization is damaged in the septic

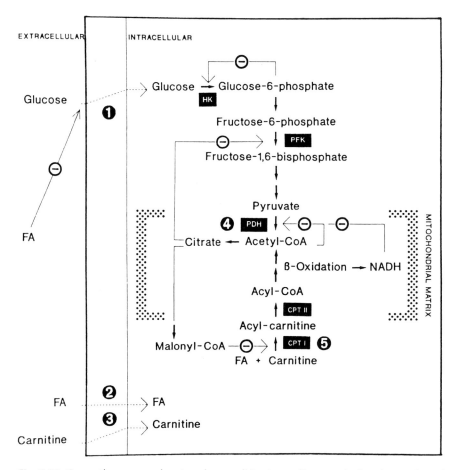

Fig. 7.10. Currently suspected major abnormalities in cardiac metabolism in sepsis and SIRS. 1 = impaired glucose uptake; 2 = impaired fatty acid uptake; 3 = impaired carnitine uptake; 4 = reduced PDH activity; 5 = reduced CPT-1 activity. (Note: This list is not considered to be complete. In particular, additional substrates typical of sepsis and SIRS, such as glutamine, have not been taken into account.) HK = hexokinase; PFK = phosphofructokinase; PDH = pyruvate dehydrogenase complex; CPT = carnitine palmitoyl transferase; FA = nonesterified free fatty acids; CoA = coenzyme A; NADH = nicotine adenine dinucleotide (Reproduced with permission from: Rupp H, Müller U, Werdan K. Metabolically deranged cardiomyopathy of the trauma-sepsis syndrome. In: Nagano M, Takeda N, Dhalla NS, eds. The Cardiomyopathic Heart. New York, Raven Press, 1994:257-267.)

heart, it could provide one explanation for why the heart fails to maintain a high cardiac output in sepsis and SIRS.

A further aspect of the deranged cardiac metabolism relates to the recent findings that subcellular organelles are affected by a shift in cardiac fuel utilization.[110-114] For example, myosin heavy chain expression is shifted in the diabetic heart, favoring myosin V_3 of a low myofibrillar adenosine triphosphatase (ATPase) activity. Furthermore, the rate of sarcoplasmic reticulum Ca^{2+}-uptake is reduced. Although such studies have not been conducted for the heart in sepsis and SIRS, it appears most likely that functionally comparable alterations occur in subcellular organelles. This contention is supported by the finding that myofibrillar ATPase was reduced in the hearts of rabbits infected with *Streptococcus viridans.*[115,116] Furthermore, sarcolemmal Na^+,K^+-ATPase and sarcolemmal Ca^{2+}-binding were reduced.[115,116] The finding that heart rate and body temperature were increased[116] indicates that a generalized

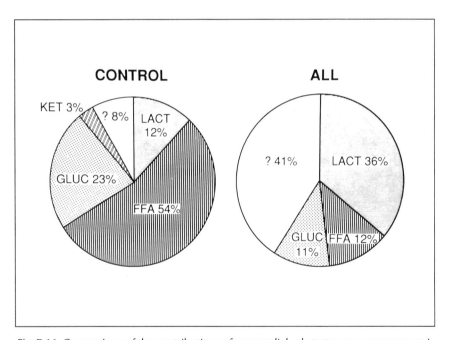

Fig. 7.11. Comparison of the contributions of myocardial substrates as energy sources in patients with septic shock (n = 40) and control patients (n = 13). The energy contribution of each myocardial substrate is expressed as percentage of measured myocardial oxygen consumption. Coronary sinus blood flow was 130 ±21 ml/min in the control group and 187 ±47 ml/min in patients with septic shock. "CONTROL" = Control patients undergoing cardiac catheterization for monovalvular dysfunction with regular ventricular function; "ALL" = All study group patients with septic shock including survivors and nonsurvivors. (Modified from Dhainaut JF, Huyghebaert MF, Monsallier JF et al. Coronary hemodynamics and myocardial metabolism of lactate, free fatty acids, glucose, and ketones in patients with septic shock. Circulation 1987; 75:533-541.)

sepsis occurred and that the changes in heart muscle might not arise solely from the observed endocarditis. In this respect, it should also be mentioned that the function of subcellular organelles is critically influenced by thyroid hormones. In sepsis, low serum triiodothyronine (T_3) and FT_3 concentrations have been observed.[117] A reduced thyroid influence is expected to slow down myocardial performance, producing, for example, a reduced expression of the sarcoplasmic reticulum Ca^{2+}-pump ATPase and the Ca^{2+}-release channel.[118] Thus, such a slow-type heart would not be well equipped for the high heart rates required in sepsis and SIRS.

MOLECULAR ASPECTS OF MYOCARDIAL PROTEIN METABOLISM IN SEPSIS

A prominent finding in sepsis is the net catabolic state with a negative nitrogen balance, as measured by an excessive excretion of urea. Nitrogen balance studies provide information regarding the whole-body response to sepsis, but they do not inform us about the dynamic changes of protein metabolism occurring in individual tissues. Only little is known about qualitative and quantitative changes in synthesis and degradation of myocardial proteins in sepsis (see above),[44,98] and even less on the molecular mechanism underlying these changes. In the opinion of the authors it is at present not possible to give a comprehensive review of this topic. Instead we will present some preliminary results on three aspects of this field which are currently under investigation.

Protein Synthesis-Inhibiting Proteins: Effects on Contractility

During sepsis, protein catabolism is enhanced, and the situation may even be aggravated in septic states in which protein synthesis is inhibited by toxins. The best characterized example is Pseudomonas (P.) exotoxin A. It inhibits protein synthesis via adenosine diphosphate (ADP) ribosylation of elongation factor 2 (EF-2) (for detailed description and discussion see chapter 4). Proteolysis already being enhanced, inhibition of protein synthesis by this toxin represents an additional detrimental factor for the heart muscle. In the case of P. exotoxin A, protein synthesis of cultured neonatal rat cardiomyocytes is inhibited by half-maximum at 10 ng/ml during a 24-hour incubation period. The consequences of partial inhibition of protein synthesis in the heart muscle cell are conspicuous with respect to the β_1-adrenoceptor/G proteins/adenylyl cyclase axis. As demonstrated in Figure 7.12, 1 ng/ml P. exotoxin A, which inhibits global protein synthesis by about 20%, had no effect on the number of β_1-adrenoceptors within two to three days of culture, and it did not interfere with the β_1-adrenoceptor-dependent and β_1-adrenoceptor-independent stimulation of adenylyl cyclase. Also, the noradrenaline-induced down-regulation of β_1-adrenoceptors that occurs independently of protein synthesis ("homologous desensitization") was not affected by P. exotoxin A (Fig. 7.12). However, when heart muscle cells were cultured in the presence of noradrenaline and P. exotoxin A, the forskolin-stimulated adenylyl cyclase activity was not reduced (loss of "heterologous desensitization"). This loss of heterologous desensitization arises from the suppression of the noradrenaline-induced rise in $G_{i\alpha2}$ and $G_{i\alpha3}$ synthesis.

The inhibition of protein synthesis affects the β_1-adrenoceptor recovery at a time when blood catecholamine levels go back to normal. Thus, in the absence of P. exotoxin A, β_1-adrenoceptors of the cardiomyocyte were found to recover within 24-48 hours following the washout of noradrenaline. However, in the presence of P. exotoxin A, synthesis of β_1-adrenoceptors was not evidenced, and the heart muscle cells were found to remain refractory toward catecholamines (Fig. 4.2). Yet the suppression of receptor recovery by P. exotoxin A equals a prolongation of the catecholamine refractory period. Noteworthy is the fact that this complete inhibition of receptor synthesis occurred even though global protein synthesis in the cardiomyocytes was only partially inhibited. The probable clinical relevance of these findings is discussed in chapter 4.

Another interesting target of P. exotoxin A in the heart is the myosin isozyme pattern: both β-adrenoceptor agonists like isoproterenol and triiodothyronine (T_3) trigger a myosin isozyme shift from V_3 to V_1 (see chapter 4). Only the isoproterenol-induced shift, but not the T_3-induced shift is inhibited by P. exotoxin A up to a concentration of 10 ng/ml (chapter 4). Although the stimuli isoproterenol and T_3 involve different signal transduction pathways for the initiation of transcription of the DNA coding for myosin,[119-122] the subsequent steps of translation might be expected to be the same. These results demonstrate that inhibition of protein synthesis at the translational level can affect T_3- and catecholamine-induced synthesis of cellular proteins in a different manner. The observed differences could be due to the fact that T_3, but not isoproterenol, stimulates the expression of elongation factor 2 (Fig. 4.11) and thereby overcomes the inhibitory action of P. exotoxin A.

A partial inhibition of basal and/or insulin-/fuel-induced protein synthesis in rat heart also occurs in hypoxia, anoxia and ischemia.[123,124] Analysis of protein synthesis at the ribosomal level during hypoxia and ischemia reveals impairment of peptide chain elongation as a causal mechanism.[124] In isolated perfused hearts from rats with P. exotoxin A injections 48 hours prior to sacrifice, the suppressive effects of hypoxia on heart rate, left ventricular systolic pressure, rates of ventricular contraction (+dP/dt) and relaxation (-dP/dt) is potentiated,[125] indicating synergistic effects. Partial inhibition of protein synthesis is also found in ATP-depleted cultured neonatal rat cardiomyocytes.[2] It is thus conceivable that the mechanisms of impaired catecholamine inotropy caused by P. exotoxin A might be relevant also for other pathological states associated with partial inhibition of protein synthesis.

Myocardial Elongation Factor 2 (EF-2)—Regulation by Metabolic Signals Relevant for Sepsis and Shock

Apart from P. exotoxin A and diphetheria toxin,[126-128] endogenous mono (ADP-ribosyl) transferases from eucaryotic cells catalyze ADP-ribosylation and thus inactivate ribosomal EF-2.[126,129] The effects brought about by P. exotoxin A as described (Fig. 7.12) might also be applicable to endogenous (ADP-ribosyl) transferases. The number and/or activity of EF-2 is physiologically modified and regulated by hormonal stimulation, by aging and neoplasia. Furthermore, the molecule is the substrate of a calmodulin-dependent protein kinase III, whereby phosphorylation results in a functional inactivation of elongation factor 2.[126] These findings point at EF-2 as a possible target of regulators of protein synthesis. So far, particularly in the heart, knowledge about EF-2 is sparse. In neonatal rat cardiomyocytes, several metabolic signals relevant for sepsis and septic shock modify the cellular content of this ribosomal EF-2 (Müller-Werdan U, Seliger C, Reithmann C et al, submitted): energy depletion with deoxyglucose (2.5 mM; 48 h) or

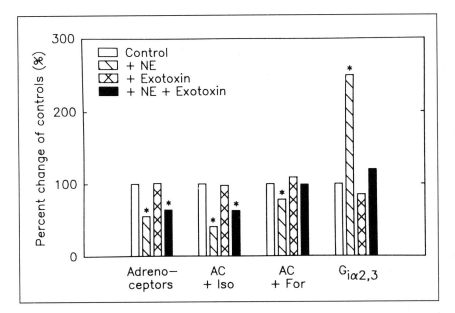

Fig. 7.12. Influence of Pseudomonas exotoxin A on the β_1-adrenoceptor/G protein/ adenylyl cyclase axis. Neonatal rat cardiomyocytes were cultured for two to three days in a serum-free medium (control) with the following additions: 1 μM norepinephrine (+NE), 1 ng/ml P. exotoxin A (+Exotoxin), 1 μM norepinephrine and 1 ng/ml P. exotoxin A (+NE+Exotoxin). The following parameters were determined; β_1-adrenoceptor number; 100 μM isoproterenol-stimulated adenylyl cyclase activity (AC+Iso), 100 μM forskolin-stimulated adenylyl cyclase activity (AC+For), and the inhibitory $G_{i\alpha2,3}$ protein synthesis. The statistical comparisons (p < 0.05) refer to heart muscle cells cultured under control conditions (Reproduced with permission from: Rupp H, Müller U, Werdan K. Metabolically deranged cardiomyopathy of the trauma-sepsis syndrome. In: Nagano M, Takeda N, Dhalla NS, eds. The Cardiomyopathic Heart. New York, Raven Press, 1994: 257-267.)

hypoxia (6 h) reduces the content of EF-2 to 76% and 62%, respectively. Tumor necrosis factor α (100 U/ml; 48 h), which is known to activate transcription, leads to an increase in EF-2 to 152%. An increased glucose oxidation resulting from an inhibition of fatty acid oxidation, mimicking an anabolic state, can experimentally be studied after inactivation of carnitine palmitoyl transferase I by etomoxir (0.01 mM; 48 h); under this condition, content of EF-2 is enhanced to 152%. At least in vitro, metabolic signals, which contribute to the pathogenesis of both septic and nonseptic forms of cardiomyopathy, regulate ribosomal EF-2 and can therefore influence induction, turnover and degradation of cellular proteins.

Alterations of Protein Pattern in Septic Cardiomyopathy

Toxins and sepsis mediators can specifically modify gene expression and protein synthesis. In the case that the induction or repression of specific proteins by one of these substances is well-known, one may look for these events in tissue samples with an established separation procedure optimized for the protein in question. On the other hand, many of the alterations of cellular protein pattern are yet unknown, necessitating some kind of analytical screening method as a first approach for clarification.

Two-dimensional polyacrylamide gel electrophorsis (2-D PAGE) is one of the high resolution methods for separation of complex protein mixtures.[130,131] With respect to the heart, several groups have applied 2-D PAGE to the investigation of protein patterns and protein metabolism under various physiological and pathophysiological conditions (for review see refs. 131-133).

As a first approach to detect probable alterations of protein pattern in septic cardioymopathy, we applied 2-D PAGE in myocardial probes from adult baboons with a 72-hour-*E. coli* sepsis,[134] with or without treatment with anti-TNF-α antibodies.[135] In the myocardial biopsy specimen of septic baboons, of septic baboons with anti-TNF-α antibodies and of sham-treated, noninfected control baboons, about 80-120 polypeptide spots can be seen under transmission light and classified according to molecular weight and isoelectric point (Fig. 7.13), with some of the spots being group-specific, others increasing and decreasing, respectively, in intensity. Further processing aims at identifying the individual protein spots of interest by amino acid microsequencing or other well-established procedures,[136,137] thereby constructing a myocardial two-dimensional electrophoresis database[133] and identifying qualitative as well as quantitative changes in the septic heart. The latter is still at its beginning, but in skeletal muscle of septic rats, first results have been obtained;[137] in gastrocnemius muscle from rats, 35 protein spots were reproducibly increased in sepsis when compared to controls, while none underwent significant down-regulation in their relative abundance. Twenty-three of these proteins were also present

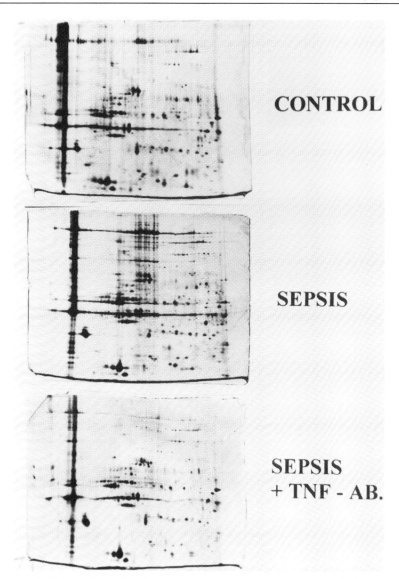

CONTROL

SEPSIS

SEPSIS + TNF - AB.

Fig. 7.13. Two-dimensional protein maps of heart specimen from baboons without sepsis, with sepsis, and with sepsis and anti-TNF-α treatment. For detection of alterations in protein pattern in acute septic cardiomyopathy, two-dimensional polyacrylamide gel electrophoresis (2-D PAGE) was applied[131] to myocardial specimen from adult baboons with E. coli sepsis[134]—either untreated ("SEPSIS") or treated with anti-TNF-α-antibodies ("SEPSIS + TNF-AB."), and for comparison, from noninfected control animals ("CONTROL"). Myocardial specimen (about 3-4 mg wet weight) were homogenized, and about 50 μg protein were applied to IPG gel strips (pH 4-7) for isoelectric focusing (starting at 300 V and finishing at 40 KVh); as second dimension, SDS polyacrylamide gel electrophoresis was applied (running conditions: 80 V (31 mA) for 2 hours and 200 V (67 mA) for 3 hours, in the stacking and separation gel, respectively; MW: 14.3-340 kDa), with subsequent silver staining of the gels. (For abstract based on these findings see Müller U, Chang He, Redl H et al. Altered protein pattern (APP) in acute septic cardiomyopathy in untreated and treated baboons: application of high resolution two-dimensional polyacrylamide gel electrophoresis (2-D PAGE). Circ Shock 1993; Suppl 1:Abstracts 31.)

in plasma, and 12 could be taken to represent skeletal muscle proteins. One of the 12 proteins was identified by immunoblot analysis to be carbonic anhydrase III. Another of the proteins was identified as triosephosphate isomerase based upon microsequencing of the N terminus.[137]

With in vitro-ex vivo analysis of 2-D PAGE protein pattern as outlined in Figure 7.14, it should be possible to clarify the specific role of individual toxins and mediators in sepsis-induced disturbance of myocardial protein pattern. Showing the preliminary results in Figures 4.17, 7.13 and 7.14, we want to emphasize that analyzing the

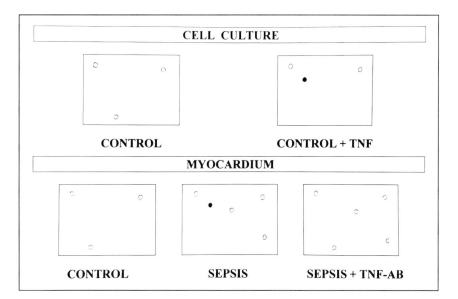

Fig. 7.14. The in vitro-ex vivo approach to study alterations in protein pattern of septic cardiomyopathy. In septic cardiomyopathy, a complex alteration of the protein pattern of the heart is expected, probably mediated by different toxins and mediators, which can be investigated by 2-dimensional polyacrylamide gel electrophoresis (2-D PAGE).

In a first step, cardiomyocytes in culture can be incubated with the respective toxin or mediator of interest; in the scheme, tumor necrosis factor α (TNF) is taken as such an example. In this hypothetical experiment, TNF exposure of the cells yields the appearance of a new protein spot (full circle) and the disappearance of a protein spot (see also Fig. 4.17). In a similar manner, the effects of other toxins and mediators can be tested.

The second step consists of 2-D PAGE protein patterns of cardiac biopsy specimen from septic animals (see also Fig. 7.13). In this hypothetical experiment, sepsis induces the appearance of several new spots and the disappearance of one spot. In septic animals treated with anti-TNF-antibodies (TNF-AB), the hypothetical 2-D maps show the disappearance of one spot seen in sepsis without TNF-AB treatment (full circle), and the reappearance of another spot seen in control animals but not in septic animals without TNF-AB-treatment. Two further spots are in common with the control group and two with the sepsis group.

By this approach, alterations of protein pattern in septic cardiomyopathy due to TNF or other sepsis mediators might be identified by the combined in vitro-ex vivo approach, with the positive control being the appearance of pattern changes induced in cardiomyocyte culture by incubation with TNF or other sepsis mediators; and the negative control consists of the disappearance of the same spots in myocardial biopsy specimen of septic animals treated with TNF-AB. This work is in progress (see Figs. 4.17 and 7.13).

changes in cardiac protein pattern in sepsis is just at its beginning: intra- and interindividual variability, probable differences in the pattern of right and left ventricles and atria, and correlation of protein data with morphological changes, biochemical findings (e.g. enzyme activities and metabolites) and functional state (cardiac output, contractility parameters) have to be worked out before definitive conclusions can be drawn concerning the sepsis-induced changes in cardiac protein pattern, its functional consequences and the influence of therapeutic measures.

NOVEL THERAPEUTIC REGIMENS DESIGNED TO TREAT THE DERANGED FUEL UTILIZATION

As glucose intolerance provides a sensitive index for the mortality rate of patients with sepsis,[138] one could speculate that improved glucose utilization might prove to be beneficial to these patients. In view of the increasing evidence that signals derived from the glycolytic flux affect gene transcription/protein translation,[102,110-114] improved glucose utilization might be helpful in normalizing protein synthesis. Among various possibilities for increasing glucose utilization, it appears that an attractive approach could involve the activation of PDH or the inhibition of carnitine palmitoyl transferase I.[139-141] Carnitine palmitoyl transferase-I inhibition has been found to increase glucose utilization in insulin-dependent diabetes[142] and to normalize both the myosin heavy chain expression as well as the sarcoplasmic reticulum Ca^{2+}-stimulated ATPase activity (Rupp H, unpublished data). Clearly, further experimental work is required to assess the potentially beneficial actions of drugs that normalize fuel utilization in sepsis and SIRS. In view of the fact that currently available pharmacologic regimens do not efficiently reduce mortality from sepsis and SIRS, alternative avenues of treatment are needed.

REFERENCES

1. Opie LH. The Heart—Physiology and Metabolism. New York: Raven Press, 1991.
2. Beuttler C. Das β-Adrenozeptor/Adenylatzyklase-System kultivierter Rattenherzmuskelzellen—Effekte chronischer Energieverarmung und erhöhter Katecholaminkonzentrationen als Teilkomponenten der chronischen Myokardischämie. Dissertationsarbeit zum Erwerb des Doktorgrades der Medizin an der Medizinischen Fakultät der Ludwig-Maximilians-Universität München, 1993.
3. Ingwall JS, Weiss RG. ^{31}P NMR spectroscopy the noninvasive tool for the study of the biochemistry of the cardiovascular system. Trends Cardiovasc Med 1993; 3:29-37.
4. Seymour A-ML. Evaluation of myocardial energy status in vivo by NMR spectroscopy. Basic Res Cardiol 1993; 88:385-395.

5. Herijgers P, Overloop K, Toshima Y et al. Ischaemic ATP degradation studied by HPLC and ^{31}P-NMR spectroscopy: Do the two techniques observe the same ATP pools? Basic Res Cardiol 1994; 89:50-60.

6. Kupriyanov VV, Lakomkin VL, Steinschneider AYa et al. Relationships between preischemic ATP and glycogen content and post-ischemic recovery of rat heart. J Mol Cell Cardiol 1988; 20:1151-1162.

7. Bittl JA, Balschi JA, Ingwall JS. Contractile failure and high-energy phosphate turnover during hypoxia: ^{31}P-NMR surface coil studies in living rat. Circ Res 1987; 60:871-878.

8. Lewandoswki ED, Johnson DL. Reduced substrate oxidation in postischemic myocardium: ^{13}C and ^{31}P NMR analyses. Am J Physiol 1990; 258:H1357-H1365.

9. Malloy CR, Thompson JR, Jeffrey FMH et al. Contribution of exogenous substrates to acetyl coenzyme: a measurement of ^{13}C NMR under non-steady-state conditions. Biochemistry 1990; 29:6756-6761.

10. Bing RJ. The metabolism of the heart. Harvey Lecture Series 50. Academic Press, Orlando, New York, London, 1954:27-70.

11. Achs MJ, Garfinkel D, Opie LH. Computer simulation of metabolism of glucose perfused rat heart in a work-jump. Am J Physiol 1982; 243:R389-R399.

12. Weiss JN, Lamp ST. Glycolysis preferentially inhibits ATP-sensitive K[+] channels in isolated guinea pig cardiac myocytes. Science 1987; 238:67-69.

13. Owen P, Dennis S, Opie LH. Glucose flux rate regulates onset of ischemic contracture in globally underperfused rat hearts. Circ Res 1990; 66:344-354.

14. Rauch B, Bode C, Piper HM et al. Palmitate uptake in calcium tolerant, adult rat myocardial single cells—evidence for an albumin mediated transport across sarcolemma. J Mol Cell Cardiol 1987; 19:159-166.

15. Camici P, Ferrannini E, Opie LH. Myocardial metabolism in ischemic heart disease: basic principles and application to imaging by positron emission tomography. Prog Cardiovasc Dis 1989; 32:217-238.

16. Armbrecht JJ, Buxton DB, Schelbert HR. Validation of (1-^{11}C)acetate as a tracer for noninvasive assessment of oxidative metabolism with positron emission tomography in normal, ischemic, postischemic, and hyperemic canine myocardium. Circulation 1990; 81:1594-1605.

17. Ferrari R, Pedersini P, Bongrazio M et al. Mitochondrial energy production and cation control in myocardial ischemia and reperfusion. Basic Res Cardiol 1993; 88:495-512.

18. Lawson JWR, Uyeda K. Effects of insulin and work on fructose 2,6-bisphosphate content and phosphofructokinase activity in perfused rat hearts. J Biol Chem 1987; 262:3165-3173.

19. McCormack JG, Edge NJ, Denton RM. Regulation of rat heart pyruvate dehydrogenase activity. Biochem J 1982; 202:419-427.

20. Weiss RG, Chacko VP, Gerstenblith G. Fatty acid regulation of glucose metabolism in the intact beating rat heart assessed by carbon-13 NMR

spectroscopy; the critical role of pyruvate dehydrogenase. J Mol Cell Cardiol 1989; 21:469-478.

21. Stacpoole PW, Wright EC, Baumgartner TG et al. A controlled clinical trial of dichloroacetate for treatment of lactic acidosis in adults. N Engl J Med 1992; 327:1564-1569.

22. Feuvray D, Plouet J. Relationship between structure and fatty acid metabolism in mitochondria isolated from ischemic rat heart. Circ Res 1981; 48:740-747.

23. Corr PB, Gross RW, Sobel BE. Arrhythmogenic amphiphilic lipids and the myocardial cell membrane. Editorial. J Mol Cell Cardiol 1982; 14:619-626.

24. Kammermeier H. Meaning of energetic parameters. Basic Res Cardiol 1993; 88:380-384.

25. Giesen J, Kammermeier H. Relationship of phosphorylation potential and oxygen consumption in isolated perfused rat hearts. J Mol Cell Cardiol 1980; 12:891-907.

26. Clarke K, Willis RJ. Energy metabolism and contractile function in rat heart during graded, isovolumic perfusion using ^{31}P nuclear magnetic resonance spectroscopy. J Mol Cell Cardiol 1987; 19:1153-1160.

27. Balaban RS. Regulation of oxidative phosphorylation in the mammalian cell. Am J Physiol 1990; 258:C377-C389.

28. Katz AM. Physiology of the Heart. New York: Raven Press,1992.

29. Camici P, Marraccinni P, Marzilli M et al. Coronary hemodynamics and myocardial metabolism during and after pacing stress in normal humans. Am J Physiol 1989; 257:E309-E317.

30. Fozzard HA, Haber E, Jennings RB et al. The Heart and Cardiovascular System—Scientific Foundations. New York: Raven Press, 1991.

31. Kübler W, Strasser RH. Signal transduction in myocardial ischemia. Eur Heart J 1994; 15:437-445.

32. Bottomley PA. Noninvasive study of high-energy phosphate metabolism in human heart by depth-resolved ^{31}P NMR spectroscopy. Science 1985; 229:769-772.

33. Bottomley PA, Hardy CJ, Roemer PB. Phosphate metabolite imaging and concentration measurements in human heart by nuclear magnetic resonance. Magn Reson Med 1990; 14:425-434.

34. Conway MA, Bristow JD, Blackledge MJ et al. Cardiac metabolism during exercise measured by magnetic resonance spectroscopy. Lancet 1988; 861:692.

35. Weiss RG, Bottomley PA, Hardy CJ et al. Regional myocardial high-energy phosphates during isometric exercise in patients with coronary artery disease. N Engl J Med 1990; 323:1593-1600.

36. Bottomley PA, Herfkens RJ, Smith LS et al. Altered phosphate metabolism in myocardial infarction: P-31 MR spectroscopy. Radiology 1987; 165:703-707.

37. Rajagopalan B, Blackledge MJ, McKenna WJ et al. Measurement of phosphocreatine to ATP ratio in normal and diseased human heart by ^{31}P

magnetic resonance spectroscopy using the rotating frame-depth selection technique. Ann NY Acad Sci 1987; 508:321-332.

38. Nascimben L, Ingwal JS. Decreased energy reserve may cause pump failure in human dilated cardiomyopathy. Circulation 1991; 84:II-563.

39. Bottomley PA, Weiss RG, Hardy CJ et al. Myocardial high-energy phosphate metabolism and allograft rejection in patients with heart transplants. Radiology 1991; 181:67-76.

40. Canby RC, Evanochko WT, Barrett LV et al. Monitoring the bioenergetics of cardiac allograft rejection using in vivo P-31 nuclear magnetic resonance spectroscopy. J Am Coll Cardiol 1987; 9:1067-1074.

41. Fraser CD, Chacko VP, Jacobus WE et al. Early phosphorus 31 nuclear magnetic bioenergetic changes potentially predict rejection in heterotopic cardiac allografts. J Heart Transplant 1990; 9:197-204.

42. American College of Chest Physicians/Society of Critical Care Medicine Consensus Conference. Definitions for sepsis and organ failure and guidelines for the use of innovative therapies in sepsis. Crit Care Med 1992; 20:864-874.

43. Parratt JR, Stoclet J-C, Fleming I. The role of the L-arginine nitric oxide pathway in sepsis and endotoxemia with special reference to vascular impairment. In: Schlag G, Redl H, eds. Pathophysiology of Shock, Sepsis, and Organ Failure. Berlin, Heidelberg, New York: Springer-Verlag, 1993:575-592.

44. Kispert P, Caldwell MD. (1990) Metabolic changes in sepsis and organ failure. In: Deitch EA, ed. Multiple Organ Failure–Pathophysiology and Basic Concepts of Therapy. New York: Thieme Medical Publishers, 1990:104-125.

45. Baracos V, Rodemann HP, Dinarello CA et al. Stimulation of muscle protein degradation and prostaglandin E_2 release by leukocytic pyrogen (interleukin-1). N Engl J Med 1983; 308:553-558.

46. Weiss RG, Chacko VP, Gerstenblith G. Fatty acid regulation of glucose metabolism in the intact beating rat heart assessed by carbon-13 NMR spectroscopy: the critical role of pyruvate dehydrogenase. J Mol Cell Cardiol 1989; 21:469-478.

47. Vary TC, Siegel JH, Nakatani T et al. Effect of sepsis on activity of pyruvate dehydrogenase complex in skeletal muscle and liver. Am J Physiol 1986; 250:E634-E640.

48. Stoner HB, Little RA, Frayn KN et al. The effect of sepsis on the oxidation of carbohydrate and fat. Br J Surg 1983; 70:32-35.

49. Scholl RA, Lang CH, Bagby GJ. Hypertriglyceridemia and its relation to tissue lipoprotein lipase activity in endotoxemic, *Escherichia coli* bacteremic, and polymicrobial septic rats. J Surg Res 1984; 37:394-401.

50. Gutierrez G. Sepsis and cellular metabolism. In: Reinhart K, Eyrich K, Sprung C, eds. Sepsis—Current Perspectives in Pathophysiology and Therapy (Update in Intensive Care and Emergency Medicine 18). Berlin, Heidelberg: Springer-Verlag, 1994:181-190.

51. Hurtado FJ, Gutierrez AM, Silva N et al. Role of tissue hypoxia as the mechanism of lactic acidosis during *E. coli* endotoxemia. J Appl Physiol 1992; 72:1895-1901.

52. Hotchkiss RS, Rust RS, Dence CS et al. Evaluation of the role of cellular hypoxia in sepsis by the hypoxic marker [^{18}F]fluoromisonidazole. Am J Physiol 1991; 261:R965-R972.

53. Tresadern JC, Threlfall CJ, Wilford K et al. Muscle adenosine 5'triphosphate and creatine phosphate concentrations in relation to nutritional status and sepsis in man. Clin Sci 1988; 75:233-242.

54. Chaudry IH, Wichtermann KA, Baue AE. Effect of sepsis on tissue adenine nucleotide levels. Surgery 1979; 85:205-211.

55. Pappova E, Urbaschek B, Heitmann L et al. Energy-rich phosphates and glucose metabolism in early endotoxin shock. J Surg Res 1971; 11:506-512.

56. Myrvold HE, Enger E, Haljamäe H. Early effect of endotoxin on tissue phosphagen levels in skeletal muscle and liver of the dog. Eur Surg Res 1975; 7:181-192.

57. Jepson MM, Cox M, Bates PC et al. Regional blood flow and skeletal muscle energy status in endotoxemic rats. Am J Physiol 1987; 253:E581-E587.

58. Gutierrez G, Dubin A. Cellular metabolism in sepsis. In: Vincent JL, ed. Update in Intensive Care and Emergency Medicine 12. Berlin, Heidelberg, New York: Springer-Verlag, 1990:227-241.

59. Illner HP, Shires GT. Membrane defect and energy status of rabbit skeletal muscle cells in sepsis and septic shock. Arch Surg 1981; 116:1302-1305.

60. Hofmann CA. Sepsis and glucose transporters. In: Gamelli RL, Dries DJ, eds. Trauma 2000—Strategies for the New Millenium. Austin: RG Landes, 1992:121-126.

61. Wolfe RR, Elahi D, Spitzer JJ. Glucose and lactate kinetics after endotoxin administration in dogs. Am J Physiol 1977; 232:E180-E185.

62. Merril GF, Spitzer JJ. Glucose and lactate kinetics in guinea pigs following *Escherichia coli* endotoxin administration. Circ Shock 1978; 5:11-21.

63. Raymond RM, Harkema JM, Emerson Jr TE. Mechanisms of increased glucose uptake by skeletal muscle during *Escherichia coli* endotoxin shock in the dog. Circ Shock 1981; 8:77-93.

64. Romanosky AJ, Bagby GJ, Bockman EL et al. Increased muscle glucose uptake and lactate release after endotoxin administration. Am J Physiol 1980; 239:E311-E316.

65. Amaral JF, Shearer JD, Mastrofrancesco B. The effect of endotoxin on glucose metabolism in skeletal muscle requires the presence of plasma. Arch Surg 1989; 124:727-732.

66. Yelich MR, Witek-Janusek L, Filkins JP. Glucose dyshomeostasis in endotoxicosis: direct versus monokine-mediated mechanisms of endotoxin action. In: Szentivanyi A, Friedman H, eds. Immunobiology and Immunopharmacology of Bacterial Endotoxins. New York: Plenum Publishing, 1986:111-132.

67. Hinshaw LB, Beller BK, Archer LT et al. Hypoglycemic response of blood to live *Escherichia coli* organisms and endotoxin. J Surg Res 1976; 21:141-150.

68. Lang CH, Dobrescu C, Meszaros K. Insulin-mediated glucose uptake by individual tissues during sepsis. Metabolism 1990; 39:1096-1107.

69. Lang CH, Dobrescu C. Gram-negative infection increases noninsulin-mediated glucose disposal. Endocrinology 1991; 128:645-653.

70. Birnbaum MJ. Identification of a novel gene encoding an insulin-responsive glucose transporter protein. Cell 1989; 57:305-315.

71. Fukumoto H, Kayano T, Buse JB et al. Cloning and characterization of the major insulin-responsive glucose transporter expressed in human skeletal muscle and other insulin-responsive tissues. J Biol Chem 1989; 264:7776-7779.

72. Lang CH, Dobrescu C. Sepsis-induced increases in glucose uptake by macrophage-rich tissues persist during hypoglycemia. Metabolism 1991; 40:585-593.

73. Shangraw RE, Jahoor F, Miyoshi H et al. Differentiation between septic and postburn insulin resistance. Metabolism 1989; 38:983-989.

74. Lang CH, Dobrescu C. In vivo insulin resistance during non lethal hypermetabolic sepsis. Circ Shock 1989; 28:165-178.

75. Zeller WP, The SM, Sweet M et al. Altered glucose transporter mRNA abundance in a rat model of endotoxic shock. Biochem Biophys Res Commun 1991; 176:535-540.

76. Lee MD, Zentella A, Pekala PH et al. Effect of endotoxin-induced monokines on glucose metabolism in the muscle cell line L6. Proc Natl Acad Sci USA 1987; 84:2590-2594.

77. Cornelius P, Marlowe M, Pekala P. Regulation of glucose transport by tumor necrosis factor-alpha in cultured murine 3T3-L1 fibroblasts. Adv Understand Trauma Burn Injury 1991; 30:S15-S20.

78. Bird TA, Davies A, Baldwin SA et al. Interleukin-1 stimulates hexose transport in fibroblasts by increasing the expression of glucose transporters. J Biol Chem 1990; 265:13578-13583.

79. Marrou A, Turner D, Oglethorpe N. Fructose 1,6-diphosphate: an agent for treatment of experimental endotoxin shock. Surgery 1981; 90:482-488.

80. Lundsgaard-Hansen P, Pappova E, Urbaschek B et al. Circulatory deterioration as the determinant of oxygen energy metabolism in endotoxin shock. J Surg Res 1972; 13:282-288.

81. Vary TC, Siegel JH, Nakatani T et al. Effect of sepsis on activity of PDH complex in skeletal muscle and liver. Am J Physiol 1986; 250:E634-E640.

82. Kilpatrick-Smith L, Erecinska M. Cellular effects of endotoxin in vitro. I. Effect of endotoxin on mitochondrial substrate metabolism and intracellular calcium. Circ Shock 1983; 11:85-99.

83. Park R, Arieff AI. Treatment of lactic acidosis with dichloroacetate in dogs. J Clin Invest 1982; 70:853-862.

84. Vary TC, Siegel JH, Tall BD et al. Metabolic effect of partial reversal of pyruvate dehydrogenase activity by dichloroacetate in sepsis. Circ Shock 1988; 24:3-38.

85. Curtis SE, Cain SM. Regional and systemic oxygen delivery/uptake relations and lactate flux in hyperdynamic, endotoxin-treated dogs. Am Rev Respir Dis 1992; 145:348-354.

86. Fink MP. Whole body and organ measures of O_2 availability. In: Sibbald WJ, Vincent J-L, eds. Clinical trials for the treatment of sepsis (Update in intensive care and emergency medicine 19). Berlin, Heidelberg: Springer-Verlag, 1995:106-121.

87. Fink MP, Cohn SM, Lee PC et al. Effect of lipopolysaccharide on intestinal intramucosal hydrogen concentration in pigs: evidence of gut ischemia in a normodynamic model of septic shock. Crit Care Med 1989; 17:641-646.

88. Mela-Riker L, Tavakoli H. Effect of endotoxin on mitochondrial function. In: Berry LJ, ed. Cellular Biology of Endotoxin (Handbook of Endotoxin 3). Amsterdam, New York, Oxford: Elsevier, 1985:166-184.

89. Poderoso JJ, Boveris A, Jorge MA et al. Function mitochondrial en el shock septico. Medicinal (Firenze) 1978; 38:371-377.

90. Mela L, Bacalzo LV, Miller LD. Defective oxidative metabolism of rat liver mitochondria in hemorrhagic and endotoxin shock. Am J Physiol 1971; 220:571-577.

91. Dawson KL, Geller ER, Kirkpatrick JR. Enhancement of mitochondrial function in sepsis. Arch Surg 1988; 123:241-246.

92. Clowes GHA, O'Donnell TF, Ryan NT et al. Energy metabolism in sepsis. Treatment based on different patterns in shock and high output stage. Ann Surg 1974; 179:684-696.

93. Hotchkiss RS, Long RC, Hall JR et al. An in vivo examination of rat brain during sepsis with ^{31}P-NMR spectroscopy. Am J Physiol 1989; 257:C1055-C1059.

94. Leon A, Boczkowski J, Dureuil B et al. Effects of endotoxic shock on diaphragmatic function in mechanically ventilated rats. J Appl Physiol 1992; 72:1466-1472.

95. Eastridge BJ, Darlington DN, Evans JA et al. A circulating shock protein depolarizes cells in hemorrhage and sepsis. Ann Surg 1994; 219:298-305.

96. Hotchkiss RS, Karl IE. Reevaluation of the role of cellular hypoxia and bioenergetic failure in sepsis. JAMA 1992; 267:1503-1510.

97. Reed PC, Erve PR, DasGupta TK et al. Endotoxemic effect of *Escherichia coli* on cardiac and skeletal muscle mitochondria. Surg Forum 1970; 21:13-14.

98. Schumer W, Erve PR. Bovine serum albumin effect on endotoxin-challenged mitochondria. Surgery 1971; 69:699-701.

99. Schumer W, Erve PR, Obernolte RP. Endotoxemic effect on cardiac and skeletal muscle mitochondria. Surg Gynecol Obstet 1971; 133:433-436.

100. Mela L, Hinshaw LB, Coalson JJ. Correlation of cardiac performance, ultrastructural morphology, and mitochondrial function in endotoxemia in the dog. Circ Shock 1974; 1:265-272.

101. Mela L. Mitochondrial metabolite alterations in experimental circulatory shock. In: Urbaschek B, Urbaschek R, Neter E, eds. Gram-negative Bacterial Infections and Mode of Endotoxin Actions. Wien: Springer-Verlag, 1975:288-295.

102. Dhainaut JF, Huyghebaert MF, Monsallier JF et al. Coronary hemodynamics and myocardial metabolism of lactate, free fatty acids, glucose, and ketones in patients with septic shock. Circulation 1987; 75:533-541.

103. Dhainaut J-F, Dall'Ava J, Mira JP. Coronary hemodynamics and myocardial metabolism in sepsis. In: Schlag G, Redl H, eds. Pathophysiology of Shock, Sepsis, and Organ Failure. Berlin, Heidelberg: Springer-Verlag, 1993:882-892.

104. McDonaugh KH, Lang CH, Spitzer JJ. The effect of hyperdynamic sepsis on myocardial performance. Circ Shock 1985; 15:247-259.

105. Pasque MK, Murphy CE, Van Trigt P et al. Myocardial adenosine triphosphate levels during early sepsis. Arch Surg 1983; 118:1437-1440.

106. Sethi R, Rupp H, Naimark BJ et al. Characteristics and mechanism of tachyphylaxis of cardiac contractile response to insulin. Int J Cardiol 1993; 38:119-130.

107. Scholl RA, Lang CH, Bagby GJ. Hypertriglyceridemia and its relation to tissue lipoprotein lipase activity in endotoxemic, *Escherichia coli* bacteremic, and polymicrobial septic rats. J Surg Res 1984; 37:394-401.

108. Dhalla NS, Elimban V, Rupp H. Paradoxical role of lipid metabolism in heart function and dysfunction. Mol Cell Biochem 1992; 116:3-9.

109. Nagano M, Dhalla NS. The Diabetic Heart. New York: Raven Press, 1991.

110. Rupp H, Elimban V, Dhalla NS. Sucrose feeding prevents changes in myosin isoenzymes and sarcoplamic reticulum Ca^{2+}-pump ATPase in pressure-loaded rat heart. Biochem Biophys Res Commun 1988; 156:917-923.

111. Rupp H, Elimban V, Dhalla NS. Diabetes-like action of intermittent fasting on sarcoplasmic reticulum Ca^{2+}-pump ATPase and myosin isoenzymes can be prevented by sucrose. Biochem Biophys Res Commun 1989; 164:319-325.

112. Rupp H, Wahl R, Hansen M. Influence of diet and carnitine palmitoyltransferase I inhibition on myosin and sarcoplasmic reticulum. J Appl Physiol 1992; 72:352-360.

113. Rupp H, Elimban V, Dhalla NS. Modification of subcellular organelles in pressure overloaded heart by etomoxir, a carnitine palmitoyltransferase I inhibitor. FASEB J 1992; 6:2349-2353.

114. Rupp H, Jacob R. Metabolically-modulated growth and phenotype of the rat. Eur Heart J 1992; 13(Suppl D):56-61.

115. Tomlinson CW, Lee SL, Dhalla NS. Abnormalities in heart membranes and myofibrils during bacterial infective cardiomyopathy in the rabbit. Circ Res 1976; 39:82-92.

116. Dhalla NS, Ziegelhoffer A, Singal PK et al. Subcellular changes during cardiac hypertrophy and heart failure due to bacterial endocardits. Basic Res Cardiol 1980; 75:81-91.

117. Dennhardt R, Gramm HJ, Meinhold K et al. Patterns of endocrine secretion during sepsis. In: Schlag G, Redl H, eds. Second Vienna Shock Forum (Progress in clinical and biological research 308). New York: Alan R Liss, 1989:751-756.

118. Arai M, Otsu K, MacLennan DH et al. Effect of thyroid hormone on the expression of mRNA encoding sarcoplasmic reticulum proteins. Circ Res 1991; 69:266-276.

119. Gupta MP, Gupta M, Stewart A et al. Activation of alpha-myosin heavy chain gene expression by cAMP in cultured fetal rat heart myocytes. Biochem Biophys Res Commun 1991; 174:1198-1203.

120. Rupp H, Berger H-J, Pfeifer A et al. Effect of positive inotropic agents on myosin isozyme population and mechanical activity of cultured rat heart myocytes. Circ Res 1991; 68:1164-1173.

121. Rupp H, Takeda N. Sympathetic nervous system activity and regulation of cardiac gene expression. In: Ganguly PK, ed. Catecholamines and Heart Disease. Boca Raton: CRC Press, 1991:217-229.

122. Morkin E, Bahl JJ, Markham BE. Control of cardiac myosin heavy chain gene expression by thyroid hormones. In: Kedes LH, Stockdale, eds. Cellular and Molecular Biology of Muscle Development. New York: Alan R Liss Inc, 1989:381-389.

123. Fuller SJ, Sugden PH. Acute inhibition of rat heart protein synthesis in vitro during β-adrenergic stimulation or hypoxia. Am J Physiol 1988; 255:E537-E547.

124. Kao R, Rannels E, Morgan HE. Effects of anoxia and ischemia on protein synthesis in perfused rat hearts. Circ Res 1976; Suppl I:I-124-I-130.

125. Kwiatkowska-Patzer B, Patzer JA, Heller LJ. *Pseudomonas aeruginosa* exotoxin A enhances automaticity and potentiates hypoxic depression of isolated rat hearts. Proc Soc Exp Biol Med 1993; 202:377-383.

126. Perentesis JP, Miller SP, Bodley JW. Protein toxin inhibitors of protein synthesis. BioFactors 1992; 3:173-184.

127. Ueda K, Hayaishi O. ADP-ribosylation. Ann Rev Biochem 1985; 54:73-100.

128. Wilson BA, Collier RJ. Diphtheria toxin and *Pseudomonas aeruginosa* exotoxin A: Active-site structure and enzymic mechanism. In: Aktories K, ed. ADP-Ribosylating Toxins (Current topics in microbiology and immunology 175). Berlin, Heidelberg: Springer-Verlag, 1992:27-41.

129. Iglewski WJ, Dehwhurst S. Cellular mono(ADP-ribosyl)transferase inhibits protein synthesis. FEBS Lett 1991; 283:235-238.

130. Görg A. Two-dimensional electrophoresis with immobilized pH gradients: current state. Biochemical Society Transaction 1993; 21:130-132.

131. Chang He, Müller U, Oberthür W et al. Application of high-resolution two-dimensional polyacrylamide gel elecrophoresis of polypeptides from cultured neonatal rat cardiomyocytes: Regulation of protein synthesis by catecholamines. Electrophoresis 1992; 13:748-754.

132. Chang He, Müller U, Werdan K. Regulation of protein biosynthesis in neonatal rat cardiomyocytes by adrenoceptor stimulation: Investigations

with high-resolution two-dimensional polyacrylamide gel electrophoresis. Electrophoresis 1992; 13:755-756.

133. Jungblut P, Otto A, Zeindl-Eberhart E et al. Protein composition of the human heart: the construction of a myocardial two-dimensional electrophoresis database. Electrophoresis 1994; 15:685-707.

134. Schlag G, Redl H, Davies J et al. Live *Escherichia coli* sepsis models in baboons. In: Schlag G, Redl H, eds. Pathophysiology of Shock, Sepsis, and Organ Failure. Berlin, Heidelberg, New York: Springer-Verlag, 1993: 1076-1107.

135. Müller U, Chang He, Redl H et al. Altered protein pattern (APP) in acute septic cardiomyopathy in untreated and treated baboons: application of high resolution two-dimensional polyacrylamide gel electrophoresis (2-D PAGE). Circ Shock 1993; Suppl 1:Abstracts 31.

136. Zeindl-Eberhart E, Jungblut PR, Otto A et al. Identification of tumor-associated protein variants during rat hepatocarcinogenesis. J Biol Chem 1994; 269:14589-14594.

137. Owens EL, Lynch CJ, McCall KM et al. Altered expression of skeletal muscle proteins during sepsis. Shock 1994; 2:171-178.

138. Dahn M, Bouwman D, Kirkpatrick JR. The sepsis-glucose intolerance riddle: a hormonal explanation. Surgery 1979; 86:423-426.

139. Wolf HPO. Aryl-substituted 2-oxirane carboxylic acids: a new group of antidiabetic drugs. In: Bailey CJ, Flatt PR, eds. New antidiabetic drugs. London:Smith-Gordon, 1990:217-229.

140. Steiner KE, Lien EL. Hypoglycemic agents which do not release insulin. Prog Med Chem 1987; 24:209-248.

141. Sherratt HSA. Inhibition of gluconeogenesis by non-hormonal hypoglycemic compounds. In: Hue L, Van de Werve G, eds. Short-term Regulation of Liver Metabolism. Amsterdam: Elsevier/North-Holland Biomedical Press, 1981:199-227.

142. Rösen P, Schmitz FJ, Reinauer H. Improvement of myocardial function and metabolism in diabetic rats by the carnitine palmitoyltransferase inhibitor etomoxir. In: Nagano M, Mochizuki S, Dhalla NS, eds. Cardiovascular Disease in Diabetes. Boston:Kluwer Academic Publishers, 1992:361-372.

143. Rupp H, Müller U, Werdan K. Metabolically deranged cardiomyopathy of the trauma-sepsis syndrome. In: Nagano M, Takeda N, Dhalla NS, eds. The Cardiomyopathic Heart. New York, Raven Press, 1994:257-267.

144. Tredget EE, Yu YM, Zhong S et al. Role of interleukin 1 and tumor necrosis factor on energy metabolism in rabbits. Am J Physiol 1988; 255:E760-E768.

145. Lancaster Jr JR, Laster SM, Gooding LR. Inhibition of target cell mitochondrial electron transfer by tumor necrosis factor. FEBS Letters 1989; 248:169-174.

146. Taylor DJ, Faragher EB, Evanson JM. Inflammatory cytokines stimulate glucose uptake and glycolysis but reduce glucose oxidation in human dermal fibroblasts in vitro. Circ Shock 1992; 37:105-110.

147. Geng Y-J, Hansson GK, Holme E. Interferon-γ and tumor necrosis factor synergize to induce nitric oxide production and inhibit mitochondrial respiration in vascular smooth muscle cells. Circ Res 1992; 71:1268-1276.

148. Schulze-Osthoff K, Bakker AC, Vanhaesebroeck B et al. Cytotoxic activity of tumor necrosis is mediated by early damage of mitochondrial functions—evidence for the involvement of mitochondrial radical generation. J Biol Chem 1992; 267:5317-5323.

149. Boekstegers P, Bauer I, Peter W et al. TNF-α induces a reversible inhibition of positive inotropic response in neonatal rat heart cells. Can J Cardiol 1994; 10(Suppl A):68A.

150. Boekstegers P, Zell R, Geck P et al. Ist die Aktivitätsabnahme der Pyruvatdehydrogenase(PDH) nach Zytokin-Exposition mit TNF-α oder IL1α die Folge der primären Hemmung der mitochondrialen Atmungskette? Z Kardiol 1995; 84(Suppl 1):559A.

151. Stadler J, Billiar TR, Curran RD et al. Effect of exogenous and endogenous nitric oxide on mitochondrial respiration of rat hepatocytes. J Appl Physiol 1991; 260:C 910-C 916.

152. Stadler J, Bentz BG, Harbrecht BG et al. Tumor necrosis factor alpha inhibits hepatocyte mitochondrial respiration. Ann Surg 1992; 216:539-546.

CHAPTER 8

DERANGEMENT OF INOTROPIC AXES OF THE CARDIOMYOCYTE

IS THE "ENDOTOXIN-TNF-α-NITRIC OXIDE-CARDIODEPRESSION CASCADE" THE WHOLE STORY?

Data obtained from septic patients and animal experiments represent the complex network of toxin and mediator sequences and interactions, leading finally to an impairment of heart function. Looking for possible mechanisms underlying this septic cardiomyopathy, one must to a great extent rely on work with isolated heart preparations and cardiomyocytes, with which "negative inotropic" cascades triggered by toxins and sepsis mediators can be identified (see chapters 3 and 4).

Since the first reports about vaguely defined circulating myocardial depressant factors almost 30 years ago, a variety of more or less well-characterized substances with negative inotropic effects have been described (Tables 8.1 and 8.2, see also chapter 4), including bacterial toxins, catecholamines, cytokines, reactive oxygen species, functionally characterized depressant factors and others.[1-3]

The presently most attractive "mechanism of myocardial depression in sepsis hypothesis" is presented in Figure 8.1; circulating endotoxin triggers mediator cells to release tumor necrosis factor α (TNF-α) and interleukin-1 (IL-1), either into the circulation or into the myocardium; TNF-α and IL-1, the latter being discussed as either important[4,5] or of less relevance,[6] then trigger the expression of an inducible nitric oxide synthase (iNOS) in the heart,[5,7,8] with the consequence of an accelerated release of nitric oxide (NO) from arginine; NO might then stimulate the activity of a soluble and probably also of a particulate form of the guanylyl cyclase of the cardiomyocyte (CM), and the consecutive rise in cyclic guanosine monophosphate (cGMP) could finally lead to an attenuation of systolic as well as of diastolic function of the heart (Fig. 8.2).[5,8-17] Both an expression of iNOS and an increase in cGMP content was described in failing hearts from septic

Table 8.1. Substances and states likely to trigger cardiac dysfunction in sepsis

Bacterial toxins
    Endotoxin
    Pseudomonas exotoxin A
    Streptolysin O
    Staphylococcal α toxin
    Fusarium fungi T-2 toxin
Catecholamines
Cytokines
    Tumor necrosis factor α (TNFα)
    Interleukin-1 (IL-1)
    Interleukin-2 (IL-2)
    Interleukin-6 (IL-6)
    Interferon-γ
Other mediators
    Nitric oxide (NO)
    Complement factors
    Platelet activating factor (PAF)
    Eicosanoids (thromboxanes, prostaglandins, leukotrienes)
    Reactive oxygen species
    Endorphins
    Renin/angiotensin II
    Atrial natriuretic factor family
    Calcitonin gene-related peptide
    Endothelin
    Serotonin
    Neuropeptide Y
    Thrombin
    Histamin
Alterations in hormone plasma levels
    Glucocorticoids
    Thyroid hormones
    Vasopressin
Toxin-/mediator-activated blood cells
    Polymorphonuclear leukocytes (PMN)
    Eosinophils
    Cytotoxic T-lymphocytes
    Platelets
Pathological states of the heart
    Energy depletion
    Hypoxia, reoxygenation and ischemia
Cardiodepressant factors
    MDF
    ECDF
    MDS
    CDF

For further information see text, especially chapter 4.

patients (72 ± 17 fmol/mg wet weight, n = 3, versus 31 ± 6.9 fmol/mg wet weight, n = 4, in nonfailing, nonseptic hearts); neither was the case in hearts failing due to dilated cardiomyopathy, ischemic heart disease, Becker muscular dystrophy or mitoxantrone-induced toxic cardiomyopathy.[8] However, it is still a matter of debate, whether the cardiodepressive effect of NO is mediated exclusively by an activation of the guanylyl cyclase.[9,10,12,16] The discussion also circles around the question, by which mechanism(s) increased cGMP depresses systolic and diastolic function of the heart: by an enhanced metabolism of cyclic adenosine monophosphate (cAMP) via stimulation of cAMP phosphodiesterases, or by an activation of cGMP-dependent protein kinases and subsequent protein phosphorylation; both could lead to an inhibition of transsarcolemmal Ca^{2+}-influx, but also to a decreased Ca^{2+} sensitivity of the contractile proteins.[12,16-19] On the one hand, measurements of Ca^{2+} current indicate that NO regulates trans-sarcolemmal calcium current by guanylyl cyclase activation of phos-phodiesterases,[12] and a similar inhibition of mammalian calcium cur-rent can apparently also be accomplished by a cGMP-dependent protein kinase.[16] On the other hand, cardiodepressive effects of cGMP can also be achieved without alteration of cellular Ca^{2+}. Enhancement of isotonic relaxation induced by 8-bromo cGMP in isolated rat ven-tricular myocytes is not accompanied by any reduction in the ampli-tude of the intracellular calcium transient, as measured by the cal-cium-sensitive fluorescent indicator indo-1.[19] This suggests that the effects of cGMP are mediated via a reduction in the response of the contractile proteins to Ca^{2+}, and argues against any mechanism in-volving alterations in Ca^{2+} flux. These effects were prevented by an inhibitor of protein kinase G, KT 5823, leading to the suggestion of a possible involvement of protein kinase G-mediated phosphorylation of troponin.[19]

For a better understanding of the role of NO in septic cardio-myopathy, the effects of NO—either applied exogenously by NO do-nors, or generated physiologically by the constitutive nitric oxide synthase (cNOS) and under various pathophysiological conditions by the in-ducible nitric oxide synthase (iNOS)—shall be briefly reviewed (see also chapter 4: Nitric Oxide).[17]

In isolated CMs, NO produced by cNOS mediates the negative chronotropic effect of the muscarinergic receptor agonist carbachol, and it partly inhibits the positive inotropic effect of β-adrenoceptor stimulation by isoproterenol, with no influence, however, on basal contractility of the CM.[9,20] Rather contradictory to the latter is the finding that authentic NO in solution inhibits basal performance of isolated guinea pig ventricular myocytes.[21] A change in relaxation pattern was not reported in this study (see also below), although this may be attributable to the lower resolution of the length measurement system used. Similar responses were also observed with bradykinin-induced

Table 8.2. Impairment of inotropic pathways in cardiomyocytes triggered by bacterial toxins and sepsis mediators

A) β_1-adrenoceptor/G proteins/adenylyl cyclase pathway
A1) Excess of catecholamines
  - decreases the number of β_1-adrenoceptors
  - increases the number of G_i-proteins
A2) Reactive oxygen species
  - impair adenylyl cyclase activity
A3) Pseudomonas exotoxin A
  - represses resynthesis of β-adrenoceptors after catecholamine-induced down-regulation
  - suppresses catecholamine-induced increase in G_i proteins
  - inhibits catecholamine-induced V_3/V_1-myosin isoenzyme shift
A4) Endotoxin
  - attenuates—in the absence of glucocorticoids—isoproterenol-induced "positive inotropy"
A5) Tumor necrosis factor α (TNFα)
  - attenuates isoproterenol-induced "positive inotropy"
  - decreases the number of β_1-adrenoceptors
  - increases G_s
  - increases G_i (α and β-unit)
  - increases the activity of the catalytic subunit
  - enhances isoproterenol-stimulated adenylyl cyclase activity
  - enhances forskolin-stimulated adenylyl cyclase activity
A6) Interleukin-1β
  - inhibits isoproterenol-stimulated cAMP formation
A7) Nitric Oxide (NO)
  - NO—generated by cNOS—attenuates isoproterenol-induced "positive inotropy"
  - NO—generated by cNOS—mediates the negative chronotropic effect of carbachol
  - N0—generated by endotoxin via iNOS—attenuates isoproterenol-induced "positive inotropy"
  - mediates—in some, but not in all conditions—the attenuating effect of TNF-α on isoproterenol-induced "positive inotropy"

B) α_1-adrenoceptor/phosphoinositide pathway
B1) Tumor necrosis factor α (TNFα)
  - inhibits basal IP_3 formation
  - inhibits α_1-adrenoceptor-stimulated IP_3 formation
  - reduces GDH activity as probable mechanism of inhibition of basal and α_1-adrenoceptor-stimulated IP_3 formation
  - reduces "positive inotropy" of α_1-adrenoceptor agonists
  - protects from α_1-adrenoceptor agonist-induced arrhythmias
B2) Platelet-activating factor (PAF)
  - stimulates the phosphoinositide pathway
  - induces a "negative inotropic" and a positve chronotropic effect by stimulation of protein kinase C via the phosphoinositide pathway
B3) Angiotensin II
  - stimulates phosphoinositide pathway

Table 8.2. Impairment of inotropic pathways in cardiomyocytes triggered by bacterial toxins and sepsis mediators (continued)

B4) Thrombin
  - stimulates phosphoinositide pathway
C) Ca^{2+}-influx/Ca^{2+}-transient
C1) Tumor necrosis factor α (TNFα)
  - depresses Ca^{2+}-transients in a NO-independent manner
C2) Cardiodepressant factor (CDF)
  - "negative inotropic" and negative chronotropic effects mediated by inhibition of Ca^{2+} inward current
C3) NO
  - regulates sarcolemmal Ca^{2+} current via cGMP
C4) Complement
  - augmentation of Ca^{2+} transients parallels a "positive inotropic" effect
  - a sharp rise in basal Ca^{2+} concentration precedes cell contracture and lysis
C5) Thrombin
  - increases both the systolic and diastolic inward Ca^{2+} current (Ca^{2+}_i), associated with a rise in force of contraction, beating frequency, and action potential duration.
C6) Reactive oxygen species
  - increase cytoplasmic Ca^{2+}
  - stimulate Ca^{2+} influx through voltage-gated Ca^{2+} channels
  - enhance Ca^{2+} release from the sarcoplasmic reticulum
  - impair cellular Ca^{2+} extrusion mechanisms
  - inhibit sarcoplasmic Ca^{2+} ATPase
  - induce delayed after-contractions attributed to a ryanodine-sensitive Ca^{2+} efflux from the sarcoplasmic reticulum

For further details see text, especially chapters 4 and 8.

NO release in coculture experiments with vascular endothelial cells.[21] NO also plays an essential role in mediating the effects of muscarinergic agonists on the rate of depolarization of sinoatrial cells.[22] In the isolated ferret papillary muscle, substance P-stimulated NO release from endothelial cells causes an earlier onset of myocardial relaxation, with little change in the maximum rate of force development, and a small reduction in peak isometric force, accompanied by an elevation of myocardial cGMP.[23] A similar response of the left ventricular waveform is exhibited by the isolated ejecting guinea pig heart to both NO from exogenous donors (sodium nitroprusside) and stimulation of endogenous NO release by substance P or bradykinin.[24,25] Left ventricular pressure, as measured by a high-fidelity micromanometer placed within the left ventricle, shows an earlier onset of relaxation, no change in +dP/dt, and a small reduction in peak left ventricular pressure. These effects are abolished by scavengers of NO (hemoglobin) and are independent of changes in coronary flow.

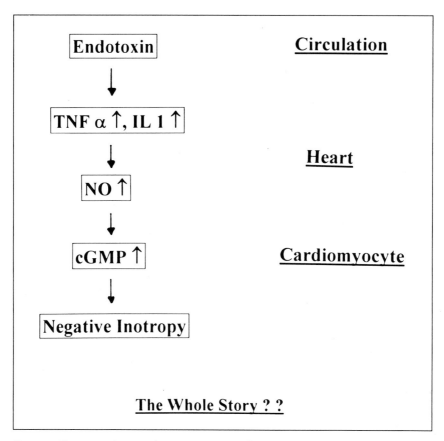

Fig. 8.1. Plasma cardiotoxic factors in sepsis—"the most attractive negative inotropic cascade."

Fig. 8.2. Opposite page: Synopsis—mechanisms of negative inotropic effects of bacterial toxins and sepsis mediators in cardiomyocytes. The scheme summarizes findings of the effects of bacterial toxins and sepsis mediators obtained in heart muscle preparations and isolated cardiomyocytes. Abbreviatons used: AC = adenylyl cyclase; 5'AMP = 5'adenosine monophosphate; ATP = adenosine triphosphate; CA = contractile apparatus; cAMP = cyclic adenosine monophosphate; CAT = catecholamines; cGMP-PK = cGMP-dependent protein kinase; DG = diacylglycerol; DR = delayed rectifier; G = guanine nucleotide-binding regulatory proteins that may stimulate (αG_s) or inhibit (αG_i) adenylyl cyclase; 5'GMP = 5'guanosine monophosphate; GTP = guanosine triphosphate; I = inositol; IP = inositol phosphate; IP_2 = inositol diphosphate; IP_3 = inositol triphophate; PDE = phosphodiesterase; pGC = particulate guanylyl cyclase; PHLB = phospholamban; PI = phosphatidylinositol; PIP = phosphatidylinositol 4-phosphate; PIP_2 = phosphatidylinositol 4,5-bisphosphate; PKA = protein kinase A; PKC = protein kinase C; PLC = phospholipase C; R_β = β_1-adrenoceptor; R_M = muscarinergic receptor; $R_{\alpha 1}$ = α_1-adrenoceptor; R_{ANF} = receptor for atrial natriuretic peptide; ROS = reactive oxygen species; sGC = soluble guanylyl cyclase; SR = sarcoplasmic reticulum. For further explanation see text. Special topics: α_1-adrenoceptor/phosphoinositide pathway;[47] impairment of positive inotropic effects;[46] Ca^{2+} transient;[51] action potential CDF;[3] action potential TNF;[44] action potential endotoxin;[35] endotoxin, NO, iNOS, sGC and pGC.[12,13,15,35,46,65,66]

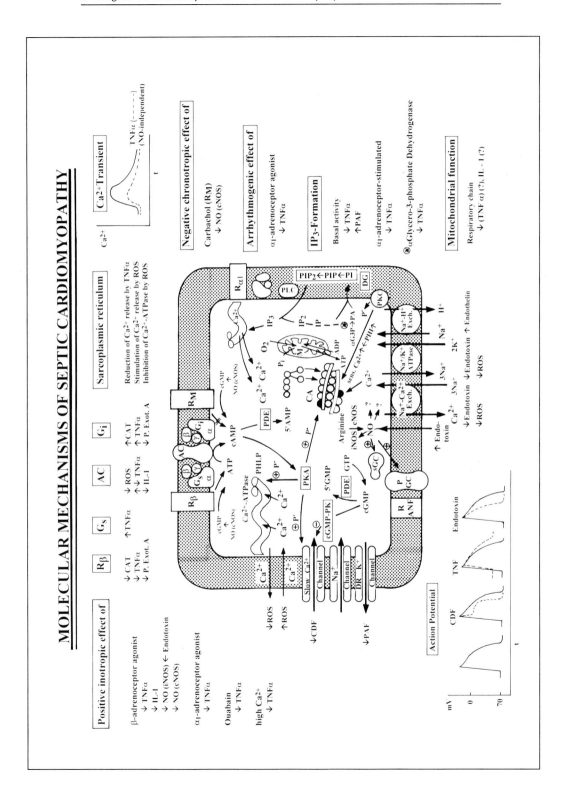

In dogs, NO mediates, at least in part, vagal inhibition of the inotropic response to β-adrenergic stimulation by dobutamine, and thus may play a role in normal physiologic regulation of myocardial autonomic response.[26] Furthermore, the conductance of the coronary vascular bed and the resting myocardial blood flow are regulated physiologically by NO, with inhibition of NOS resulting in a 30%-50% reduction of coronary blood flow.[27,28]

Recently, effects have been also shown in the human heart in vivo in response to intracoronary infusions of sodium nitroprusside.[29] Bicoronary infusion of nitroprusside at a dose of ≤ 4 µg/min (previously shown to be too low to cause systemic vasodilation) was performed in 13 patients with normal epicardial coronary angiograms with high-fidelity measurement of left ventricular pressure. Nitroprusside infusion resulted in a reduction of peak left ventricular (LV) pressure and an earlier onset of relaxation. Contrary to what would be expected from an increase in coronary flow, nitroprusside also caused an increase in LV distensibility, as revealed by a reduction in LV end-diastolic pressure accompanied by an increase in end-diastolic volume, an effect which would be expected to facilitate LV filling. Right atrial infusions of the same dose of nitroprusside failed to reproduce these findings, suggesting that they were indeed a result of direct action of NO on the myocardium.

This short overview outlines some negative chronotropic, inotropic and lusitropic acute effects of NO in various species including men, and it documents the important regulatory role of this molecule. It is well understandable that the enhanced production of NO by iNOS in sepsis might even more profoundly alter the function of the heart.

NO produced by iNOS partly reduces the positive inotropic effect of the β-adrenergic agonist isoproterenol, while basal contractility and the contractile response to high extracellular Ca^{2+} are not affected.[10] In the ferret papillary muscle, induction of iNOS by interleukin-1β produces negative inotropic effects similar to those of endothelium-derived NO, although of much greater magnitude,[30] and the endotoxin-mediated induction of iNOS in guinea pigs significantly reduces peak shortening of isolated CMs in a manner that was sensitive to dexamethasone and an NOS antagonist.[31]

However, this "endotoxin-TNF-α-NO-cardiodepression cascade" does not probably make up the whole story, as will be discussed in the following chapters.

IS ALL ENDOTOXIN CARDIODEPRESSION MEDIATED BY TNF-α AND IL-1?

Endotoxin injection in animals as well as in human volunteers clearly impairs cardiac function,[32-34] with the maximum of cardiodepression (reduction in ejection fraction) occurring in the dog 48 hours after endotoxin clot implantation.[33] In addition, in endotoxin-treated animals, both the hearts in vivo as well as the CMs ex vivo-in vitro exhibit depressed contractility.[31,35] Endotoxin injection in rats time-dependently induces NOS activity and raises cyclic cGMP content in the left ventricular wall.[4] Furthermore, endotoxin results in a shortening of the action potential of the heart muscle cell,[35] an impaired sarcoplasmic reticulum Ca^{2+}-ATPase activity, a reduced Ca^{2+}-induced Ca^{2+} release from the sarcoplasmic reticulum, an altered Na^+-Ca^{2+} exchange and an inhibition of (Na^++K^+)-ATPase, the latter two effects being probably due to changes in the cell membrane microenvironment in response to phospholipase A activation (Fig. 8.2).[35,36] Endotoxin also disrupts the myocardial response to direct β-receptor stimulation, but not to adenylyl cyclase stimulation in the isolated rat heart.[34] At least part of these effects can be overcome by inhibition of NOS induction and/or activity,[31,38,39] arguing for an indirect, NO-mediated effect of endotoxin on the heart.

Although there are many arguments for a TNF-α- and probably also for an IL-1-mediated cardiodepression of endotoxin in sepsis,[4,32-34] some other modes of action might exist, with a probable direct depressive effect of endotoxin on CMs being one example.

Even at very high concentrations (up to 10 μg/ml), endotoxin does neither impair viability nor beating of adult and neonatal rat CMs (for review see chapter 4: Bacterial and Fungal Toxins: Endotoxin). All the more surprising was the finding that endotoxin can indeed exert direct effects in heart muscle cells, when the glucocorticoid dexamethasone is omitted from the culture medium; under this condition, endotoxin induces NO production both in cultured heart muscle cells as well as in heart nonmuscle cells from neonatal rats (Table 4.5), and it unequivocally suppresses the "positive inotropic" effect of isoproterenol in these cardiomyocytes (Fig. 4.8). Addition of dexamethasone, which suppresses the formation of iNOS, both inhibits endotoxin-induced NO synthesis and derepresses isoproterenol-inotropy (Fig. 4.8, ref. 46). In view of the only weak stimulation of NO production by IL-1 and the complete lack of stimulation by TNF-α at low concentrations (Table 4.6), an indirect endotoxin effect mediated by one of these cytokines seems unlikely. Therefore, not only TNF-α/IL-1-dependent, but also TNF-α/IL-1-independent iNOS stimulation by endotoxin may occur. The putative endotoxin receptors of the heart await identification.

IS ALL TNF-α CARDIODEPRESSION MEDIATED BY NITRIC OXIDE?

Infusion of TNF-α in humans and animals results in a profound and long-lasting (up to several days) depression in left ventricular ejection fraction,[33,40-42] with no change in coronary blood flow,[42] but probably with an increase in coronary microvascular permeability,[43] and with the maximum depression in TNF-α-challenged dogs occurring between 8 and 48 hours.[33,40] In view of the increased levels of TNF-α and soluble TNF receptors in septic shock, these findings argue for a relevant role of TNF-α in the pathogenesis of septic cardiomyopathy.

ACUTE VERSUS CHRONIC CARDIODEPRESIVE TNF-α EFFECTS: WHICH ARE CLINICALLY RELEVANT?

In a variety of heart muscle preparations, cardiodepressant effects of TNF-α were described (Table 4.5) in combination with transient positive inotropic effects.[44] Acute depressive effects within minutes, requiring high TNF-α concentrations, must be discerned from more chronic effects, which become evident only after several hours, yet with much lower concentrations being necessary to produce profound negative inotropy (Table 4.5).[45,46] In view of the powerful interplay of TNF-α with gene expression, the chronic TNF-α effects at low, clinically relevant concentrations seem the more likely mode of action. In agreement with this hypothesis, interaction with protein expression of the inotropic machinery was documented for TNF-α in CMs (Fig. 8.2, Table 8.2), including nitric oxide synthase, the β_1-adrenoceptor/G proteins/adenylyl cyclase pathway and the α_1-adrenoceptor/phosphoinositide cascade (for review see chapter 4 and also next paragraph).[5,7,47,56]

DOES TNF-α INDUCE NITRIC OXIDE PRODUCTION IN CARDIOMYOCYTES AT REALLY RELEVANT CONCENTRATIONS?

The group of TW Smith recently described the characterization and regulation of the inducible nitric oxide synthase in primary cultures of inflammatory cytokine-pretreated adult rat ventricular myocytes.[5] They amplified a 217-base pair cDNA by reverse transcriptase-polymerase chain reaction from these cells that was nearly identical to other iNOScDNA sequences. Using this 217-base pair cDNA as a probe in Northern blots, they found no evidence of iNOSmRNA in control myocytes, but both interleukin-1β and interferon-γ individually increased iNOSmRNA in these cells, with maximal expression at 12 hours. The half-life of iNOSmRNA in actinomyocin C1-treated cells was 4 hours. Both dexamethasone and transforming growth factor-β attenuated the induction of iNOSmRNA abundance and enzyme activity by IL-1β and interferon-γ. Pretreatment with dexamethasone also abolished the induction of iNOSmRNA, but not the increase in mRNA of GTP cyclohydrolase—the rate-limiting enzyme of tetrahydrobiopterin (cofactor of NOS) synthesis—in purified cardiac myocytes from lipopolysaccharide-injected rats. With an NO-specific porphyrinic/NaF ion-coated microsensor, NO release in adult rat ventricular CMs pretreated with IL-1β and IFN-γ in arginine-depleted medium could be detected following microinjection of L-arginine in the vicinity of the cell juxtaposed to the NO microsensor, but not following microinjection of D-arginine, and not from these CMs pretreated with L-N-mono-methylarginine. Cytokine-preincubated adult rat heart muscle cells that had been maintained in L-arginine-depleted medium also exhibited a depressed contractile response to isoproterenol after addition of L-arginine, but not D-arginine. Taken together, the results of TW Smith's group indicate that altered contractile function of CMs following exposure to specific inflammatory cytokines is due at least in part to induction of myocyte iNOS.

So, undoubtedly, cytokines including TNF-α, IL-1[48] and IL-6[49] can trigger the expression of iNOS in CMs, the question is: does this occur indeed at the lowest concentrations of cytokines with clearly documented cardiodepressive effects? With this respect, several publications can be discussed. Finkel and colleagues[50] reported in hamster papillary muscle a concentration-dependent, reversible inhibition of contractility by TNF-α (59% and 44% of baseline tension at 900 and 3200 U/ml, respectively), IL-2 (62% and 50% of baseline tension at 66 and 1000 U/ml, respectively) and IL-6 (70% and 55% of baseline tension at 900 and 3200 U/ml, respectively), but not by IL-1 (87% of baseline tension at 3200 U/ml). The inhibition could be overcome by the NOS inhibitor N^G-monomethyl-L-argine (L-NMMA). Therefore, the authors argued for a direct negative inotropic effect of cytokines mediated through a myocardial NOS. However, the cytokine concentrations necessary to achieve this cardiodepression were very high. Furthermore, the fact that these cytokine effects postulated to be mediated by NO become apparent within 2 to 3 minutes and are maximal after 5 minutes is in obvious contradiction with the classical time dependence of hours for iNOS expression; it may instead point to a possible activation of a constitutively expressed cNOS by inflammatory mediators, however, at clinically less relevant concentrations. Schulz and colleagues[7] found an expression of iNOS in adult rat CMs by incubating them for 24 hours in the presence of TNF-α (20 ng/ml, estimated as ≥ 400 U/ml) plus IL-1β (5 ng/ml). In isolated working rat hearts incubated for 2 hours in the presence of TNF-α (20 ng/ml, estimated as ≥ 400 U/ml) plus IL-1β (5 ng/ml), the depression in contractility observed within 1 to 2 hours could be attributed at least in part to a myocardial iNOS activity.[4] In adult rat CMs, induction of iNOS activity could be achieved by a 24-hour-incubation of the cells either in the presence of rhTNF-α (100 ng/ml, estimated as ≥ 2000 U/ml) plus rhIL-1β (2 ng/ml) plus rmIFN-γ (500 U/ml), or by the combination of IL-1β and IFN-γ in the combination mentioned.[5] The expression of iNOSmRNA in these cells has been found again after a 24 hour-cell exposure to the cytokine double and triple combinations mentioned, but also after exposure to IL-1β (2 ng/ml) or IFN-γ (500 U/ml) alone.[5] And with the same experimental setting, the authors found a depression of isoproterenol-induced increase in amplitude of shortening in these adult rat cardiomyocytes pretreated for 24 hours in the presence of TNF-α (100 ng/ml, estimated as ≥ 2000 U/ml) plus IL-1β (2 ng/ml) plus IFN-γ (500 U/ml).[5]

On the other hand, documented negative inotropic effects of TNF-α in CMs at the lowest concentrations (0.1-10 U/ml) reported[46] are clearly NO-independent (Tables 4.5 and 4.6), as well as the found depression of the Ca^{2+}-transient in these cells at 100 U/ml TNF-α.[51]

Also in case of the described chronotropic effects of cytokines in CMs, both NO-dependent a well as NO-independent actions were reported: in neonatal rat CMs, TNF-α (1000 U/ml), IL-1β (500 U/ml), IL-6 (1000 U/ml), but also the NOS inhibitor L-NMMA (10^{-5} M and 10^{-3} M), significantly increased frequency of spontaneous beating of the cells during an incubation period of 48 hours, while only IL-1 stimulated NO production in these cultures, as measured by the release of nitrite.[52] On the other hand, in the experiments from Roberts and colleagues,[53,54] addition of IL-1β for at least 24 hours to neonatal rat CMs decreased the spontaneous beating rate of these cells, a change that could be reversed by addition of a NOS antagonist, the L-arginine analog L-NMMA. This effect of IL-1β was associated with the expression of iNOS protein in these primary isolates and was antagonized by cotreatment with transforming growth factor β.

What conclusions can we draw at the moment? Cytokine-induced expression of NOSmRNA and enzyme activity in the heart, coupled with attenuation of β-adrenoceptor-mediated positive inotropy, are well documented phenomena, best investigated in rat heart. For induction, relatively high cytokine concentrations are necessary, with optimum results achieved when IL-1, IFN-γ and probably also TNF-α play in concert. Also in the hearts of patients with sepsis, iNOS was found,[8] pointing to its clinical relevance in sepsis.

On the other hand, there is also no doubt that TNF-α can exert negative inotropic effects at much lower concentrations (Table 4.5) than those necessary or at least documented to induce iNOS in the heart. If NO-mediated cardiodepression of TNF-α is relevant in sepsis, then also these NO-independent negative inotropic effects must be discussed as probable mechanisms of septic cardiomyopathy (see next paragraph).

LOOKING FOR A TNF-α TARGET BEYOND NO/cGMP ACTIVATION: THE PHOSPHOINOSITIDE CASCADE AND THE Ca²⁺ TRANSIENT

Most work on TNF-α-induced cardiodepression focuses on the impairment of the positive inotropic effect of catecholamines mediated by β-adrenoceptors (β-ARs).[55-57] However, the negative inotropic effect of TNF-α is not confined to the β-AR-mediated inotropy. TNF-α also impairs and abolishes—in an NO-independent manner—the "inotropic" response of rat CMs to the cardiac glycoside ouabain, to high Ca²⁺, and also to α₁-AR agonists (Table 4.16; Fig. 8.2).[45-47] This argues for an interference of TNF-α with some final steps of the inotropic cascade, common to positive inotropic agents acting via α₁- and β₁-ARs, as well as via inhibition of Na⁺/K⁺-ATPase in case of ouabain. With this respect, interference of TNF-α with the phosphoinositide pathway and the Ca²⁺ transient of the CM could explain the cardiodepressive action of this cytokine (see also chapter 4: Cytokines; Tumor Necrosis Factor α). The positive inotropic and also the toxic, arrhythmogenic effects of α_1-AR stimulation in the heart are mediated at least in part by the phosphoinositide pathway (Fig. 8.3): α_1-AR occupation activates a phosphoinositol (PI)-specific phospholipase C. The substrate of this enzyme is phosphoinositol bisphosphate (PIP$_2$). It is cleaved to diacylglycerol and the calcium mobilizing inositol triphosphate (IP$_3$), which leads to a release of Ca^{2+} from the sarcoplasmic reticulum into the cytosol. This signal transduction pathway is one of the targets of TNF-α action in CMs. Both basal and α_1-AR-mediated formation of IP$_3$ is reduced by chronic exposure (3 days) of CMs to low TNF-α concentrations. This reduction is due to a diminished synthesis of PIP$_2$. As one likely mechanism of TNF-α induced lowering of PIP$_2$ formation, inhibition of the activity of a key enzyme of lipogenesis, glycerol-3 phosphate dehydrogenase (GDH), was identified (Fig. 4.25; Fig. 8.3).[47] TNF-α concentrations necessary to impair the phosphoinositide pathway of CMs can be found in plasma of patients with septic or cardiogenic shock. incubation of rat CMs with patient plasma inhibits GDH activity of the cells, and this GDH inhibition correlates well with the ratios of TNF-α to soluble TNF receptors (p55 and p75) in patient plasma (Fig. 4.26). The results document biological activity of free TNF-α in plasma of patients with sepsis and heart

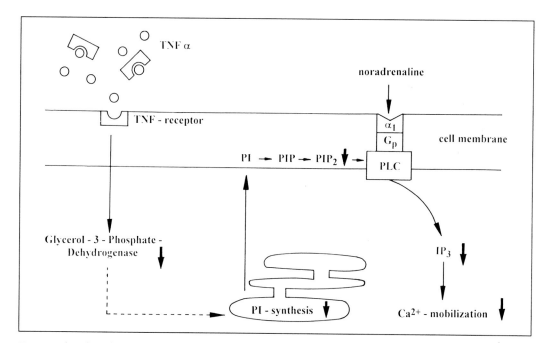

Fig. 8.3. The phosphoinositide pathway in the heart. (Reproduced with permission from: Werdan K, Müller-Werdan U, Reithmann C et al. Nitric oxide-dependent and independent effects of tumor necrosis factor-α on cardiomyocyte beating activity and signal transduction pathways. In: Schlag G, Redl H, eds. Shock, Sepsis, and Organ Failure–Nitric Oxide. 4th Wiggers Bernard Conference 1994. Berlin. Springer-Verlag, 1995:286-309.)

diseases high enough to interfere with an important signal transduction pathway in CMs.

This impairment of the phosphoinositide pathway has functional consequences. TNF-α (10 U/ml) exposure of rat CMs for 3 days does not only attenuate the "positive inotropic effect" of α_1-AR stimulation by noradrenaline (Fig. 4.23), it also prevents noradrenaline-induced arrhythmias seen at high α_1-AR occupancy (Fig. 4.24). α_1-AR-mediated arrhythmias are thought to play a prominent role in reperfusion injury of the heart (see ref. 47). The suppression of these arrhythmias by TNF-α as documented in CMs points to the fact that this cytokine might not only be harmful, but also beneficial under certain circumstances. This should be taken into consideration when applying anti-TNF-α-antibodies in patients with sepsis.

At present, phosphoinositide signaling is thought to be primarily involved in α_1-AR-mediated positive inotropy, which is of minor importance in human heart. However, chronic inhibition of this pathway by TNF-α should lower intracellular Ca^{2+} and thereby impair the Ca^{2+} transient. Therefore, not only α_1-AR-mediated positive inotropy, but also basal contractility, as well as other inotropic pathways with the Ca^{2+} transient as a final step might be impaired by TNF-α. The documented, NO-independent lowering of the Ca^{2+} transient by TNF-α[51] in conjunction with the described TNF-α production of cultured mouse heart cells after endotoxin stimulation[11] might favor this assumption.

PSEUDOMONAS EXOTOXIN A: CARDIODEPRESSION BY INHIBITION OF PROTEIN SYNTHESIS

Pseudomonas (P.) exotoxin A is a prominent virulence factor of *P. aeruginosa sepsis* (for a detailed discussion see chapter 4: Bacterial and Fungal Toxins). It exerts its cytotoxic action by inhibition of protein synthesis via ADP-ribosylation of the elongation factor 2. Also, inhibition of protein synthesis was documented for the heart in experimental P. sepsis in the burned mouse. Hearts from P. exotoxin A treated rats show a pronounced increase in excitability and an enhanced vulnerability to hypoxic insults.[58]

In neonatal rat CMs in culture, P. exotoxin A is cytotoxic at high concentrations, with the chance of cellular restitution when the toxin is washed out from the medium or is neutralized by an immunoglobulin rich in P. exotoxin A-antibodies. At low concentrations (1-10 ng/ml), neither gross cytotoxic effects nor impairment of spontaneous beating are observed. However, these low concentrations partially inhibit protein synthesis by ADP-ribosylation of elongation factor 2.[59] The consequence is a lowered rate of protein synthesis, affecting especially rapid regulatory processes, as given in case of catecholamine desensitization and resensitization of the β-AR/G proteins/adenylyl cyclase axis (Table 8.2). Suppression of the rise of inhibitory G_i proteins during desensitization and inhibition of the resynthesis of β-adrenoceptors by the toxin in the recovery phase after desensitization was documented in neonatal rat CMs (Fig. 4.9). The clinical relevance of these partially antagonistic effects on catecholamine inotropy remains to be established (Fig. 4.13).

CDF: BLOCKAGE OF CA²⁺ CURRENT AS A MECHANISM OF ACTION

CDF is one of the myocardial depressant factors described with yet nonidentified structure, but the only one whose mechanism of action has been clarified (for a detailed discussion see chapter 4: Cardiodepressant Factors). Primarily isolated from blood of dogs in hypovolemic-traumatic shock, it also was found in hemofiltrates of patients with septic and/or cardiogenic shock; at our present knowledge, CDF represents a family of low molecular weight ($\leq$ 1000 Da) N-terminally blocked peptides, with plasma concentrations of $\leq$ 1 to 2 nmol/l.[60] Its documented negative inotropic and chronotropic effect is sufficiently explained by blockage of the calcium inward current seen in adult guinea pig CMs (Fig. 4.28), as well as in neonatal rat heart muscle cells. However, not only the CM, but also the vascular smooth muscle cell might be a target for CDF, thereby possibly contributing to the refractory vasodilatation in septic shock.

DISTURBANCE OF MITOCHONDRIAL FUNCTION, ENERGY METABOLISM AND CELLULAR GLUTATHIONE POOL

The most likely candidates to impair glycolytic and oxidative substrate utilization at distinct levels are reactive oxygen species (ROS). Inhibition of a mitochondrial key enzyme, the pyruvate dehydrogenase complex by H_2O_2 in adult rat CMs could well explain an O_2 consumption defect at the cellular level, often discussed, and also supported by the finding of high O_2 partial pressures in skeletal muscle of patients in sepsis (see also chapter 7: Metabolically Deranged Cardiomyopathy of Sepsis and SIRS—a preliminary draft).

In this respect the data of Dhainaut and colleagues[61] are worthwhile mentioning, showing that in patients with septic shock the myocardial substrate utilization of energy metabolism is shifted, with 41% of myocardial O_2 consumption not being explained by the utilization of commonly available substrates extracted from the coronary circulation.

Neonatal rat CMs tolerate a 30-50% fall in cellular ATP relatively well, induced by metabolic inhibitors, with no gross impairment of spontaneous beating. As, at best, only a modest fall in myocardial ATP content might occur in sepsis, ATP depletion per se does not seem to play a prominent causative role in myocardial depression in sepsis. However, one must be aware that ATP depletion also triggers additional events such as inhibition of protein synthesis and impairment of adenylyl cyclase activity, with possible consequences on regulation of inotropy in CMs.

Oxidation of cellular glutathione (GSH) is a relatively early event in the sequence of cytotoxic effects mediated by ROS in CMs. However, severe depletion of GSH per se is apparently without a negative effect on contractility, at least within a period of several days (for a more detailed discussion see chapter 4).

CELL MEMBRANE DAMAGE AND ITS FUNCTIONAL CONSEQUENCES

Not surprisingly, the cell membrane of the CM is one of the main subcellular targets of substances relevant to sepsis (Fig. 8.2); however, it is surprising that apparently not the unspecific membrane damage (membrane leakiness) is well to the fore, but relatively specific functional impairments of channels, receptors and transporter molecules. A reduction in activity by ROS has been described for active Na^+/K^+ transport and passive (ouabain-insensitive) K^+ efflux, for the Na^+/Ca^{2+} exchanger, for cellular Ca^{2+} extrusion mechanisms, and for the glucose transporter. In the case of the Ca^{2+} channel and Ca^{2+} current, the data are equivocal. In a descriptive manner, a characteristic pattern of membrane potential derangement is the result, with final depolarization and inexcitability of the cells. These electrophysiological alterations are accompanied by an (inconsistently reported) initial increase in contractility, with aftercontractures and a decreased contractility later on and final standstill of the cells. Distinct effects on membrane function involve flickering and depression of the inwardly rectifying K^+ channels I_{k1} by PAF, inhibition of active and passive K^+ flux by staphylococcal α toxin, a modulation of Na^+ channel activity and an augmentation of the Ca^{2+} current by angiotensin, an attenuation of the L-type Ca^+ current by cytotoxic T-lymphocytes, and a stimulation of the Na^+/H^+ exchanger, with the consequence of a positive inotropic effect, by endothelin (for a more detailed review see chapter 4). The list can be continued with a significant decrease in resting membrane potential of the CM, a lowering of the action potential amplitude and a prolongation of its duration by TNF-α,[44] without effect of this cytokine on calcium inward current.[51] Also in skeletal muscle, TNF-α decreases the resting membrane potential in a dose-related fashion.[62] On the other hand, the most prominent effect of in vivo application of endotoxin is a shortening of the action potential duration of isolated CMs, which might well explain the observed myocardial depression, while sarcoplasmic reticulum function is at best mildly suppressed by endotoxin.[35] No shortening of the action potential duration, but a lowering of the resting membrane potential was found in CMs obtained from rats with abdominal sepsis (cecal ligation and puncture (CLP)).[63] These CLP CMs responded adequately to isoproterenol with an increase in L-type calcium current.

Two cardiodepressant shock substances of protein nature not yet identified in structure can also derange the membrane potential of the cardiomyocyte. The first, named circulating shock protein (CSP), appears in rat plasma drawn after hemorrhage; it depolarizes a variety of cells and has a negative inotropic and chronotropic effect in rat heart and rat CMs.[64] The second, CDF (see chapter 4: Cardiodepressant Factors) exerts its cardiodepressant action by blocking calcium inward current (Fig. 4.28). At present, human CDF is the only substance the electrophysiological effect of which is documented with concentrations found in plasma of patients with septic and/or cardiogenic shock.[60]

So far, only an incomplete, merely descriptive characterization of electrophysiological effects of toxins and mediators with respect to the CM can be given at the moment. A more general pathophysiological understanding awaits further clarification.

PARACRINE EFFECTS OF ENDOTHELIAL CELLS AND OF LEUKOCYTES ON CARDIOMYOCYTE FUNCTION

Several recent reviews have stressed the importance of these cell-cell interactions with respect to cardiodepression in sepsis.[17,65-67]

Endothelial cells of both endocardial and coronary vascular origin can exercise substantial influences on myocardial contractile function. Endothelin, NO, with its release stimulated by peptides such as bradykinin and substance P, and a "myofilament desensitizing factor" (see below) seem to represent the major members in this endothelium/myocardium interplay, with adenylpurines like adenosine, prostanoids such as prostacyclin and thromboxane A_2, angiotensin II and factors unidentified in structure being further candidates. Endothelin acts as a "positive inotropic" agent, while NO and the "myofilament desensitizing factor" reduce peak contraction and modify relaxation. In case of NO, depression has been shown also for the human heart in vivo (see above).[17,29]

The information regarding the "myofilament desensitizing factor" comes from experiments where isolated adult rat CMs were superfused with the supernatants of endocardial endothelial and vascular endothelial cells.[66] Endothelial cell superfusate induced a potent negative inotropic effect with a rapid reversible decrease in myocyte twitch amplitude, earlier twitch relaxation and a significant increase in diastolic length. This effect was not associated with significant changes in intracellular calcium nor pH; it was not attributable to nitric oxide, prostanoids, cGMP or protein kinase C activation; and it did not involve pertussis toxin-sensitive G proteins. Its activity was stable at 37°C for several hours, was not destroyed by protease treatment and was found to be in the low-molecular-weight (< 1 kDa) superfusate fraction. These data suggest the tonic release by endothelial cells of a novel, stable factor that acts predominantly by reducing the response of cardiac myofilaments to calcium (i.e. "desensitizes" them). This "desensitizing" factor could rapidly modulate cardiac contraction-relaxation coupling and diastolic tonus and exert distant effects because of its stability.

Viewing this work on paracrine effects of endothelial cells on the beating of CMs one can state that there is no doubt that endothelial cells may strongly affect contractility of the heart under both physiological as well as pathological conditions. Though endothelial cells are vividly activated in septic state their contribution, in a quantitative sense, to myocardial depression in this state remains to be elucidated.

Sepsis is also associated with stiffening of neutrophils and up-regulation of adhesion molecules on leukocytes and endothelium which may slow leukocyte transit thus allowing increased time for leukocyte-myocardium interaction. After endotoxin infusion in pigs, a significant increase in the myocardial capillary leukocyte transit time of the endotoxin group (39.1 ± 20.6 s; $p < 0.05$) versus the vehicle group (5.0 ± 1.4 s) can be observed, with no significant difference in red blood cell transit time between the endotoxin (0.36 ± 0.13 s) and the vehicle group (0.45 ± 0.13 s).[68] Assuming a mediator-triggered activation of leukocytes during this prolonged transit time, these cells might contribute significantly to myocardial depression in sepsis, by mechanisms already described in chapter 4. Walley[67] nicely describes, in the frame of a broader concept, the potentially very prominent harmful effects of leukocytes in septic cardiomyopathy: "In the context of the entire inflammatory cascade, the myocardial depression of sepsis could be imagined as follows. Endotoxin or other products of infecting organisms trigger TNF-α and IL-1 release by monocytes/macrophages. Circulation of these early mediators of the inflammatory response activates neutrophils and other inflammatory cells. Activated neutrophils become stiffer and therefore plug the myocardial capillary bed. Activated leukocytes also express adhesion proteins to a greater degree and endothelial cells up-regulate expression of adhesion proteins. The net effect is that neutrophils and other leukocytes slow and marginate, plug capillaries, adhere and release damaging products within capillaries, or migrate and release damaging products directly into myocardial tissue. Circulating levels of TNF-α, IL-2 and IL-6 as well as other cytokines may achieve concentrations sufficient to cause a decrease in left ventricular contractility via stimulation of iNOS activity of endothelial cells and cardiomyocytes, and via other mechanisms. Continued secretion of TNF-α and other cytokines from intramyocardial monocytes/macrophages and neutrophils could result in very high local concentrations of TNF-α, IL-2 and IL-6 resulting in an even greater cytokine-mediated decrease in left ventricular contractility. Migration of neutrophils and release of digestive enzymes and oxygen-free radicals during an oxidative burst would result in high local concentrations of cytotoxic substances. Therefore patchy obstruction of capillary bed and patchy areas of myocardial damage would be expected. The endocardium is more susceptible to ischemic damage possibly because the endocardium is at a higher hydrostatic pressure than the epicardium and therefore not as easily perfused. Therefore, the endocardium may be even more involved in patchy damage. Endothelial cells, damaged by inflammatory mediators and cells, probably lose their neural transmission capacity so that local capillary matching of oxygen delivery to consumption would be lost. Like pulmonary V/Q mismatch, this would result in impaired gas exchange and therefore a decreased myocardial oxygen extraction as observed during human sepsis, with the possibility of patchy regional ischemia of some poorly regulated capillary beds. Decreased systolic contractility would occur as a result of circulating cytokine-mediated myocardial depression, local monocyte/macrophage secreted cytokine-mediated myocardial depression, cell mediated myocardial damage, and patchy ischemia/reperfusion-induced necrosis. Normal diastolic dilation in response to decreased systolic contractility would not occur if the inflammatory response were severe enough to result in significant myocardial edema, contraction band formation, and myocyte necrosis. Just as with other tissues healing from the inflammatory response would be expected to take one to two weeks or more."

A black box continues to be the relevance of the many final mediators of the sepsis cascade (see chapter 4 and Figure 11.1), from whom many bear the potential of a negative inotropic effector.

CARDIODEPRESSION IN SEPSIS: "THE MOST PROVEN CONCEPTS" IN PERSPECTIVE

It would be presumptuous to postulate a proven uniform concept of the mechanism of cardiodepression in sepsis. However, some picture in diversity emerges (Table 4.4; Figs. 8.2 and 8.4.).

Though endotoxin is thought to represent the main trigger toxin of cardiodepression in Gram-negative sepsis,[34] the situation is much less clear in Gram-positive sepsis, where endotoxin is not required for the onset of the disease,[69] and toxins acting as superantigens may play a dominant role. The well-documented similar degree of myocardial depression in Gram-positive in comparison to Gram-negative sepsis (Fig. 2.3) might come about either by toxins which can directly inhibit myocardial function, like toxic shock syndrome toxin-1[70] and the alpha toxin from *Clostridium perfringens*;[71] more likely, however, cytokine release (TNF-α, IL-1, IL-6) is causative, which is as common in Gram-positive infection as it is in Gram-negative infection.[69] Therefore, TNF-α and other cytokines might mediate myocardial depression not only in Gram-negative, but also in Gram-positive sepsis. It may also be a point of interest that toxins, as shown for endotoxin, do not exclusively depress contractility of the cardiac muscle, but also that of skeletal muscle, a yet unknown mechanism.[72]

By which mediator(s) do cytokines exert their cardiodepressive action? Unequivocally, an activation of the NO/cGMP pathway in the heart is induced by cytokines; arguments in favor of this pathway are the induction of iNOS in CMs by IL-1β/IFN-γ/TNF-α exposure, however at relatively high concentrations (see above), as well as the expression of iNOS and increased cGMP levels in the hearts of septic patients.[8] Activation of this axis could also well explain not only the impairment in systolic, but also in diastolic function of the heart in sepsis.

But are there also other mechanisms of cytokine cardiodepression which may also play a role? In our opinion, the answer is "yes"; there are NO-independent mechanisms, which may come into play even at much lower cytokine concentrations as documented to be necessary for the NO/cGMP pathway. Both the observed TNF-α-induced impairment of Ca^{2+}-transient as well as the inhibition of phosphoinositide pathway with a reduced IP_3 release could very well explain the TNF-α-induced attenuation of basal contractility, as well as the lowering of the positive inotropic effects of α- and β-AR agonists, of digitalis and also of high Ca^{2+}. In contrast, in case of cytokine-mediated activation of the NO/cGMP pathway, only an attenuation of the β-AR agonist inotropy has been consistently described.

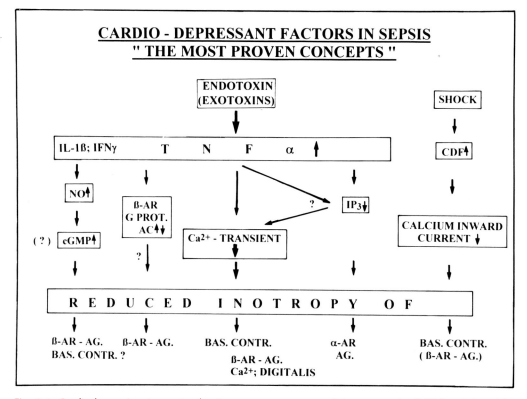

Fig. 8.4. Cardiodepression in sepsis: the "most proven concepts" in perspective. "NO" = nitric oxide; "cGMP" = cyclic guanosine monophosphate; "G PROT" = G protein; "AC" = adenylyl cyclase; "AR-AG." = adrenoceptor agonist; "IP_3" = inositol triphosphate; "CDF" = cardiodepressant factor; "BAS.CONTR." = basal contractility; "TNF-α" = tumor necrosis factor α.

An attractive unique hypothesis could postulate that a TNF-α-induced impairment of the phosphoinositide pathway with the consequence of a reduced IP_3 release would also explain the reduction in the TNF-triggered Ca^{2+} transient. Whether impairment of IP_3 release and of Ca^{2+} transient may also give an explanation, for the observed negative lusitropy in sepsis remains to be clarified. Finally, it should be emphasized that the described impairment of the phosphoinositide pathway in rat CMs can be induced even with very low TNF concentrations which can be found in the plasma of septic patients, while for the other TNF-α effects (impairment of the Ca^{2+}-transient, activation of the NO/cGMP pathway) much higher TNF-α concentrations are necessary in vitro.

With respect to the cytokine-induced impairment of the β-AR/G protein/adenylyl cyclase axis, controversial results have been obtained in in vitro studies (see chapter 4: Catecholamines, Cytokines). Regardless of these controversial results an attenuation of this axis has been found in a number of animal sepsis models; as to patients with sepsis and septic shock, the findings of Silverman and colleagues[73] also argue for a myocardial hyporesponsiveness to catecholamines due to an impaired β-adrenergic receptor stimulation of cyclic adenosine monophosphate.

Of course, many questions remain open, including the role of only recently described cytokines with effects on the heart like cardiotrophin 1,[74] the reversal of potentially harmful effects of NO and IL-1 on the CM by transforming growth factor,[75,76] and also the role of the population of NO-sensitive neurons in the intrinsic cardiac nervous system that are involved in cardiac regulation.[77]

REFERENCES

1. Parrillo JE. Pathogenetic mechanisms of septic shock. N Engl J Med 1993; 328:1471-1477.
2. Vincent JL, Berlot G. Cardiac effects of the mediators of sepsis. In: Lamy M, Thijs LG, eds. Mediators of Sepsis (Update in Intensive Care and Emergency Medicine 16). Berlin, Heidelberg, New York: Springer-Verlag, 1992:255-266.
3. Hallström S, Koidl B, Müller U et al. Cardiodepressant factors. In: Schlag G, Redl H, eds. Pathophysiology of Shock, Sepsis, and Organ Failure. Berlin, Heidelberg: Springer-Verlag, 1993: 200-214.
4. Schulz R, Panas DL, Catena R et al. The role of nitric oxide in cardiac depression induced by interleukin-1β and tumor necrosis factor-α. Br J Pharmacol 1994; 114:27-34.
5. Balligand J-L, Ungureanu-Longrois D, Simmons WW et al. Cytokine-inducible nitric oxide synthase (iNOS) expression in cardiac myocytes, characterization and regulation of iNOS expression and detection of iNOS activity in single cardiac myocytes in vitro. J Biol Chem 1994; 44:27580-27588.

6. Natanson C, Eichacker PQ, Hoffman WD et al. Human recombinant interleukin-1 (IL-1) produced minimal effects on canine cardiovascular (CV) function. Clin Res 1989; 37:346A.

7. Schulz R, Nava E, Moncada S. Induction and potential biological relevance of a Ca^{2+}-independent nitric oxide synthase in the myocardium. Br J Pharmacol 1992; 105:575-580.

8. Thoenes M, Förstermann U, Rüdiger J et al. Expression of inducible nitric oxide synthase in failing and non-failing human heart. Naunyn-Schmiedeberg's Arch Pharmacol 1995; 351:R112.

9. Balligand J-L, Kelly RA, Marsden PA et al. Control of cardiac muscle cell function by an endogenous nitric oxide signalling system. Proc Natl Acad Sci USA 1993; 90:347-351.

10. Balligand J-L, Ungureanu D, Kelly RA et al. Abnormal contractile function due to induction of nitric oxide synthesis in rat cardiac myocytes follows exposure to activated macrophage-conditioned medium. J Clin Invest 1993; 91:2314- 2319.

11. Giroir BP, Johnson JHZ, Brown T et al. The tissue distribution of tumor necrosis factor biosynthesis during endotoxemia. J Clin Invest 1992; 90:693-698.

12. Mery P-F, Pavoine C, Belhassen L et al. Nitric oxide regulates cardiac Ca^{2+} current, involvement of cGMP-inhibited and cGMP-stimulated phosphodiesterase through guanylyl cyclase activation. J Biol Chem 1993; 268:26286-26295.

13. Murad F. Regulation of cytosolic guanylyl cyclase by nitric oxide: the NO-cyclic GMP signal transduction system. Adv Pharmacol 1994; 26:19-33.

14. Szabo C, Wu C-C, Gross SS et al. Interleukin-1 contributes to the induction of nitric oxide synthase by endotoxin in vivo. Eur J Pharmacol 1993; 250:157-160.

15. Thiemermann C. The Role of the L-arginine: nitric oxide pathway in circulatory shock. Adv Pharmacol 1994; 28:45-79.

16. Wahler GM, Dollinger SJ. Nitric oxide donor SIN-1 inhibits mammalian cardiac calcium current through cGMP-dependent protein kinase. Am J Physiol 1995; 268:C45-C54.

17. Pepper CB, Shah AM. Endothelial modulation of myocardial contraction: a novel cardioregulatory mechanism? In: Vincent J-L, ed. Yearbook of Intensive Care and Emergency Medicine 1995. Berlin, Heidelberg, New York: Springer-Verlag, 1995:493-504.

18. Lohmann SM, Fischmeister R, Walter U. Signal transduction by cGMP in the heart. Basic Res Cardiol 1991; 86:503-514.

19. Shah AM, Spurgeon HA, Sollott SJ et al. 8-Bromo-cGMP reduces the myofilament response to Ca^{2+} in intact cardiac myocytes. Circ Res 1994; 74:970-978.

20. Weyrich AS, Ma X-L, Buerke M et al. Physiological concentrations of nitric oxide do not elicit an acute negative inotropic effect in unstimulated cardiac muscle. Circ Res 1994; 75:692-700.

21. Brady AJB, Warren JB, Poole-Wilson PA et al. Nitric oxide attenuates cardiac myocyte contraction. Am J Physiol 1993; 265:H176-H182.

22. Han X, Shimomi Y, Giles WR. An obligatory role for nitric oxide in autonomic control of the mammalian heart rate. J Physiol 1994; 476:309-314.

23. Smith JA, Shah AM, Lewis MJ. Factors released from endocardium of the ferret and pig modulate myocardial contraction. J Physiol 1991; 439:1-14.

24. Grocott-Mason R, Fort S, Lewis MJ et al. Myocardial relaxant effect of exogenous nitric oxide in isolated ejecting hearts. Am J Physiol 1994; 266:H1699-H1705.

25. Grocott-Mason R, Anning P, Evans H et al. Modulation of left ventricular relaxation in the isolated ejecting heart by endogenous nitric oxide. Am J Physiol 1994; 267:H1804-H113.

26. Hare JM, Keaney Jr J, Balligand J-L et al. Role of nitric oxide in parasympathetic modulation of β-adrenergic myocardial contractility in normal dogs. J Clin Invest 1995; 95:360-366.

27. Benyo Z, Kiss G, Szabo C et al. Importance of basal nitric oxide synthesis in regulation of myocardial blood flow. Cardiovasc Res 1991; 25:700-703.

28. Wang J, Zhao G, Shen W et al. Effects of an orally active NO- releasing agent, CAS 936, and its active metabolite, 3754, on cardiac and coronary dynamics in normal conscious dogs and after pacing-induced heart failure. J Cardiovasc Pharmacol 1993; 22(suppl 7):S51-S58.

29. Paulus WJ, Vantrimpont PJ, Shah AM. Acute effects of nitric oxide on left ventricular relaxation and diastolic distensibility in humans. Assessment by bicoronary sodium nitroprusside infusion. Circulation 1994; 89:2070-2078.

30. Evans HG, Lewis MJ, Shah AM. Interleukin-1β modulates myocardial contraction via dexamethasone sensitive production of nitric oxide. Cardiovasc Res 1993; 27:1486-1490.

31. Brady AJB, Poole-Wilson PA, Harding SE et al. Nitric oxide production within cardiac myocytes reduces their contractility in endotoxemia. Am J Physiol 1992; 263:H1963-H1966.

32. Martich GD, Boujoukos AJ, Suffredini AF. Response of man to endotoxin. Immunobiol 1993; 187:403-416.

33. Natanson C, Eichenholz PW, Danner RL et al. Endotoxin and tumor necrosis factor challenges in dogs simulate the cardiovascular profile of human septic shock. J Exp Med 1989; 169:823-832.

34. Suffredini AF, Fromm RE, Parker MM et al. The cardiovascular response of normal humans to the administration of endotoxin. N Engl J Med 1989; 321:280-287.

35. Hung J, Lew WYW. Cellular mechanisms of endotoxin-induced myocardial depression in rabbits. Circ Res 1993; 73:125-134.

36. Liu M-S. Mechanisms of myocardial membrane alterations in endotoxin shock: roles of phospholipase and phosphorylation. Circ Shock 1990; 30:43-49.

37. Bensard DD, Banerjee A, McIntyre RC et al. Endotoxin disrupts β-adrenergic signal transduction in the heart. Arch Surg 1994; 129:198-205.

38. Meyer J, Lentz CW, Stothert JC et al. Effects of nitric oxide synthesis inhibition in hyperdynamic endotoxemia. Crit Care Med 1994; 22:306-312.

39. Smith REA, Palmer RMJ, Moncada S. Coronary vasodilatation induced by endotoxin in the rabbit isolated perfused heart is nitric oxide-dependent and inhibited by dexamethasone. Br J Pharmacol 1991; 104:5-6.

40. Eichenholz PW, Eichacker PQ, Hoffman WD et al. Tumor necrosis factor challenges in canines: patterns of cardiovascular dysfunction. Am J Physiol 1992; 263:H668-H675.

41. Schirmer WJ, Schirmer JM, Fry DE. Recombinant human tumor necrosis factor produces hemodynamic changes characteristic of sepsis and endotoxemia. Arch Surg 1989; 124:445-448.

42. Pagani FD, Baker LS, Hsi C et al. Left ventricular systolic and diastolic dysfunction after infusion of tumor necrosis factor-α in conscious dogs. J Clin Invest 1992; 90:389-398.

43. Hansen PR, Sveendsen JH, Hoyer S et al. Tumor necrosis factor-α increases myocardial microvascular transport in vivo. Am J Physiol 1994; 266:H60-H67.

44. DeMeules JE, Pigula FA, Mueller M et al. Tumor necrosis factor and cardiac function. J Trauma 1992; 32:686-692.

45. Boekstegers P, Bauer I, Peter W et al. TNF-α induces a reversible inhibition of positive inotropic response in neonatal rat heart cells. Can J Cardiol 1994; 10(suppl A):68A(Abst).

46. Werdan K, Müller-Werdan U, Reithmann C et al. Nitric oxide-dependent and independent effects of tumor necrosis factor-α on cardiomyocyte beating activity and signal transduction pathways. In: Schlag G, Redl H, eds. Shock, Sepsis, and Organ Failure—Nitric Oxide. 4th Wiggers Bernard Conference 1994. Berlin. Springer-Verlag, 1995:286-309.

47. Reithmann C, Werdan K. Tumor necrosis factor α decreases inositol phosphate formation and phosphatidylinositolbisphosphate (PIP$_2$) synthesis in rat cardiomyocytes. Naunyn Schmiedeberg's Arch Pharmacol 1994; 349:175-182.

48. Tsujino M, Hirata Y, Imai T et al. Induction of nitric oxide synthase gene by interleukin-1β in cultured rat cardiocytes. Circulation 1994; 90:375-383.

49. Kinugawa K, Takahashi T, Kohmoto O et al. Nitric oxide-mediated effects of interleukin-6 on (Ca^{2+})i and cell contraction in cultured chick ventricular myocytes. Circ Res 1994; 75:285-295.

50. Finkel MS, Oddis CV, Jacob TD et al. Negative inotropic effects of cytokines on the heart mediated by nitric oxide. Science 1992; 257:387-389.

51. Yokoyama T, Vaca L, Rossen RD et al. Cellular basis for the negative inotropic effects of tumor necrosis factor-α in the adult mammalian heart. J Clin Invest 1993; 92:2303-2312.

52. Oddis C, Simmons RL, Hattler BG et al. Chronotropic effects of cytokines and the nitric oxide synthase inhibitor, L-NMMA, on cardiac myocytes. Biochem Biophys Res Commun 1994; 205:992-997.

53. Roberts AB, Vodovotz Y, Roche NS et al. Role of nitric oxide in antagonistic effects of transforming growth factor-β and Interleukin-1 β on the beating rate of cultured cardiac myocytes. Mol Endocrinol 1992; 6:1921-1939.

54. Roberts AB, Roche NS, Winokur TS et al. Role of transforming growth factor-β in maintenance of function of cultured neonatal cardiac myocytes—Autocrine action and reversal of damaging effects of interleukin-1. J Clin Invest 1992; 90:2056-2062.

55. Chung MK, Gulick TS, Rotondo RE et al. Mechanism of cytokine inhibition of beta-adrenergic agonist stimulation of cyclic AMP in rat cardiac myocytes—impairment of signal transduction. Circ Res 1990; 67:753-763.

56. Reithmann C, Gierschik P, Werdan K et al. Tumor necrosis factor α upregulates $G_{i\alpha}$ and G_β proteins and adenylate cyclase responsiveness in rat cardiomyocytes. Eur J Pharmacol—Mol Pharmacol Section 1991; 206:53-60.

57. Reithmann C, Gierschik P, Jakobs KH et al. Regulation of adenylyl cyclase by noradrenaline and tumor necrosis factor α in rat cardiomyocytes. Eur Heart J 1991; 12(suppl F):139-142.

58. Kwiatkowska-Patzer B, Patzer JA, Heller LJ. *Pseudomonas aeruginosa* exotoxin A enhances automaticity and potentiates hypoxic depression of isolated rat hearts. Proc Soc Exp Biol Med 1993; 202:377-383.

59. Reithmann C, Gierschik P, Müller U et al. Pseudomonas exotoxin A prevents β-adrenoceptor-induced upregulation of G_i protein α-subunits and adenylyl cyclase desensitization in rat heart muscle cells. Mol Pharmacol 1990; 37:631-638.

60. Hallström S, Bernhart E, Müller U et al. A cardiodepressant factor (CDF) isolated from hemofiltrates of patients in septic and /or cardiogenic shock blocks calcium inward current in cardiomyocytes. Shock 1994; suppl. to Vol 2:abstract 1 (Abst).

61. Dhainaut JF, Huyghebaert MF, Monsallier JF et al. Coronary hemodynamics and myocardial metabolism of lactate, free fatty acids, glucose and ketones in patients with septic shock. Circulation 1987; 75:533-541.

62. Tracey KJ, Lowry SF, Beutler B et al. Cachectin/tumor necrosis factor mediates changes of skeletal muscle plasma membrane potential. J Exp Med 1986; 164:1368-1373.

63. Wu S-N, Lue S-I, Yang S-L et al. Electrophysiological properties of isolated adult cardiomyocytes from septic rats. Circ Shock 1993; 41:239-247.

64. Jones RO, Carlson DE, Gann DS. A circulating shock protein that depolarizes cells in vitro depresses myocardial contractility and rate in isolated rat hearts. J Trauma 1994; 37:752-758.

65. Mebazaa A, Shah AM. "Obligatory role of endothelial cells in regulating myocardial contraction?" In: Vincent J-L, ed. Yearbook of Intensive Care and Emergency Medicine 1995. Berlin, Heidelberg, New York: Springer 1995: 485-492.

66. Shah AM, Mebazaa A, Wetzel RC et al. Novel cardiac myofilament desensitizing factor released by endocardial and vascular endothelial cells. Circulation 1994; 89:2492-2497.

67. Walley KR. Ventricular dysfunction during sepsis. In: Vincent J-L, ed. Yearbook of Intensive Care and Emergency Medicine 1995. Berlin, Heidelberg, New York: Springer-Verlag, 1995:505-517.

68. Goddard CM, Allard MF, Hogg JC et al. Myocardial leukocyte transit time is increased after endotoxin. Clin Intens Care 1995; 6(suppl):62.

69. Bone R. How gram-positive organisms cause sepsis. J Crit Care 1993; 8:51-59.

70. Olson RD, Stevens DL, Melish ME. Direct effects of purified staphylococcal toxic shock syndrome toxin 1 on myocardial function of isolated rabbit atria. Rev Infect Dis 1989; 11(suppl 1):S313-S315.

71. Stevens DL, Troyer BE, Merrick DT et al. Lethal effects and cardiovascular effects of Clostridium perfringens. J Infect Dis 1988; 157:272-279.

72. Gutierrez G, Hurtado FJ, Fernandez E. Inhibitory effect of *Escherichia coli* endotoxin on skeletal muscle contractility. Crit Care Med 1995; 23:308-315.

73. Silverman HJ, Penaranda R, Orens JB et al. Impaired β-adrenergic receptor stimulation of cyclic adenosine monophosphate in human septic shock: association with myocardial hyporesponsiveness to catecholamines. Crit Care Med 1993; 21:31-39.

74. Pennica D, King KL, Shaw KJ et al. Expression cloning of cardiotrophin 1, a cytokine that induces cardiac myocyte hypertrophy. Proc Natl Acad Sci USA 1995; 92:1142-1146.

75. Pinsky DJ, Cal B, Yang X et al. The lethal effects of cytokine-induced nitric oxide on cardiac myocytes are blocked by nitric oxide synthase antagonism or transforming growth factor β. J Clin Invest 1995; 95:677-685.

76. Roberts AB, Roche NS, Winokur TS et al. Role of transforming growth factor-β in maintenance of function of cultured neonatal cardiac myocytes—Autocrine action and reversal of damaging effects of interleukin-1. J Clin Invest 1992; 90:2056-2062.

77. Armour JA, Smith FM, Losier AM et al. Modulation of intrinsic cardiac neuronal activity by nitric oxide donors induces cardiodynamic changes. Am J Physiol 1995; 268:R403-R413.

═══ CHAPTER 9 ═══

CYTOKINES IN NON-SEPTIC HEART DISEASES

INCREASED CIRCULATING CYTOKINES IN PATIENTS WITH NON-SEPTIC HEART DISEASES

In a variety of non-septic heart diseases, increased circulating cytokine levels can be found (Tables 9.1, 9.2, Fig. 9.1). Taking into account the described cardiodepressive effects of some of these cytokines at relatively low concentrations (see chapters 4 and 8), then either pathogenetic roles or at least additive detrimental effects of some of them might be likely in several forms of cardiac impairment, like myocarditis, dilated and hypertrophic cardiomyopathy, myocardial infarction, heart failure, post-pump inflammatory response, allograft rejection and others (see also below). However, it remains to be clarified, whether cytokines play causal roles or only represent epiphenomena in the course of these diseases. Their importance in infective endocarditis and pericarditis is even less clear.

CYTOKINE EFFECTS IN NON-SEPTIC HEART DISEASES

In the following chapter, only a very incomplete mosaic of information can be presented, as the data available are still scarce.

In the cardiovascular field the relevance of these findings for the pathogenesis of cardiac disease remains to be clarified.[1,2]

MYOCARDITIS

Increased circulating inflammatory cytokines like IL-1α, IL-1β, IL-6 and TNF-α can be found in some patients with—mostly viral—myocarditis (Fig. 9.1, Table 9.1), whereby no clear correlation between clinical variables and increased concentrations of cytokines can be made.[3]

The pathogenetic role of TNF and interferon-γ in this process was studied in a murine model of autoimmune myocarditis, mediated by T lymphocytes:[4] neutralizing monoclonal antibodies against TNF-α/β and IFNγ were administered to myosin-immunized mice developing

Table 9.1. Frequency of detectable plasma cytokines in cardiac patients

	Acute myocarditis (n = 13)	Dilated cardiomyopathy (n = 23)	Hypertrophic cardiomyopathy (n = 51)	Acute myocardial infarction (n = 9)	Angina pectoris (n = 18)	Essential hypertension (n = 12)	Healthy volunteers (n = 17)	Detectable concentration
Interleukin-1 α	23·1%* (25 (11))	4·3% (14)	7·8% (38(15))	0%	11·1% (31)	0%	0%	> 10 pg/ml
Interleukin-1 β	30·8%*† (56 (34))	0%	9·8% (96 (68))	0%	0%	0%	0%	> 20 pg/ml
Interleukin-2	7·7% (109)	4·3% (301)	13·7% (2318 (4378))	0%	0%	0%	0%	> 78 pg/ml
Interleukin-6	7·7% (145)	4·3% (36)	3·9% (231 (186))	0%	0%	0%	0%	> 32 pg/ml
Tumour necrosis factor-α	46·1%*‡ (61 (31))	30·4%* (402 (555))	19·6%* (992 (1517))	11·1% (113)	16·7% (146 (159))	0%	0%	> 20 pg/ml
Tumour necrosis factor-β (U/ml)	7·7% (2·2)	4·3% (1·8)	3·9% (1·7 (0·8))	0%	0%	0%	0%	> 1 U/ml
Granulocyte macrophage colony stimulating factor	7·7% (100)	4·3% (29)	9·8% (92 (16))	11·1 (102)	5·5% (164)	8·3% (50)	0%	> 20 pg/ml
Granulocyte colony stimulating factor	46·1%* (18 (10))	65·2%* (28 (30))	58·8%* (37 (89))	22·2%* (20 (11))	44·4%* (38 (48))	8·3% (84)	5·9% (13)	> 10 pg/ml
Macrophage colony stimulating factor (ng/ml)	2·5† (1·8)	1·5 (0·4)	1·9 (0·4)	3·3*†‡ (1·1)	2·4 (0·9)	14 (0·4)	1·9 (0·4)	> 0·2 g/ml
Interferon-α	7·7% (171)	0%	3·9% (447 (474))	0%	0%	0%	0%	> 100 pg/ml
Interferon-γ	7·7% (18)	4·3% (19)	3·9% (34 (11))	0%	5·5% (21)	0%	0%	> 10 pg/ml

Data are given as mean ± SD of detectable values (pg/ml except for tumor necrosis factor β and macrophage colony stimulating factor). "*" $P < 0.05$ versus healthy volunteers; "†" $P < 0.05$ versus dilated cardiomyopathy; "‡" $P < 0.05$ versus hypertrophic cardiomyopathy. Concentrations of macrophage colony stimulating factor were above the detectable value in all individuals .(Reproduced with permission from Matsumori A, Yamada T, Suzuki H et al. Increased circulating cytokines in patients with myocarditis and cardiomyopathy. Br Heart J 1994; 72:561-566.)

autoimmune myocarditis. Anti-TNF treatment significantly reduced the severity of myocarditis when given before myosin immunization. Myosin-specific lymph node T cell proliferation studies showed no difference in the proliferative response between the anti-TNF-treated mice and controls. Administration of anti-TNF to mice after myosin immunization had no effect on the severity of inflammation. This argues for TNF-α as an important mediator early in the pathogenesis of myocardial inflammation in this model of myocarditis.

Neutralization of IFN-γ significantly increased the severity of myocarditis, suggesting that IFN-γ may function as a relevant regulatory cytokine early in the pathogenesis of myocardial inflammation.

The probable pathogenetic role of cytokines in viral and autoimmune myocarditis is further substantiated by the findings that administration of IL-1 or TNF-α promotes Coxsackie virus B3 myocarditis in genetically resistant B10A mice,[5,6] and that exogenously applied recombinant human TNF-α exacerbates myocardits due to encephalomyocarditis virus.[7] The increased circulating levels of cytokines in myocarditis (Table 9.1, Fig. 9.1)[3] may find explanation by a virus-induced production of TNF-α, IL-1β and IL-6 in human monocytes in vitro.[8]

A better understanding of cytokine function in the inflammatory response to myocardial injury may provide important information on possible therapeutic strategies to limit myocardial damage in myocarditis.

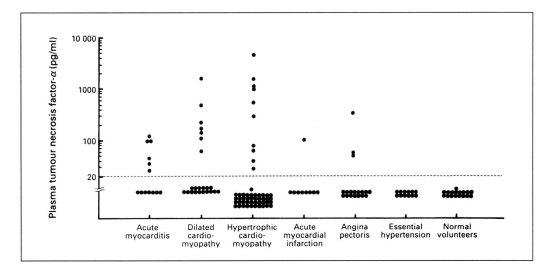

Fig. 9.1. *Plasma tumor necrosis factor α in patients with non-septic heart diseases. Plasma concentrations of TNF-α were more frequently raised in acute myocarditis than in the other groups, but the values were higher in patients with dilated cardiomyopathy or hypertrophic cardiomyopathy. (Reproduced with permission from: Matsumori A, Yamada T, Suzuki H et al. Increased circulating cytokines in patients with myocarditis and cardiomyopathy. Br Heart J 1994; 72:561-566.)*

DILATED CARDIOMYOPATHY

One out of three patients with dilated cardiomyopathy has elevated TNF-α levels (Fig. 9.1), with no clear-cut correlation of TNF-α plasma concentration and severity of heart failure.[3] As in myocarditis, dilated cardiomyopathy plasma levels of granulocyte colony stimulating factor (G-CSF) are increased in about 65% of all patients (Table 9.1), with no correlation to the number of circulating leukocytes.[3] A possible explanation for this finding is the fact that IL-1 and TNF-α are able to induce the production of G-CSF not only in bone marrow stromal cells, but also in endothelial cells and fibroblasts.[9] The other cytokine levels exhibit no consistent rise (Table 9.1, Fig. 9.1).

Table 9.2. Cytokines and non-septic heart diseases—a brief overview

Heart Disease	Cytokines/Mediators	Findings	Refs.
Myocarditis	IL-1α, IL-1β, IL-6, TNF-α	Increased plasma/serum levels in some patients	3
	TNF-α; IL-1, IL-6	Pathogenetic role in experimental myocarditis	4-7
	IFN-γ	Regulatory beneficial cytokine in autoimmune myocarditis	4
	Anti-TNF-α-AB	Improvement in autoimmune myocarditis	4,7
Dilated cardiomyopathy	iNOS↑↑/cNOS↓↓	Reversed ratio in comparison to ischemic heart disease	10
Hypertrophic cardiomyopathy	G-CSF↑, TNF-α↑	Involvement of immunological mechanisms in pathogenesis?	3
Acute myocardial infarction and unstable angina	TNF-a	Plasma level ↑, especially in severe cases	11-13
	sTNFRtI, IL-1Ra, IL-6	Plasma/serum levels ↑	11, 14
	IL-1β, IL-8	not found in plasma	11
Post-pump inflammatory response in patients undergoing cardiac surgery	TNF, IL-6, IL-8	Elevated arterial plasma levels after hypothermic CPB, may contribute to post-operative myocardial ischemia and segmental wall motion abnormalities	16, 18
	TNF, IL-1β, Endotoxin	No significant rise in arterial plasma after normothermic CPB	17
	IL-6, IL-8	Elevated arterial plasma levels after normothermic CPB; IL-8 may play a role in lung and heart reperfusion injury	17
Myocardial ischemia-induced arrhythmias	Endotoxin	Preconditioning reduced arrhythmia severity probably via induction of iNOS	19

Human myocardium, in addition, has the capacity to produce nitric oxide (NO) from arginine, by both the constitutive nitric oxide synthase (cNOS) as well as by the inducible nitric oxide synthase (iNOS): atrial appendages of seven patients with ischemic heart disorder show a clear predominance of cNOS activity (15.4 ± 2.0 pmol/mg/min by the citrulline assay and 30.4 ± 2.4 fmol/mg/min by the cGMP assay) over iNOS activity (2.5 pmol/mg/min by the citrullin assay and not detectable by the cGMP assay).[10] In dilated cardiomyopathy, this ratio

Table 9.2. Cytokines and non-septic heart diseases—a brief overview (continued)

Heart Disease	Cytokines/Mediators	Findings	Refs.
Myocardial ischemia and ischemia-reperfusion injury	Adhesion molecules	Expression triggers leukocyte endothelial interaction	21
	TNF-α	Mediates at least in part myocardial reperfusion injury	22
	NO	Reduced release or action in coronary vessels	24-27
Severe heart failure	TNF-α, IL-6	Increased serum levels in some patients	29
	IL-1, IFN-γ	Serum levels not increased	29
	TNF-α	Increased levels correlate with cardiac cachexia	31-32
	NO	Vascular release of NO: Basal release: preserved or even enhanced; ACH-stimulated release: reduced	36, 37
Essential hypertension	G-CSF, GM-CSF	Plasma levels slightly increased in a small percentage of patients	3
	Reactive oxygen species	Production increased in peripheral blood neutrophils	38, 39
	NO	NOS activity decreased in peripheral blood neutrophils	1, 38, 39
Heart allograft rejection	TNF-α	Plasma level ↑	
	TNF-α	Expression of TNF-α-positive inflammatory cells	42
	IL-2	Plasma level ↑, expression of CD4-IL-2 receptor positive cells	16, 17 in 41
Kawasaki disease	TNF-α	Serum levels in acute and subacute disease states significantly higher than in convalescence	43
	TNF-α, IL-1, IFN-γ	Possible role in the mechanism of vascular injury; circulating antibodies that are cytotoxic for endothelial cell antigens inducible by these cytokines	43

For further explanation see text and also Fig. 9.1 and Table 9.1. Abbreviations used: IL-1 = interleukin-1; IL-1α = interleukin-1α; IL-1β = interleukin-1β; IL-2 = interleukin-2; IL-6 = interleukin-6; IL-8 = interleukin-8; TNF-α = tumor necrosis factor-α; IFN γ = interferon γ; anti-TNF-α-AB = anti-tumor necrosis factor-α antibodies; NO = nitric oxide; NOS = nitric oxide synthase; iNOS = inducible nitric oxide synthase; cNOS = constitutive nitric oxide synthase; G-CSF = granulocyte colony stimulating factor; GM-CSF = granulocyte macrophage colony stimulating factor; sTNFRtI = soluble tumor necrosis factor receptor type I; IL-1Ra = interleukin-1 receptor antagonist; CPB = cardiopulmonary bypass.

is reversed: right ventricular biopsy specimens from 17 patients with dilated cardiomyopathy reveal a significant iNOS activity (13.7 ± 3.0 pmol citrulline/mg/min and 26.0 ± 10.3 fmol cyclic GMP/mg/min), while cNOS activity was 10- to 11-fold lower (1.2 ± 0.3 citrulline/mg/min) or not detectable (cyclic GMP assay).[10]

The consequences of myocardial iNOS expression remain to be clarified. One may speculate that an increased production of TNF-α could induce iNOS activity; the NO produced might then attenuate inotropy of the heart (see chapter 4).

HYPERTROPHIC CARDIOMYOPATHY

Surprising findings in patients with hypertrophic cardiomyopathy include the high percentage (65%) of raised plasma levels of G-CSF (Table 9.1) and the high plasma levels of TNF-α in every fifth patient (Fig. 9.1). The genes encoding TNF-α and TNF-β are situated within the major histocompatibility complex locus. Familial hypertrophic cardiomyopathy has been shown to be associated with HLA-DR4 and with other major histocompatibility complex haplotypes (see ref. 3). The raised concentrations of these cytokines suggest that an immunological mechanism may be involved in the pathogenesis of hypertrophic cardiomyopathy.[3]

ACUTE MYOCARDIAL INFARCTION AND UNSTABLE ANGINA

TNF-α enhances leukocyte adherence to vascular endothelium and increases procoagulant activity in the endothelial cells. Thus it may be implicated in the pathogenesis of acute vascular occlusion syndromes. In agreement with this suggestion, increased plasma/serum TNF-α levels can be found in about 11-25-50% of patients with acute myocardial infarction (range: < 20-1510 pg/ml) and in up to 25% of patients with unstable angina (range: < 20-240 pg/ml).[3,11-13] Serial measurements of TNF-α revealed that peak values were reached within 6 hours and disappeared after 24 hours,[11,12] with a second peak between 48 and 96 hours reported by one group.[13]

Analyzing the data of about 80 patients with unstable angina and myocardial infarction,[11-13] respectively, a clear-cut correlation of high TNF-α levels with large, complicated infarctions was described in two of the three reports.[11,13] High TNF-α levels were present in plasma (peak plasma levels (pg/ml): 1094 ± 1177 (SD), 180-3600, n = 7) of 6 out of 7 patients with severe acute myocardial infarction (Killip class 3 or 4), while no TNF-α (< 50 pg/ml) was detected in the group of 11 patients with an uncomplicated course (Killip class I).[11] On the other hand, Basaran and colleagues[12] could not see any correlation between the serum TNF levels and the occurrence of complications and the extent of myocardial damage; CRP response was also unrelated to TNF levels.

Soluble TNF receptor type I and IL-1 receptor antagonist were also significantly increased in the group with severe acute myocardial infarction (peak plasma concentrations (pg/ml): sTNFRtI: 1184 ± 404, 740-1640, n = 5; IL-1Ra: 4766 ± 2953, 1580-8500, n = 5) compared with those with an uncomplicated course (peak plasma concentrations (pg/ml): sTNFRtI: 162 ± 160, <125-364, n = 5; IL-1Ra: 2026 ± 1271, 570-4100, n = 5) or in control patients without acute myocardial infarction (peak plasma concentrations (pg/ml): sTNFRtI: 62 ± 139, <125-310, n = 5; IL-1Ra: 219 ± 89, 115-345, n = 5; TNF: <50, n = 5).[11] No IL-1β and no IL-8 could be detected in plasma of these patients,[11] but serum levels of IL-6 were reported to be elevated in patients after myocardial infarction.[14]

At the present it remains unclear whether the high TNF-α plasma/serum levels in the course of acute myocardial infarction represent an overspilling of a causative inflammatory substance worsening the course of the disease, whether high TNF-α levels only indicate a high degree of derangement of the physiological state of the patient due to a large myocardial infarction and its complications, or whether they reflect an epiphenomenon. As TNF-α can be effectively antagonized by antibodies and soluble TNF receptors, a therapeutic approach would be available, if the first option holds true. It is also worthwhile mentioning that medications for treatment of myocardial infarction can interfere with the cytokine cascade: heparin infusions in human volunteers were reported to bind TNF and to induce the release of a soluble form of the TNF receptor into the circulation.[15]

As to activities of cNOS and iNOS in atrial tissue of patients with ischemic heart disease, please refer to paragraph "dilated cardiomyopathy".

POST-PUMP INFLAMMATORY RESPONSE IN PATIENTS UNDERGOING CARDIAC SURGERY

Both cardiopulmonary bypass (CPB) and extracorporeal membrane oxygenation induce a systemic inflammatory response characterized by the activation of chemotactic factors, reactive oxygen species and proinflammatory cytokines. This so-called post-pump inflammatory response has been linked to stunned myocardium, respiratory distress syndrome, renal failure, pancreatitis and neurologic injury (for discussion see refs. 16 and 17).

Looking for postoperatively elevated cytokine levels in 22 patients having undergone uncomplicated coronary bypass grafting with moderate systemic hypothermia, Hennein and colleagues[16] found a bimodal peaking of arterial TNF-α at 2 and 18 to 24 hours after the operation (20.2 ± 6.4 pg/ml and 5.8 ± 1.6 pg/ml, respectively; before CPB: 0.90 ± 0.20 pg/ml) and thereafter a progressive decline to levels before bypass. Arterial IL-6 was maximally elevated immediately on termination of CPB and peaked again at 12 to 18 hours thereafter (7520 ± 2439 pg/ml and 6216 ± 1928 pg/ml, respectively; before bypass

746 ± 187 pg/ml). As well, very high IL-6 levels were found in pulmonary effluents of patients immediately after bypass grafting (n = 7: 686-4686 U/ml) and in coronary sinus effluents (n = 4:164-3869 U/ml).[18] The IL-6 concentrations encountered are high enough to depress contractility of both hamster papillary muscles and human pectinate muscles dissected from atrial appendages at the time of bypass surgery.[18] Arterial IL-8 levels were more variable but followed a similar pattern, peaking in the early period after CPB and again at 16 to 18 hours after the operation (4110 ± 1403 pg/ml and 1760 ± 1145 pg/ml, respectively; before bypass: 461 ± 158 pg/ml). Aortic crossclamp time was independently predictive of postoperative cytokine levels. Left ventricular wall motion abnormalities were associated with both IL-6 and IL-8 levels, worsening scores being correlated with increasing levels. Postoperative ischemic episodes were associated with IL-6 levels, six of seven (85%) with episodes of myocardial ischemia after a peak in IL-6 concentrations. Though other groups have documented not such a clear-cut picture (see discussions in refs. 16-18), at least the findings of Hennein and colleagues[16] document that proinflammatory cytokines are elevated after uncomplicated coronary revascularization and that they may contribute to postoperative myocardial ischemia with stunning and segmental wall motion abnormalities.

Not only in hypothermic[16] but also in normothermic CPB[17] elevated arterial plasma levels of IL-6 and IL-8 were seen in 10 patients from 2 until 24 hours after the start of bypass, with a peak at 4 and 12 hours respectively after the beginning of bypass (IL-6: 268.1 ± 131.4 pg/ml; IL-8: 370 ± 420 pg/ml). However, peak values were not correlated with the duration of aortic crossclamping or the bypass procedure nor with the hemodynamic parameters recorded at the same times. And also in contrast to patients undergoing hypothermic cardiopulmonary bypass (see above) traces of TNF-α were detected only in three out of the ten patients at times independent of the cardiopulmonary bypass procedure. Also no circulating IL-1β and endotoxin was found in the plasma of these patients. The authors[17] come to the conclusion that normothermic cardiopulmonary bypass triggers a similar pattern of IL-6 and IL-8 release when compared with the release during hypothermic CPB. Furthermore, they suggest that IL-8, an important chemotactic neutrophil factor, might play a role in reperfusion injuries observed in lungs and hearts after CPB.

MYOCARDIAL ISCHEMIA-INDUCED VENTRICULAR ARRHYTHMIAS

The administration of endotoxin to rats markedly reduces the severity of life-threatening ischemia-induced ventricular arrhythmias that occur when a major coronary artery is occluded.[19] The time course of this pronounced protection (reduction in the incidence of ventricular fibrillation from 54% to 4% and in the number of ventricular premature beats during the occlusion period by more than 90%) follows almost precisely the induction of NOS, which results from endotoxin administration and which is most pronounced between 3 and 10 hours; accordingly, the protection is not apparent two hours after administration, is maximum at 8 hours, and is much reduced at 24 and 48 hours. The fact that this protection is not seen in hearts from rats given dexamethasone one hour prior to endotoxin administration again suggests a likely role for iNOS.[19]

A nontoxic analog of the lipid A component of endotoxin reduces infarct size in a canine model of ischemia.[20] However, arrhythmias were not assessed in this study.

MYOCARDIAL ISCHEMIA AND ISCHEMIA-REPERFUSION INJURY

Early reperfusion represents one of the most effective means of reducing myocardial damage in acute myocardial infarction.

However, even under these conditions there often persists a marked cardiac injury which is attributed at least in part to a reperfusion-induced damage of the heart. Interactions of endothelial cells with leukocytes, with the expression of adhesion molecules[21] (see also chapter 4) and subsequent binding of leukocytes to endothelial cells trigger a cascade of detrimental effects in the heart with the release of aggressive mediators like reactive oxygen species, thromboxane A_2, platelet activating factor and cytokines (for discussion see refs. 22 and 23).

Probably one of the earliest events in this detrimental cascade is a marked reduction in endothelium-dependent relaxation (EDR) due to a reduced release or action of endothelium-derived relaxing factor (EDRF) whose active form is NO. The findings of the group of Lefer clarified the sequence of events:[24] reduced EDR activity occurs in coronary rings isolated from cats 2.5 min after reperfusion and in isolated perfused cat hearts 2.5 min after reperfusion. No decrease in EDR activity occurs before reperfusion in the coronary ligation phase in either preparation, suggesting that this impairment takes place during reperfusion. The decrease in EDR activity occurs soon after the generation of superoxide radicals by the reperfused coronary endothelium. Accumulation of neutrophils and myocardial cell injury does not occur until 3-4.5 hours after reperfusion. Thus, endothelial generation of superoxide radicals acts as a trigger mechanism for endothelial dysfunction which is then amplified by neutrophil adherence and diapedesis into the ischemic region[25] enhancing postreperfusion ischemic injury. The most causal therapeutic approach is represented by a supply of the coronary vasculature with nitric oxide; in cats, intravenous nitric oxide infusions ($1-2 \times 10^{-9}$ M) started 30 min after occlusion of the left anterior descending coronary artery and continued through reperfusion one hour later up to 5.5 hours, significantly reduced the myocardial infarction area and lowered the number of neutrophils attracted to the necrotic myocardial zone.[26] Also two NO donors in a 6 hour model of a feline myocardial ischemia-reperfusion model significantly decreased the myocardial necrotic area/area-at-risk ratio from $29 \pm 3\%$ in the placebo group to 9 ± 2 and $11 \pm 5\%$ in the NO donor groups.[27] Both substances also significantly attenuated coronary endothelial dysfunction, while the accumulation of neutrophils in the necrotic area was not reduced.[27] Also agents that reserve endothelial function or inhibit neutrophil activation (e.g. superoxide dismutase, prostacyclin analogs, transforming growth factor β, antibodies to adhesive proteins) can protect against endothelial dysfunction and myocardial injury if administered before reperfusion.[24]

Besides NO, TNF-α also seems to play a role in reperfusion injury of the heart; in a rat model of coronary artery ligation (60 min) and reperfusion, serum TNF-α was undetectable during the occlusion period, but increased significantly upon release of the coronary artery;[22] at the end of reperfusion, macrophage TNF-α was also increased. Passive immunization with a hyperimmune serum containing antibodies against murine TNF-α significantly increased survival rate (80%), lowered myocardial necrosis, reduced the increase in serum creatine kinase activity and decreased myeloperoxidase activity in the area-at-risk and in the necrotic area. These data are consistent with an involvement of TNF-α in myocardial ischemia-reperfusion injury. It remains to be clarified whether a reduced formation and release of EDRF by TNF-α with resulting endothelial dysfunction, as shown for carotid arteries,[28] is responsible for the detrimental effect of this cytokine during myocardial reperfusion.

SEVERE HEART FAILURE

In severe heart failure, TNF-α and IL-6 levels can, but must not, be increased; in a well defined population of 16 patients with heart failure[29] of high degree (New York Heart Association functional class III of IV; average ejection fraction $28 \pm 2\%$; cause of heart failure: in eight patients coronary artery disease, in one patient end stage valvular heart disease, and in seven patients primary dilated cardiomyopathy; 14 men, 2 women; mean age 63 ± 4 years), circulating levels of TNF-α were higher (24 ± 4 pg/ml) than those of the 11 control subjects (11 ± 2 pg/ml). Independently, also, the IL-6 levels were higher in 11 of these patients with heart failure (36 ± 13 pg/ml) than in the 11 control subjects (4 ± 1 pg/ml). However, serum levels of TNF-α and IL-6 were not elevated in all patients with heart failure. Ten patients had TNF-α serum levels ≥ 15 pg/ml, whereas six patients had serum levels < 15 pg/ml. Serum levels of IL-6 > 7 pg/ml were found in 10 of the 11 patients studied. No elevation was seen for IL-1 and for interferon γ. On the other hand, circulating levels of neopterin produced by activated monocytes and macrophages were also increased. Concerning the activity of neutrophils, basal and phorbolester-triggered release of oxygen radicals was not affected in neutrophils from patients with heart failure; however, formylpeptide-stimulated release of oxygen radicals was significantly reduced. Wiedermann and colleagues[29] interpret these findings in the way that suppressed neutrophil function in patients with heart failure exhibiting elevated levels of TNF-α may indicate self-protection against the deleterious effects of neutrophil-derived oxygen radicals. Through induction of synthesis of tetrahydrobiopterin, a co-factor required for synthesis of NO and reflected by increased neopterin, TNF-α may affect NO synthesis.

Since the time of Hippocrates, cachexia has been recognized as a prominent feature of patients with end-stage heart failure.[30] Although cachexia often accompanies advanced heart failure, little is known about the causes of this cachectic state.

Two groups now have presented evidence that TNF-α may play a role in cardiac cachexia. In 33 patients with chronic heart failure, mean serum levels of TNF-α (115 ± 25 U/ml) were higher than in the healthy controls (9 ± 3 U/ml).[31] Nineteen of these patients had serum levels of TNF-α ≥ 39 U/ml, whereas the remaining 14 patients had serum TNF-α levels below this value. Patients with high levels of TNF-α were more cachectic than those with low levels and had more advanced heart failure, as evidenced by their higher values for plasma renin activity. In the second study,[32] 26 patients with cardiac failure were prospectively identified as "cachectic" (body fat < 27% in men and < 29% in women) or "non cachectic". All were in New York Heart Association class III or IV. In 9 of the 16 cachectic patients concentrations of TNF-α were increased (72 ± 20, mean ± SEM, pg/ml) compared with one of the ten "non cachectic" patients (22 pg/ml), with TNF-α in the other 9 "non cachectic" patients below the detection limit (<15 pg/ml). Patients with a raised circulating concentration of TNF-α weighed significantly less (55.6 ± 3.5 kg) than those in whom the concentration of TNF-α was normal (69.0 ± 4.1 kg).

Both studies demonstrate that circulating concentrations of TNF-α are increased in a significant portion of cachectic patients with heart failure. TNF-α stimulates catabolism experimentally and it may be a factor in the weight loss seen in patients with "cardiac cachexia".[32] TNF-α elevation is also associated with a marked activation of the renin-angiotensin system seen in patients with end-stage cardiac disease.[31]

What about the consequences of the impaired heart function on the systemic circulation and the role of NO? NO co-regulates basal systemic and pulmonary vascular resistance in healthy humans.[33] Increased NO production occurs in healthy individuals in response to acute volume loading; there is arteriolar vasodilation in the forearm vascular bed when healthy subjects are volume expanded with an intravenous infusion of normal saline,[34] with no change in blood pressure under these conditions. This vasodilation is abolished by preinfusion of L-N^G-monomethyl-arginine (L-NMMA), an inhibitor of NOS, suggesting that the vasodilation is mediated, at least in part, by NO. In congestive heart failure, this NO-mediated regulation of vascular tone seems to be dysranged. Plasma nitrate, the stable end product of NO production, is significantly increased in patients with heart failure compared to those of controls (means 51.3 and 24.6 µmol/l, respectively).[35] In patients with congestive heart failure, NO release stimulated by acetylcholine is reduced in the forearm resistance vessels;[36] in contrast, basal release of NO is preserved or may even be enhanced.[36,37] This probably enhanced basal NO release may play an important compensatory role by antagonizing vasoconstrictor forces, which are pathologically enhanced in congestive heart failure.

Essential Hypertension

In patients with essential hypertension, no elevation of plasma cytokine levels can be observed, with the exception of a small percentage of slightly raised plasma levels of colony stimulating factors (Table 9.1). However, an increased production of reactive oxygen species and a decreased NOS activity in peripheral blood neutrophils may play a role in the pathogenesis of essential hypertension.[1,38,39] This fits into the finding that inhibition of NO synthesis in healthy humans increases blood pressure.[40]

Heart Allograft Rejection

Human heart allograft rejection leads to a rise in plasma levels of TNF-α. In the series of Chollet-Martin and colleagues[41] TNF-α levels during eight episodes of rejection in six heart recipient patients were considerably higher (607 ± 42 pg/ml, range 210-1200 pg/ml) than the low, even in some measurements nondetectable (detection limit 100 pg/ml) levels of 34 healthy subjects (≤ 124.1 ± 5, 8 pg/ml (mean ± SEM)). The elevation of plasma TNF-α was an early event of the rejection period, preceding the pathomorphological changes in the endomyocardial biopsies in four out of eight cases. When high plasma levels of TNF-α persisted despite antirejection therapy, then also persistent abnormalities in endomyocardial biopsy and echocardiography were associated.

TNF-α immunoreactivity can be found in endomyocardial biopsies from human cardiac allografts (n = 43),[42] in 45% of biopsies with mild acute rejection, in 83% of biopsies with focal moderate rejection, in 80% of biopsies with diffuse moderate rejection, and in 45% of biopsies with resolving rejection. Biopsies with absent rejection do not show cells with TNF-α immunoreactivity. In mild rejection, positive cells were few and monocytes, macrophages and T lymphocytes (up to 20% of all infiltrating cells) were scanty. Expression of major histocompatibility complex (MHC) class II antigens on infiltrating and endothelial cells occurred earlier and independent of reactivity. The number of immunoreactive cells increased in moderate rejection (up to 50%).

Also high levels of IL-2 and CD4-IL-2 receptor positive cells were observed during heart transplant rejection; however, the association between increased numbers of such activated lymphocytes and tissue rejection in terms of endomyocardial biopsy is, at present, controversial.[41]

Taking the findings together, increased TNF-α and IL-2 plasma levels are associated with acute heart allograft rejection. Such increases occurred at an early stage of rejection and persisted for as long as abnormalities on endomyocardial biopsy and echocardiography were present. The pathomorphological correlate are TNF-α-positive inflammatory cells in the heart which rise in number with increasing severity of the rejection reaction. Therefore, measurement of TNF-α plasma levels could be of considerable clinical interest in assisting with the early detection and monitoring of heart transplantation rejection.

KAWASAKI DISEASE

Kawasaki disease, the mucocutaneous lymph node syndrome, has aroused great scientific interest because of the occurrence of coronary arteritis in early childhood, accompanied by myocardial infarction, coronary aneurysm and thrombosis. It is an acute illness of unknown pathogenesis, characterized by fever, mucosal inflammation, skin changes, and lymphadenopathy. Histopathological examination reveals panvasculits with endothelial necrosis, immunoglobulin deposition and mononuclear cell infiltration. Recent studies suggested a role for circulating antibodies that are cytotoxic for endothelial cell antigens inducible by cytokines (see discussion in ref. 43). Increased plasma/serum levels of these cytokines in debate (TNF-α, IL-1, IFNγ) would support this hypothesis; in 39 children with Kawasaki disease (mean age 2.9 years, range 2 months to 9 years), the TNF-α levels in sera from the acute and subacute phases of the disease are significantly higher (acute phase: 33.2 ± 17 pg/ml) than in sera taken in the convalescence phase (13.7 ± 11.5 pg/ml) or in sera from children without inflammatory disease (< 7 pg/ml (detection limit)).[43] Patients who developed coronary aneurymsms (n = 4) were among those who had the highest levels of circulating TNF-α during the acute and subacute phase (51.1 ± 13.6 pg/ml) in comparison to patients without coronary aneurysms (30.4 ± 15.8 pg/ml). No differences in circulating TNF-α levels were observed between patients who received as treatment aspirin plus intravenous immunoglobulin and those who received aspirin alone. The results show that the levels of circulating TNF-α are increased in acute Kawasaki disease and support the hypothesis that this cytokine may be involved in the pathogenesis of the vascular injury of the disease.[43]

MYOCARDIAL DEPRESSION IN STATES OF SIRS

A generalized inflammatory host response to noninfectious stimuli has been classified as "systemic inflammatory response syndrome" (SIRS).[44]

Though this term is discussed controversially,[45] it is nonetheless widely used. It includes such heterogenous stimuli like hypovolemia, trauma, burns, pancreatitis, reperfusion and resuscitation injury, with a postulated relatively monotonous response reaction similar to that triggered by infectious agents, including elevations of cytokines and of other inflammatory mediators. Cardiodepressant factors, alterations of pre- and afterload, of contractility and of compliance, myocardial ischemia, adrenergic unresponsiveness, release of oxygen free radicals, leukotrienes and thromboxanes have been identified or claimed as pathogenically important (see also chapter 4),[46-48] yet without a clear-cut picture of the molecular mechanisms involved.

CARDIOVASCULAR IMPAIRMENT DURING CYTOKINE TREATMENT OF CANCER PATIENTS

Cytokines are applied to patients in pharmacological doses as anticancer treatment. Impairment of myocardial function is well known as side effect of treatment with TNF-α-, IL-2- and IFN-γ.

TNF-α

Looking on the reported side effects in 88 TNF-treated cancer patients,[49-51] dose-dependent development of hypotension persisting for up to 36 hours, requiring fluid management and also vasopressor (dopamine) treatment in some cases, is frequent at doses of $\geq$ 545 $\mu g/m^2$;[50] less frequent TNF treatment is combined with fluid retention, dyspnea, pulmonary congestion and edema. No data are given favoring either a vascular leakage syndrome or myocardial depression as underlying mechanism.

Hegewisch and coworkers[52] reported about a 44-year-old man with renal cell carcinoma whom has been given 17 courses of TNF in intervals of 3 weeks. During the last five courses he had substernal pressure, and from the eleventh cycle ST-segment depression was seen on the ECG. On day two of the fifteenth cycle TNF was discontinued because of severe chest pain, and a nontransmural myocardial infarction was diagnosed. Arteriography revealed no significant signs of coronary artery disease. Two more cycles were then administered, substernal pressure appearing whenever TNF was infused. The patient presented 3 months after TNF therapy had been discontinued with respiratory distress and the symptoms of cardiac failure, due to an enlarged heart with severe depression, without the signs of active myocarditis. The patient quickly responded to digitalis and diuretics and when discharged he no longer had pulmonary congestion or right heart failure, and cardiac enlargement was reduced.[52]

INTERLEUKIN 2

Cardiovascular toxicity occurs in approximately 5% of patients receiving high-dose IL-2 therapy, most frequently consisting of hypotension and tachycardia.[53,54] Acute myocardial infarction was documented in at least four patients, two of whom clearly had antecedent hypotension. Atrial and ventricular arrhythmias were noted as well,[54] and also a case report of eosinophilic myocarditis associated with high-dose IL-2 therapy was reported.[53]

Despite the well-documented nature of IL-2-induced cardiovascular toxicity, there were few data reported regarding specific hemodynamic consequences of such therapy. Gaynor and colleagues[55] monitored the systemic hemodynamics of 13 patients receiving IL-2 therapy. In 12 of the 13 patients, IL-2 administration produced a significant reduction in mean arterial pressure and in systemic vascular resistance, requiring use of pressor support in 9, associated with an increased heart rate and cardiac output. No consistent or significant change in pulmonary capillary wedge pressure was observed. The similarity of IL-2-induced impairment of the cardiovascular system and those of septic shock is further substantiated by the findings of Ognibene and co-workers.[56] In addition to the vascular changes described, IL-2 treatment in five patients resulted in tachycardia (84.0 ± 3.5/min before treatment and 138 ± 6.9/min at day four of therapy), an increase in cardiac index (4.27 ± 0.49 l/min/m^2 vs 5.88 ± 0.66 l/min/m^2), a fall in left ventricular ejection fraction ($58.0 \pm 4.7\%$ vs $36.4 \pm 4.0\%$), a trend toward left ventricular dilatation and a depression of left ventricular stroke work index (57.0 ± 8.1 g x m/m^2 vs $31.7 \pm 3,8$ g x m/m^2; $0.05 < p < 0.10$). There is experimental evidence that IL-2-induced cardiovascular impairment is not the result of a direct effect of IL-2 but is instead mediated by other cytokines, with interferon-γ, TNF-α and IL-1 being likely candidates.[57] These substances then trigger the cytokine-inducible NO synthesis, as reflected by a striking increase in serum nitrate levels and 24-hour-urinary nitrate excretion,[57] with all its detrimental effects on the vasculature and probably also on the heart. Thus, IL-2 induces multiple reversible cardiovascular abnormalities that are similar to the hemodynamic manifestations of human septic shock.

INTERFERON

The side effects of interferon treatment are generally mild and disappear after treatment is stopped.[58] Fortunately, drug-induced cardiac impairment seems to be rare, as only few case reports dealt with this topic:

A case of cardiomyopathy due to interferon after one week of therapy and confirmed at necropsy was reported by Cohen and colleagues.[59] Another case report deals with a reversible cardiac dysfunction associated with interferon treatment in a patient with AIDS.[60] The potential cardiotoxicity of interferon was attributed in this patient to a synergistic interaction with HIV infection. Sonnenblick and colleagues[58] described a case of severe cardiomyopathy—cardiomegaly, pulmonary congestion, large pleural effusions shown to be transudate, lowered left ventricular ejection fraction of 18% with severe diffuse hypokinesis—induced by interferon α_2 in a patient who had a complete clinical recovery two months after interferon treatment was withdrawn.

THE EVOLVING KNOWLEDGE ABOUT THE ROLE OF CYTOKINES IN HEART DISEASES

Investigating the pathophysiology of sepsis and SIRS has gained a lot of information about the detrimental effects of a deranged cytokine/mediator network in these states, including septic cardiomyopathy. In addition, we have learned a lot about the physiological importance of these substances. And furthermore, all these findings gave interest to look for some role of cytokines and inflammatory mediators also in nonseptic heart diseases. Surprisingly, increased circulating levels of these compounds are not only found in the "classical" inflammatory heart diseases like myocarditis, but also in states of cardiac impairment where such a role is at the first glance unlikely, like myocardial infarction, heart failure, dilated and hypertrophic cardiomyopathy. At the present findings are still very scarce, and one can, at best, give some descriptional information. However, with an ongoing interest in this field and a better understanding of the mechanisms underlying the cardiodepressive action of cytokines and mediators, a clearer picture of the role of cytokines and inflammatory mediators in various forms of heart disease may emerge within the next few years.

REFERENCES

1. Warren JB, Pons F, Brady AJB. Nitric oxide biology: implications for cardiovascular therapeutics. Cardiovasc Res 1994; 28:25-30.
2. Topol EJ, ed. Current Opinion in Cardiology 1994; 9/3:255-400 and B89-B127.
3. Matsumori A, Yamada T, Suzuki H et al. Increased circulating cytokines in patients with myocarditis and cardiomyopathy. Br Heart J 1994; 72:561-566.
4. Smith SC, Allen PM. Neutralization of endogenous tumor necrosis factor ameliorates the severity of myosin-induced myocarditis. Circ Res 1992; 70:856-863.
5. Lane JR, Neumann DA, Lafond-Walker A et al. Interleukin 1 or tumor necrosis factor can promote coxsackie B3-induced myocarditis in resistant B10.A mice. J Exp Med 1992; 175:1123- 1129.
6. Neumann DA, Lane JR, Allen GS et al. Viral myocarditis leading to cardiomyopathy: do cytokines contribute to pathogenesis? Clin Immunol Immunopathol 1993; 68:181-190.
7. Yamada T, Matsumori A, Sasayama S. Therapeutic effect of anti-tumor necrosis factor-α antibody on the murine model of viral myocarditis induced by encephalomyocarditis virus. Circulation 1994; 89:846-851.
8. Henke A, Mohr C, Sprenger H et al. Coxsackievirus B3-induced production of tumor necrosis factor-α, IL-1β, and IL-6 in human monocytes. J Immunol 1992; 148:2270-2277.
9. Koeffler HP, Gasson J, Ranyard J et al. Recombinant human TNF-α stimulates production of granulocyte colony-stimulating factor. Blood 1987; 70:55-59.

10. De Belder A, Why HJF, Bucknall CA et al. Nitric oxide synthase activities in human myocardium. Lancet 1993; 341:84-85.

11. Latini R, Bianchi M, Correale E et al. Cytokines in acute myocardial infarction: selective increase in circulating tumor necrosis factor, its soluble receptor, and interleukin-1 receptor antagonist. J Cardiovasc Pharmacol 1994; 23:1-6.

12. Basaran Y, Basaran MM, Babacan KF et al. Serum tumor necrosis factor levels in acute myocardial infarction and unstable angina pectoris. Angiology 1993; 44:332-337.

13. Maury CPJ, Teppo A-M. Circulating tumour necrosis factor-α (cachectin) in myocardial infarction. J Int Med 1989; 225:333-336.

14. Ikeda U, Ohkawa F, Seino Y et al. Serum interleukin 6 levels become elevated in acute myocardial infarction. J Mol Cell Cardiol 1992; 24:579-584.

15. Lantz M, Thysell H, Nilsson E et al. On the binding of tumor necrosis factor (TNF) to heparin and the release in vivo of the TNF-binding protein I by heparin. J Clin Invest 1991; 88:2026-2031.

16. Hennein HA, Ebba H, Rodriguez JL et al. Relationship of the proinflammatory cytokines to myocardial ischemia and dysfunction after uncomplicated coronary revascularization. J Thorac Cardiovasc Surg 1994; 108:626-635.

17. Frering B, Philip I, Dehoux M et al. Circulating cytokines in patients undergoing normothermic cardiopulmonary bypass. J Thorac Cardiovasc Surg 1994; 108:636-641.

18. Finkel MS, Hoffman RA, Shen L et al. Interleukin-6 (IL-6) as a mediator of stunned myocardium. Am J Cardiol 1993; 71:1231-1232.

19. Song W, Furman BL, Parratt JR. Attenuation by dexamethasone of endotoxin protection against ischemia-induced ventricular arrhythmias. Br J Pharmacol 1994; 113:1083-1084.

20. Yao Z, Auchampach JA, Pieper GM et al. Cardiodeprotective effects of monophosphoryl lipid A, a novel endotoxin analogue, in the dog. Cardiovasc Res 1993; 27:832-838.

21. Smith CW, Anderson DC, Taylor AA et al. Leucocyte adhesion molecules and myocardial ischemia. Trends Cardiovasc Med 1991; 1:167-170.

22. Squadrito F, Altavilla D, Zingarelli B et al. Tumor necrosis factor involvement in myocardial ischemia-reperfusion injury. Eur J Pharmacol 1993; 237:223-230.

23. Nose PS. Cytokines and reperfusion injury. J Card Surg 1993; 8(Suppl):305-308.

24. Lefer AM, Tsao PS, Lefer DJ et al. Role of endothelial dysfunction in the pathogenesis of reperfusion injury after myocardial ischemia. FASEB J 1991; 5:2029-2034.

25. Ma X-l, Weyrich AS, Lefer DJ et al. Diminished basal nitric oxide release after myocardial ischemia and reperfusion promotes neutrophil adherence to coronary endothelium. Circ Res 1993; 72:403-412.

26. Johnson G, Tsao PS, Lefer AM. Cardioprotective effects of authentic nitric oxide in myocardial ischemia with reperfusion. Crit Care Med 1991; 19:244-252.

27. Siegfried MR, Erhardt J, Rider T et al. Cardioprotection and attenuation of endothelial dysfunction by organic nitric oxide donors in myocardial ischemia-reperfusion. J Pharmacol Exp Ther 1992; 260:668-675.

28. Aoki N, Siegfried M, Lefer AM. Anti-EDRF effect of tumor necrosis factor in isolated perfused cat carotid arteries. Am J Physiol 1989; 256:H1509-H1512.

29. Wiedermann CJ, Beimpold H, Herold M et al. Increased levels of serum neopterin and decreased production of neutrophil superoxide anions in chronic heart failure with elevated levels of tumor necrosis factor-alpha. J Am Coll Cardiol 1993; 22:1897-1901.

30. Katz AM, Katz PB. Diseases of the heart in works of Hippocrates. Br Heart J 1962; 24:257-264.

31. Levine B, Kalman J, Mayer L et al. Elevated circulating levels of tumor necrosis factor in severe chronic heart failure. N Engl J Med 1990; 323:236-241.

32. McMurray J, Abdullah I, Dargie HJ et al. Increased concentrations of tumour necrosis factor in "cachectic" patients with severe chronic heart failure. Br Heart J 1991; 66:356-358.

33. Stamler J, Roddy MA, Currie KE et al. Nitric oxide regulates basal systemic and pulmonary vascular resistance in healthy humans. Circulation 1994; 89:2035-2040.

34. Calver A, Green D, Collier J et al. The effect of acute plasma volume expansion on peripheral arteriolar tone in healthy volunteers. Clin Sci 1992; 83:541-547.

35. Winlaw D, Smythe GA, Keogh AM. Increased nitric oxide production in heart failure. Lancet 1994; 344:373-374.

36. Drexler H, Hayoz D, Münzel T et al. Endothelial function in chronic congestive heart failure. Am J Cardiol 1992; 69:1596- 1601.

37. Habib F, Dutka D, Crossman D et al. Enhanced basal nitric oxide production in heart failure: another failed counter-regulatory vasodilator mechanism? Lancet 1994; 344:371-373. Letter to the editor: 887-888.

38. Mehta JL, Lopez LM, Cheng L et al. Alterations in nitric oxide synthase activity, superoxide anion generation, and platelet aggregation in systemic hypertension, and effects of celiprolol. Am J Cardiol 1994; 74:901-905.

39. MacAllister R, Vallance P. Nitric oxide in essential and renal hypertension. J Am Soc Nephrol 1994; 5:1057-1065.

40. Haynes WG, Noon JP, Walker BR et al. Inhibition of nitric oxide synthesis increases blood pressure in healthy humans. J Hypertension 1993; 11:1375-1380.

41. Chollet-Martin S, Depoix JP, Hvass U et al. Raised plasma levels of tumor necrosis factor in heart allograft rejection. Transplant Proc 1990; 22:283-286.

42. Arbustini E, Grasso M, Diegoli M et al. Expression of tumor necrosis factor in human acute cardiac rejection. Am J Pathol 1991; 139:709-715.

43. Maury CPJ, Salo E, Pelkonen P. Elevated circulating tumor necrosis factor-α in patients with Kawasaki disease. J Lab Clin Med 1989; 113:651-654.

44. ACCP/SCCM Concensus Conference. Definitions of sepsis and multiple organ failure. Crit Care Med 1992; 20:864-874.

45. Vincent J-L. Sepsis and septic shock: update of definitions. In: Reinhart K, Eyrich K, Sprung C, eds. Sepsis—Current Perspectives in Pathophysiology and Therapy (Update in Intensive Care and Emergency Medicine 18). Berlin, Heidelberg: Springer-Verlag, 1994:3-15.

46. Traber DL, Meyer J, Traber LD. Cardiac function during hypovolemia. In: Schlag G, Redl H, eds. Pathophysiology of Shock, Sepsis, and Organ Failure. Berlin, Heidelberg, New York: Springer-Verlag, 1993:194-199.

47. Law WR. Myocardial depression. In: Gamelli RL, Dries DJ, eds. Trauma 2000—Strategies for the New Millenium. Austin: Landes, 1992:30-35.

48. Jones RO, Carlson DE, Gann DS. A circulating shock protein that depolarizes cells in vitro depresses myocardial contractility and rate in isolated rat hearts. J Trauma 1994; 37:752-758.

49. Selby P, Hobbs S, Viner C et al. Tumour necrosis factor in man: clinical and biological observations. Br J Cancer 1987; 56:803-808.

50. Spriggs DR, Sherman ML, Michie H et al. Recombinant human tumor necrosis factor administered as a 24-hour intravenous infusion. A phase I and pharmacologic study. J Natl Cancer Institute 1988; 80:1039-1044.

51. Blick M, Sherwin SA, Rosenblum M et al. Phase I study of recombinant tumor necrosis factor in cancer patients. Cancer Res 1987; 47:2986-2989.

52. Hegewisch S, Weh H-J, Hossfeld DK. TNF-induced cardiomyopathy. Lancet 1990; 335:295-296.

53. Schuchter LM, Hendricks CB, Holland KH et al. Eosinophilic myocarditis associated with high-dose interleukin-2 therapy. Am J Med 1990; 88:439-440.

54. Isner JM, Dietz WA. Cardiovascular consequences of recombinant DNA technology: interleukin-2. Ann Int Med 1988; 109:933-935.

55. Gaynor ER, Vitek L, Sticklin L et al. The hemodynamic effects of interleukin-2 and lymphokine-activated killer cells. Ann Intern Med 1988; 109:953-958.

56. Ognibene FP, Rosenberg SA, Lotze M. Interleukin-2 administration causes reversible hemodynamic changes and left ventricular dysfunction similar to those seen in septic shock. Chest 1988; 94:750-754.

57. Hibbs JB, Westenfelder C, Taintor R. Evidence for cytokine-inducible nitric oxide synthesis from L-arginine in patients receiving interleukin-2 therapy. J Clin Invest 1992; 89:867- 877.

58. Sonnenblick M, Rosenmann D, Rosin A. Reversible cardiomyopathy induced by interferon. Brit Med J 1990; 300:1174-1175.

59. Cohen MC, Huberman MS, Nesto RW. Recombinant α-2 interferon related cardiomypathy. Am J Med 1988; 85:549-550.

60. Deyton LR, Walker RE, Kovacs JA et al. Reversible cardiac dysfunction in patients with Kaposi's sarcoma. N Engl J Med 1989; 321:1246-1249.

CHAPTER 10

TOWARDS A MORE CAUSAL TREATMENT OF SEPTIC CARDIOMYOPATHY

M any new insights into the mechanisms underlying myocardial depression in sepsis were gained in the last years, enabling first attempts of a more causal treatment, though, at present, still with very limited success. As the merely symptomatic therapy with fluids and catecholamines is only of limited success,[1-6] about 15% of all deaths in septic shock are due to refractory pump failure of the heart,[7] a more causal treatment of septic cardiomyopathy may help improve prognosis. Some of these therapeutic approaches in the nascent state will be outlined in this chapter.

CATECHOLAMINE TREATMENT OF SEPTIC VERSUS NON-SEPTIC HEART FAILURE: IS DESENSITIZATION DIFFERENT?

In nonseptic heart failure, plasma catecholamine levels, predominantly noradrenaline, are more increased, the more severe myocardial function is impaired. This catecholamine excess induces a down-regulation of β_1-adrenoceptors and an up-regulation of inhibitory G_i proteins of the adenylyl cyclase system of the heart,[8] with both factors contributing to catecholamine tolerance, i.e., an attenuation of the positive inotropic effect of catecholamines (see also chapter 4: Catecholamines). Ex vivo-in vitro data[9] indicate that this catecholamine tolerance also develops in patients with septic shock under therapy with noradrenaline (Table 10.1; see also chapter 4: Catecholamines—Catecholamine-Induced Desensitization of Adenylyl Cyclase in an Experimental "Ex Vivo-In Vitro" System).

Patients with clinically well-characterized septic shock were treated either with dopamine (group III in Table 10.1) or predominantly with noradrenaline (group IV in Table 10.1). Patients with cardiogenic shock treated with adrenaline (group II in Table 10.1) and cardiac patients without shock (group I in Table 10.1) served as nonseptic control groups. Plasma levels of the pharmacologically applied catecholamines were increased in the expected manner (Table 10.1; see also Fig. 4.4.).

To maintain the positive inotropic effect, as measured by left ventricular stroke work index, in the noradrenaline group (III), the dosage had to be more than doubled from day 1 to day 2 and could be kept constant thereafter (Table 10.1; see also Fig. 4.7). In the case of the dopamine group (group III), no increase in dosage was necessary.[9]

To compare catecholamine desensitization in treated patients with cardiogenic and septic shock, neonatal rat cardiomyocytes—with at least 90% of β-adrenoceptors belonging to the β_1-subtype[10]—were incubated for 48 hours with the plasma of these patients. In these rat cardiomyocytes, the plasma of noradrenaline-treated patients with septic shock led to a down-regulation of β-adrenoceptors by 35%, an increase in

Table 10.1. Catecholamine desensitization in patients with cardiogenic or septic shock: Effects of patient plasma on the β-adrenoceptor/ G proteins/adenylyl cyclase system of neonatal rat cardiomyocytes during a 48 h-incubation period

Group	I "Cardiac disease" n = 5	II "Cardio- genic shock" n = 6	III "Septic Shock" n = 7	IV "Septic Shock" n = 8
Patient data				
Catecholamine dosage (μg/min)				
Dopamine	200	200	671 ± 237	200
Noradrenaline				13,1 ± 8,6
Adrenaline		17,1 ± 7,9		3,3 ± 4,9
Plasma levels				
Dopamine (ng/ml)	49,3 ± 26,1	38,8 ± 15,5	169,0 ± 74,8	25,0 ± 14,8
Noradrenaline (pg/ml)	1309 ± 703	964 ± 837	689 ± 487	8117 ± 5866
Adrenaline (pg/ml)	178 ± 112	8487 ± 4218	98,6 ± 7,0	1391 ± 1258
Ex vivo - in vitro data (rat cardiomyocytes incubated with patient plasma)				
β-Adrenoceptors (%)	87,6 ± 10,0	76,9 ± 9,6	94,3 ± 19,0	63,0 ± 17,1
$G_{i\alpha}$ proteins	120,9 ± 22,7	147,6 ± 26,5	97,1 ± 25,8	160,9 ± 35,8
Isoproterenol- stimulated adenylyl cyclase activity (%)	98,2 ± 27,4	71,6 ± 25,8	81,8 ± 15,4	51,5 ± 31,5

For further explanation see text. The values for β-adrenoceptors and for stimulated adenylyl cyclase activity are calculated as percentage of control values obtained from cardiomyocytes exposed to the respective patient's plasma in the presence of 10^{-7} M timolol (for further explanation see ref. 9).

the level of inhibitory G_i protein α-subunits by 60%, and a decrease in isoproterenol-stimulated adenylyl cyclase activity by 50%. The higher the noradrenaline plasma concentration, the lower was the number of β-adrenoceptors (see also Fig. 4.4). Similar alterations were observed following pretreatment of the cells with plasma of adrenaline-treated patients in cardiogenic shock. Binding affinity of myocardial β-adreno-ceptors for ligands and the potency of catecholamines in stimulating cAMP formation and contractile response are very similar in human cardiac preparations and in cultured neonatal rat cardiomyocytes.[8,10-12] Therefore, it can be inferred that noradrenaline treatment of septic patients may induce a similar pattern of catecholamine desensitization in human heart as in the in vitro model of rat cardiomyocytes.

In contrast, exposure of the cardiomyocytes to plasma of intensive care cardiac patients without shock (group I in Table 10.1), and to plasma of dopamine-treated patients with septic shock (group III in Table 10.1) did not induce alterations of the cardiomyocytes' adenylyl cyclase system. This lack of desensitization by the plasma of dopam-ine-treated patients can be easily explained by the low affinity of dopam-ine for β-adrenoceptors ($K_D > 10^{-4}M$) both in human heart[12] and in rat cardiomyocytes in comparison to the noradrenaline and adrenaline af-finities ($K_D = 2.4 \times 10^{-6}M$ and $1.1 \times 10^{-6}M$)[9]; also, the plasma levels of noradrenaline and adrenaline are much lower in the dopamine-treated patients in comparison to the noradrenaline/adrenaline treated group (Table 10.1).

While the ex vivo-in vitro data of group IV in Table 10.1 exclude a clinically relevant direct stimulation of myocardial β-adrenoceptors by dopamine high enough to induce catecholamine tolerance, the pos-sibility cannot be ruled out that this might occur in vivo due to a dopamine-induced release of myocardial noradrenaline into the synap-tic cleft.[9]

In experimental studies on endotoxemia and sepsis, cardiac adenylyl cyclase stimulation was shown to be markedly depressed, concomitant with an increase in the level of circulating catecholamines, whereas the down-regulation of β-adrenoceptors in these cardiac preparations was relatively small (about 25% at maximum).[13] It has, therefore, been suggested that the mechanisms leading to agonist-induced β-adrenoceptor down-regulation (phosphorylation, sequestration, internalization) may be altered in endotoxemia and sepsis (for review see chapter 4: Cat-echolamines). The results of Table 10.1, however, indicate that the β-adrenoceptor down-regulation and the G_i up-regulation induced by the plasma of patients with septic shock amounts to a similar or even higher degree than the regulatory steps induced by the plasma of pa-tients with cardiogenic shock. Thus, the mechanisms of agonist-in-duced β-adrenoceptor down-regulation (about 2/3 of total effect) and G_i up-regulation (about 1/3 of total effect) are apparently not altered by long living ($\geq$ 48 hours) factors present in the plasma of the patients with septic shock.[9] Therefore, similar to development of tolerance during catecholamine treatment of cardiogenic shock,[14] also in septic shock a tolerance to β-adrenoceptor stimulation occurs during noradrenaline and probably dobutamine therapy within the initial 48 hours.

CAN WE IMPROVE SEPTIC CARDIOMYOPATHY BY EXTRACORPOREAL MEASURES?

If myocardial depressant factors circulate in sepsis, then the elimination of these factors by extracorporeal measures like hemofiltration, hemodialysis or plasmapheresis would be an attractive approach.

In a dog model of sepsis, left ventricular dysfunction could be reversed by hemofiltration.[15] In human sepsis, elimination of potentially cardiodepressive mediators like TNF-α and other cytokines by hemofiltration was described,[16,17] but was not necessarily accompanied by a fall in the respective plasma cytokine levels.[17] Also, the cardiodepressant factor CDF can be eliminated by hemofiltration (Chapter 4: Cardiodepressant Factors).[18] However, in observational studies, no relevant improvement of myocardial contractility, as measured by left ventricular stroke work index, has been observed in septic patients in the course of either hemofiltration or plasmapheresis (Table 10.2).

ANTIBODIES AGAINST TOXINS AND MEDIATORS: FIRST ATTEMPTS OF A CAUSAL TREATMENT OF SEPTIC CARDIOMYOPATHY

Vincent and coworkers were the first who demonstrated a slight improvement of the impaired heart function in 10 septic patients by a single dose of anti-TNF-α antibodies.[19] We could confirm this finding in 20 patients with severe sepsis who were repetitively treated with a murine monoclonal anti-TNF-α antibody (Fig. 10.1; Table 10.2).[20] In comparison to the achievable improvement witnessed after the administration of catecholamines, the increase in left ventricular stroke work index by anti-TNF-α antibodies is only modest. However, one should bear in mind that this improvement adds to the positive inotropic effect of catecholamines (Table 10.2).

Up to now, two antiendotoxin antibodies (HA-1A, E 5) have been tested in placebo-controlled sepsis trials (for review see ref. 21). Data concerning the effects of these antibodies on the impaired heart function are scarce. In the few patients which we treated with the antiendotoxin antibody HA-1A (Centoxin®), we could see no improvement of septic cardiomyopathy (Table 10.2). In a canine model of experimental septic shock, even a detrimental effect of this antibody on the heart has been described.[22] It is interesting to note that an endotoxin analog, monophosphoryl lipid A, with significantly less activity than endotoxin in producing circulatory shock and death, can exert a potentially beneficial effect in acute myocardial infarction.[23]

Inhibitors of the NO/guanylyl cyclase pathway like N^G-monomethyl-L-arginine (L-NMMA), N^G-nitro-L-arginine methyl ester (NAME) or methylene blue undoubtedly improve blood pressure by increasing systemic vascular resistance. With respect to the heart, however, the data available are in favor of deterioration (fall in cardiac output) rather than of improvement of heart function by these substances,[24] both in animal models[25-27] and in patients,[28-30] with the potential risk of coronary vasoconstriction[31] and pulmonary hypertension.[32] However, one cannot exclude that the induced rise in afterload achieved by NO inhibition may mask a potential beneficial effect of these substances on myocardial function.

All results presented in this chapter arise from animal and from clinical observational studies, but not from placebo-controlled trials. Therefore, they are only of preliminary value.

Table 10.2. Aiming at a causal therapy of acute septic cardiomyopathy: Effect of supplemental sepsis therapies on left ventricular stroke work index in observational studies

Supplemental therapy	Patients	Left ventricular stroke work index (LVSWI; g x m/m²)		
	n	day 0	→ day 4 (1*)	Δ LVSWI
Anti-endotoxin-antibody (Centoxin®)	6	42 ± 8	→ 43 ± 9	+ 1
Anti-TNFα-antibody	20	33 ± 12	→ 41 ± 11	+ 8
Immunoglobulin (IgG)	57	40 ± 2	→ 43 ± 3	+ 3
Hemofiltration	8	17 ± 1	→ 23 ± 6	+ 6
Plasmapheresis	11	43 ± 7	→ 50 ± 8	+ 7
(Noradrenaline (6,6 µg/min)	5	22 ± 7	→ 35 ± 12*	+ 13)

In addition to standard therapy including catecholamines, patients with sepsis or septic shock were treated with the supplemental sepsis therapies indicated. For comparison, the effect of noradrenaline treatment on left ventricular stroke work index is shown in addition. Left ventricular stroke work index was calculated as "cardiac index x mean blood pressure x 13.6/heart rate (mean ± SD). "*": In case of noradrenaline, the change in left ventricular stroke work index was calculated from day 0 to day 1. Calculation of systemic vascular resistance (dynes x sec x cm^{-5}) are available for the plasmapheresis group (day 0: 397 ± 48 day 4: 405 ± 59) and the hemofiltration group (day 0:716 ± 66; day 4: 780 ± 122); in case of anti-TNF-α-antibody-treatment, the systemic vascular resistance indices (dynes x sec x cm^{-5} x m^{-2}) were calculated as 1202 ± 227 on day 0 and 1466 ± 274 on day 4. (Data were obtained in collaboration with Dr. P. Boekstegers, Dr. S. Fateh-Moghadam, Dr. S. Kääb, Dr. G. Pilz. For further details see refs. 6 and 20.)

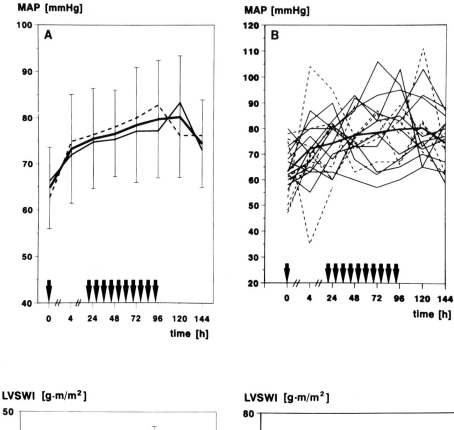

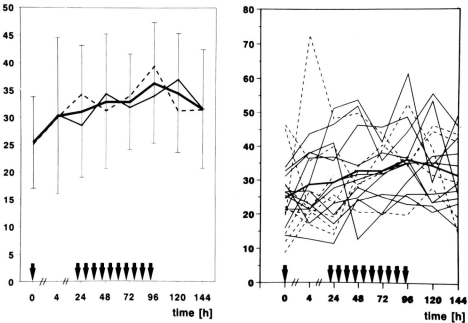

TREATMENT OF VASCULAR AND CARDIAC DYSFUNCTION IN SEPSIS MAY REQUIRE DIFFERENTIAL CAUSAL APPROACHES

Vascular and cardiac dysfunction in sepsis can show a different response pattern to therapy. In a canine model of septic shock, norepinephrine is similarly effective in raising blood pressure as in control animals, but its potential to improve cardiac performance is diminished; dopamine, in contrast, loses some of its vasoconstrictive efficacy, but retains the capacity to enhance cardiac performance.[33] In another dog model of sepsis, left ventricular dysfunction can effectively be treated by hemofiltration, while hypotension is refractory.[15] In rats, TNF-α exerts a rapid attenuation of catecholamine inotropy within 60 minutes, while the attenuation of α-adrenoceptor agonist-induced vasoconstriction only emerges at 24 hours.[34]

An impressive confirmation of this hypothesis of differential therapeutic approaches is given in a recent paper from Kilbourn and colleagues.[25] By the combination of N^G-methyl-L-arginine (L-NMMA) and dobutamine, complete restoration of blood pressure could be obtained in endotoxemic dogs, with L-NMMA improving the vascular and dobutamine the cardiac dysfunction.

Some information is also available for septic patients. In the case of anti-TNF-α-antibody treatment both myocardial and vascular impairment improve (Table 10.2 and legend to Table 10.2);[6,20] on the other hand, hemofiltration and plasmapheresis are of little effect on systemic vascular resistance, but these measures moderately increase left ventricular stroke work index (Table 10.2 and legend to Table 10.2).[6] Inhibitors of the NO/guanylyl cyclase pathway unequivocally improve vascular dysfunction and hypotension in septic shock, but their effect on cardiac function is rather detrimental than beneficial (see above). In an observational study with septic patients treated with polyvalent immunoglobulin G, a rapid increase in the lowered systemic vascular resistance was observed within 4 days (Fig. 10.2); heart function, however, remained constantly impaired in these patients (Fig. 10.2), with the induced increase in afterload possibly masking an actual small improvement of myocardial contractility.

Fig. 10.1 Opposite page: Effects of the anti-TNF-α antibody MAK 195F on cardiovascular impairment in patients with severe sepsis. Changes in mean arterial pressure (MAP; upper graphs) and in left ventricular stroke work index (LVSW; lower graphs) are given, measured during the application of the anti-TNF-α antibody MAK 195F (arrows) to patients with severe sepsis. Graphs on the left: all patients surviving more than 2 days (heavy solid line; n=16); patients which received 1 mg antibody/kg per dose (light solid line; n=9); patients which received 3 mg antibody/kg per dose (dashed line; n=7). Data are given as mean ± SD. Graphs on the right: 28 day survivors (light solid line); 28 day nonsurvivors (dashed line); mean of all patients (heavy solid line; n=20). (Reproduced with permission from: Boekstegers P, Weidenhöfer S, Zell R et al. Repeated admini stration of a F(ab')$_2$ fragment of an anti-tumor necrosis factor α monoclonal antibody in patients with severe sepsis: effects on the cardiovascular system and cytokine levels. Shock 1994; 1:237-245.)

With these findings in mind, it is fair to speculate that there might be no unique mediator cascade being responsible for cardiac as well as for vascular impairment in sepsis, probably necessitating different causal therapeutic approaches.

PERSPECTIVES

Treatment of septic cardiomyopathy has regained special interest in the context of the "pathological oxygen supply/demand in sepsis" discussion. In a recent trial,[35] attempts to increase cardiac index by dobutamine in severely ill, mostly septic patients, to a desired goal of 4.5 l/m² x min did not result in a better prognosis, but even led to a higher mortality. These data question a possible benefit of a symptomatic treatment with catecholamines of myocardial depression in sepsis beyond the level necessary to maintain a sufficiently high blood pressure. On the other hand, in the same trial all patients survived, in whom the cardiac index limit could be achieved solely by volume substitution. Therefore, accomplishing a high cardiac output in patients with sepsis might, in principle, be beneficial, but not at the cost of additionally stressing a severely damaged heart by catecholamines. An effective causal treatment of septic cardiomyopathy, based on a better understanding of the underlying pathophysiological mechanisms, might be preferable to achieve this goal than a symptomatic support with catecholamines.

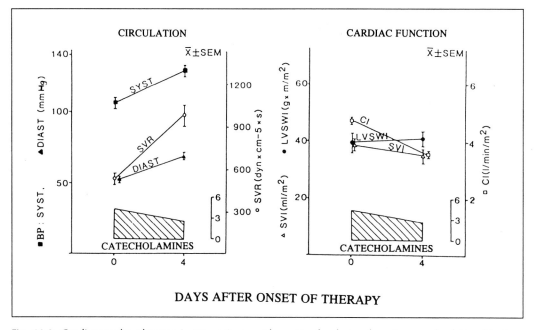

Fig. 10.2. Cardiovascular changes in 22 patients with septic shock, in close temporal relationship to a supplemental therapy with polyvalent immunoglobulin G on day 0 and 1. For further experimental details see text and ref. 6. SVR = systemic vascular resistance; CI = cardiac index; LVSWI = left ventricular stroke work index; SVI = stroke volume index.

QUESTIONNAIRE

Receive a FREE BOOK of your choice

Please help us out—Just answer the questions below, then select the book of your choice from the list on the back and return this card.

R.G. Landes Company publishes five book series: *Medical Intelligence Unit, Molecular Biology Intelligence Unit, Neuroscience Intelligence Unit, Tissue Engineering Intelligence Unit* and *Biotechnology Intelligence Unit.* We also publish comprehensive, shorter than book-length reports on well-circumscribed topics in molecular biology and medicine. The authors of our books and reports are acknowledged leaders in their fields and the topics are unique. Almost without exception, there are no other comprehensive publications on these topics.

Our goal is to publish material in important and rapidly changing areas of bioscience for sophisticated scientists. To achieve this goal, we have accelerated our publishing program to conform to the fast pace in which information grows in bioscience. Most of our books and reports are published within 90 to 120 days of receipt of the manuscript.

Please circle your response to the questions below.

1. We would like to sell our *books* to scientists and students at a deep discount. But we can only do this as part of a prepaid subscription program. The retail price range for our books is $59-$99. Would you pay $196 to select four *books* per year from any of our Intelligence Units–$49 per book–as part of a prepaid program?

    Yes   No

2. We would like to sell our *reports* to scientists and students at a deep discount. But we can only do this as part of a prepaid subscription program. The retail price range for our reports is $39-$59. Would you pay $145 to select five *reports* per year–$29 per report–as part of a prepaid program?

    Yes   No

3. Would you pay $39–the retail price range of our books is $59-$99–to receive any single book in our Intelligence Units if it is spiral bound, but in every other way identical to the more expensive hardcover version?

    Yes   No

To receive your free book, please fill out the shipping information below, select your free book choice from the list on the back of this survey and mail this card to:

R.G. Landes Company, 909 S. Pine Street, Georgetown, Texas 78626 U.S.A.

Your Name _____

Address _____

City _____ State/Province:_____

Country: _____ Postal Code:_____

My computer type is Macintosh_____ ; IBM-compatible _____ ; Other _____

Do you own ____ or plan to purchase ___ a CD-ROM drive?

Available Free Titles

☐ Water Channels
*Alan Verkman,
University of California-San Francisco*

☐ The Na,K-ATPase:
Structure-Function Relationship
J.-D. Horisberger, University of Lausanne

☐ Intrathymic Development of T Cells
*J. Nikolic-Zugic,
Memorial Sloan-Kettering Cancer Center*

☐ Cyclic GMP
Thomas Lincoln, University of Alabama

☐ Primordial VRM System and the Evolution
of Vertebrate Immunity
John Stewart, Institut Pasteur-Paris

☐ Thyroid Hormone Regulation
of Gene Expression
Graham R. Williams, University of Birmingham

☐ Mechanisms of Immunological Self Tolerance
*Guido Kroemer, CNRS Génétique Moléculaire et
Biologie du Développement-Villejuif*

☐ The Costimulatory Pathway
for T Cell Responses
Yang Liu, New York University

☐ Molecular Genetics of Drosophila Oogenesis
Paul F. Lasko, McGill University

☐ Mechanism of Steroid Hormone Regulation
of Gene Transcription
M.-J. Tsai & Bert W. O'Malley, Baylor University

☐ Liver Gene Expression
*François Tronche & Moshe Yaniv,
Institut Pasteur-Paris*

☐ RNA Polymerase III Transcription
R.J. White, University of Cambridge

☐ src Family of Tyrosine Kinases in Leukocytes
Tomas Mustelin, La Jolla Institute

☐ MHC Antigens and NK Cells
*Rafael Solana & Jose Peña,
University of Córdoba*

☐ Kinetic Modeling of Gene Expression
James L. Hargrove, University of Georgia

☐ PCR and the Analysis of the T Cell Receptor
Repertoire
*Jorge Oksenberg, Michael Panzara & Lawrence
Steinman, Stanford University*

☐ Myointimal Hyperplasia
Philip Dobrin, Loyola University

☐ Transgenic Mice as an In Vivo Model
of Self-Reactivity
*David Ferrick & Lisa DiMolfetto-Landon,
University of California-Davis and Pamela Ohashi,
Ontario Cancer Institute*

☐ Cytogenetics of Bone and Soft Tissue Tumors
*Avery A. Sandberg, Genetrix & Julia A. Bridge ,
University of Nebraska*

☐ The Th1-Th2 Paradigm and Transplantation
Robin Lowry, Emory University

☐ Phagocyte Production and Function Following
Thermal Injury
*Verlyn Peterson & Daniel R. Ambruso,
University of Colorado*

☐ Human T Lymphocyte Activation Deficiencies
*José Regueiro, Carlos Rodríguez-Gallego
and Antonio Arnaiz-Villena,
Hospital 12 de Octubre-Madrid*

☐ Monoclonal Antibody in Detection and
Treatment of Colon Cancer
Edward W. Martin, Jr., Ohio State University

☐ Enteric Physiology of the Transplanted Intestine
Michael Sarr & Nadey S. Hakim, Mayo Clinic

☐ Artificial Chordae in Mitral Valve Surgery
Claudio Zussa, S. Maria dei Battuti Hospital-Treviso

☐ Injury and Tumor Implantation
*Satya Murthy & Edward Scanlon,
Northwestern University*

☐ Support of the Acutely Failing Liver
A.A. Demetriou, Cedars-Sinai

☐ Reactive Metabolites of Oxygen and Nitrogen
in Biology and Medicine
Matthew Grisham, Louisiana State-Shreveport

☐ Biology of Lung Cancer
*Adi Gazdar & Paul Carbone,
Southwestern Medical Center*

☐ Quantitative Measurement
of Venous Incompetence
*Paul S. van Bemmelen, Southern Illinois University
and John J. Bergan, Scripps Memorial Hospital*

☐ Adhesion Molecules in Organ Transplants
Gustav Steinhoff, University of Kiel

☐ Purging in Bone Marrow Transplantation
*Subhash C. Gulati,
Memorial Sloan-Kettering Cancer Center*

☐ Trauma 2000: Strategies for the New Millennium
*David J. Dries & Richard L. Gamelli,
Loyola University*

REFERENCES

1. Conrad SA, Finkelstein JL, Madden MR et al. Cardiovascular dysfunction in multiple organ failure. In: Deitch EA, ed. Multiple Organ Failure, Pathophysiology and Basic Concepts of Therapy. New York: Thieme, 1990:172-191.

2. Groeneveld ABJ, Schneider AJ, Thijs LG. Cardiac alterations in septic shock: pathophysiology, diagnosis, prognostic and therapeutic implications. In: Vincent JL, ed. Update 1991 (Update in Intensive Care and Emergency Medicine 15). Berlin Heidelberg: Springer-Verlag, 1991:126-136.

3. Parrillo JE. Pathogenetic mechanisms of septic shock. N Engl J Med 1993; 328:1471-1477.

4. Vincent JL, Berlot G. Cardiac effects of the mediators of sepsis. In: Lamy M, LG Thijs LG, eds. Mediators of Sepsis (Update in Intensive Care and Emergency Medicine 16). Berlin, Heidelberg: Springer-Verlag, 1992:255-266.

5. Sibbald WJ, Vincent J-L, eds. Clinical Trials for the Treatment of Sepsis (Update in Intensive Care and Emergency Medicine 19). Berlin, Heidelberg: Springer 1995.

6. Werdan K. Therapie der akuten septischen Kardiomyopathie. In: Schuster H-P, ed. Intensivtherapie bei Sepsis und Multiorganversagen. Berlin Heidelberg: Springer-Verlag, 1993:164-197.

7. Parrillo JE. The cardiovascular pathophysiology of sepsis. Ann Rev Med 1989; 40:469-485.

8. Reithmann C, Werdan K. Noradrenaline-induced desensitization in cultured heart cells as a model for the defects of the adenylate cyclase system in severe heart failure. Naunyn-Schmiedeberg's Arch Pharmacol 1989; 339:138-144.

9. Reithmann C, Hallström S, Pilz G et al. Desensitization of rat cardiomyocyte adenylyl cyclase stimulation by plasma of noradrenaline-treated patients with septic shock. Circ Shock 1994; 41:48-59.

10. Reithmann C, Wieland F, Jakobs KH et al. Intrinsic sympathomimetic activity of β-adrenoceptor antagonists: Down-regulation of cardiac β_1- and β_2-adrenoceptors. Eur J Pharmacol 1989; 170:243-255.

11. Böhm M, Gierschik P, Jakobs KH et al. Increase of $G_{i\alpha}$ in human hearts with dilated but not in ischemic cardiomyopathy. Circulation 1990; 82:1249-1265.

12. Brown L, Lorenz B, Erdmann E. Reduced positive inotropic effects in diseased human ventricular myocardium. Cardiovasc Res 1986; 20: 516-520.

13. Jones SB, Romano FD. Myocardial beta adrenergic receptor coupling to adenylate cyclase during developmental septic shock. Circ Shock 1990; 30:51-60.

14. Unverferth DV, Blanford M, Kates RE et al. Tolerance to dobutamine after a 72 hour continuous infusion. Am J Med 1980; 69:262-266.

15. Gomez A, Wang R, Unruh H et al. Hemofiltration reverses left ventricular dysfunction during sepsis in dogs. Anesthesiology 1990; 73:671-685.

16. Bellomo R, Tipping P, Boyce N. Continuous veno-venous hemofiltration with dialysis removes cytokines from the circulation of septic patients. Crit Care Med 1993; 21:522-526. Letter: 1994; 22:715-716.

17. Tonnesen E, Hansen MB, Hohndorf K et al. Cytokines in plasma and ultrafiltrates during continuous arteriovenous haemofiltration. Anaesth Intensive Care 1993; 21:752-758.

18. Hallström S, Bernhart E, Müller U et al. A cardiodepressant factor (CDF) isolated from hemofiltrates of patients in septic and/or cardiogenic shock blocks calcium inward current in cardiomyocytes. Shock 1994; suppl. to Vol 2: abstract 1.

19. Vincent JL, Bakker J, Marecaux G et al. Administration of anti-TNF antibody improves left ventricular function in septic shock patients. Results of a pilot study. Chest 1992; 101:810-815.

20. Boekstegers P, Weidenhöfer S, Zell R et al. Repeated administration of a F(ab')$_2$ fragment of an anti-tumor necrosis factor α monoclonal antibody in patients with severe sepsis: effects on the cardiovascular system and cytokine levels. Shock 1994; 1:237-245.

21. Natanson CN, Hoffman WD, Suffredini AF et al. Selected treatment strategies for septic shock based on proposed mechanisms of pathogenesis. Ann Intern Med 1994; 120:771-783.

22. Quezado ZM, Natanson C, Alling DW et al. A controlled trial of HA-1A in a canine model of gram-negative septic shock. JAMA 1993; 269: 2221-2227.

23. Yao Z, Auchampach JA, Pieper GM et al. Cardioprotective effects of monophosphoryl lipid A, a novel endotoxin analog, in the dog. Cardiovasc Res 1993; 27:832-838.

24. Thiemermann C. The Role of the L-Arginine: Nitric Oxide Pathway in Circulatory Shock. Adv Pharmacol 1994; 28:45-79.

25. Kilbourn RG, Cromeens DM, Chelly FD et al. N^G-methyl-L-arginine, an inhibitor of nitric oxide formation, acts synergistically with dobutamine to improve cardiovascular performance in endotoxemic dogs. Crit Care Med 1994; 22:1835-1840.

26. Klabunde RE, Ritger RC. N^G-monomethyl-L-arginine (NMA) restores arterial blood pressure but reduces cardiac output in a canine model of endotoxic shock. Biochem Biophys Res Commun 1991; 178:1135-1140.

27. Statman R, Cheng W, Cunningham JN et al. Nitric oxide inhibition in the treatment of the sepsis syndrome is detrimental to tissue oxygenation. J Surg Res 1994; 57:93-98.

28. Petros A, Bennett D, Vallance P. Effect of nitric oxide synthase inhibitors on hypotension in patients with septic shock. Lancet 1991; 338:1557-1558.

29. Petros A, Lamb G, Leone A et al. Effects of a nitric oxide synthase inhibitor in humans with septic shock. Cardiovasc Res 1994; 28:34-39.

30. Schilling J, Cakmakci M, Bättig U et al. A new approach in the treatment of hypotension in human septic shock by N^G- monomethyl-L-arginine, an inhibitor of the nitric oxide synthase. Intensive Care Med 1993; 19:227-231.

31. Benyo Z, Kiss G, Szabo C et al. Importance of basal nitric oxide synthesis in regulation of myocardial blood flow. Cardiovasc Res 1991; 25:700-703.

32. Robertson FM, Offner PJ, Ciceri DP et al. Detrimental hemodynamic effects of nitric oxide synthase inhibition in septic shock. Arch Surg 1994; 129:149-156.

33. Natanson C, Reilly JM, Hoffman WD et al. Effect of septic shock on cardiovascular responses to dopamine (DA) and norepinephrine (NE) in a conscious canine model. Crit Care Med 1993; 21(Suppl):S 277.

34. Foulkes R, Shaw S. The cardiodepressant and vasodepressant effects of tumor necrosis factor in rat isolated atrial and aortic tissues. Br J Pharmacol 1992; 106:942-947.

35. Hayes MA, Timmins AC, Yau EHS et al. Elevation of systemic oxygen delivery in the treatment of critically ill patients. N Engl J Med 1994; 330:1717-1722.

CHAPTER 11

SYNOPSIS: HYPOTHETICAL VERSUS PROVEN MOLECULAR MECHANISMS OF SEPTIC CARDIOMYOPATHY IN HUMANS

With every year of intensive sepsis research the complexity of sepsis pathophysiology increases (Fig. 11.1), with the first concepts of a one-way toxin/mediator cascade turning more and more to an even much more complicated network of an inflammatory response syndrome as a redundant, highly integrated, self-regulating system of proinflammatory and counteracting anti-inflammatory responses including repair mechanisms.

How does this knowledge help us to better understand the molecular mechanisms of septic cardiomyopathy? At the present, we know a lot about probable candidates mediating this cardiodepression, and we also know a lot about the ways these candidates in principle could interfere with the contractility of the heart (see chapters 4 and 8). But where is the problem? The problem lies in the question of which place the individual toxin and/or mediator has in the various forms of microbial sepsis. Solving this problem is difficult enough in animal-sepsis-models, and it is even more difficult in septic patients.

What are the facts? We know that some substances can impair heart function in humans when given to volunteers or as treatment regimens mostly applied to cancer patients; as shown in the previous chapters 4, 8 and 9, this holds true for endotoxin, TNF-α, IL-2 and IFN (Table 11.1). Of course, this does not imply that these substances indeed play a role in septic cardiomyopathy in humans.

Nevertheless, we have at least some information concerning the pathophysiology of septic cardiomyopathy in humans: we know that the response of the heart to β-adrenoceptor agonists is diminished in patients with sepsis, arguing for a β-adrenoceptor desensitization under these circumstances.[1] Baseline hemodynamic values for mean arterial pressure, cardiac index, left ventricular stroke work index and oxygen delivery index at approximately 2 days after the onset of sepsis are significantly lower in septic shock patients compared with septic (nonshock) patients. Myocardial responsiveness to dobutamine was better in septic nonshock than shock patients. Dobutamine produced significantly greater increases in heart rate, cardiac index and left ventricular stroke work index in the septic patients compared with the septic shock patients. As an equivalent to a hyporesponsiveness of the β_2-adrenoceptor/adenylyl cyclase system, both the isoproterenol-stimulated (β_2-adrenoceptor-dependent) as well as the sodium fluoride-stimulated (acting on the nucleotide regulatory protein) cyclic adenosine monophosphate accumulation in lymphocytes were significantly reduced in septic shock patients compared with those accumulations observed in septic patients. The authors concluded that in patients with septic shock, impaired β-adrenergic receptor stimulation of cyclic adenosine monophosphate is associated with myocardial hyporesponsiveness to catecholamines, and that this β-adrenergic receptor dysfunction may contribute to the reduced myocardial performance observed in this shock state. Though these data point to the importance of catecholamine tolerance in sepsis and even more so in septic shock, methodological limitations are unavoidable.[2] It remains to be clarified whether this catecholamine desensitization is either due to a receptor defect based on the high endogenous catecholamine levels in sepsis, whether the phar-

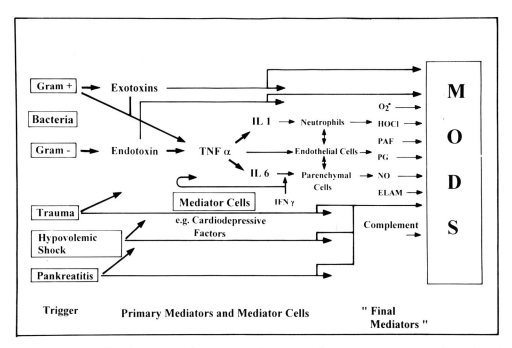

Fig. 11.1. Toxin and mediator networks in sepsis and systemic inflammatory response syndrome (SIRS).

macologically applied catecholamines are responsible for that,[3] or whether indeed a cytokine-mediated desensitization of the β-adrenoceptor/ G proteins/adenylyl cyclase system accounts for the attenuation of the catecholamine inotropy (see chapters 4 and 8). Also, the extrapolation of cAMP assays from lymphocytes to myocytes is inherently problematic.[2]

Despite all these possible limitations of Silverman's study,[1] further support for an impairment of a specific component of this signal transduction system in septic shock comes from another observation:[4] in patients having died from catecholamine-refractory septic shock or septic multiorgan failure an increase in myocardial inhibitory $G_{i\alpha}$ was observed (by 62% of immunological $G_{i\alpha}$, by 221% of pertussis toxin substrate). The increases were greater than those found in chronic heart failure reported earlier. Such an increase in the expression of $G_{i\alpha}$ could also play a pathophysiologically relevant role in catecholamine refractoriness in septic shock. One should, however, be aware that the reported increase in $G_{i\alpha}$ does not necessarily mean an attenuation of the catecholamine response; if not only the $G_{i\alpha}$, but also the Gβ subunit

---

Table 11.1. Substances proven to impair heart function in humans

Endotoxin

Tumor necrosis factor α

Interleukin-2

Interferon

For further explanation see text.

Table 11.2. Myocardial alterations probably contributing to septic cardiomyopathy in humans

Decreased responsiveness of the heart to β-adrenoceptor agonists

Increase in myocardial inhibitory $G_{i\alpha}$ proteins

TNF-α induced myocardial impairment: Improvement of reduced left ventricular stroke work index by anti-TNFα antibodies

Increased iNOS and increased myocardial levels of cGMP

CDF obtained from hemofiltrates of patients with septic shock: documented depression of calcium inward current in cardiomyocytes

"CDF" = Cardiodepressant factor, "$G_{i\alpha}$" = inhibitory guanine nucleotide binding protein—α subunit, "iNOS" = inducible nitric oxide synthase. For further explanation see text.

rises, as this is the case as a response of cardiomyocytes to TNF-α,[5] then no attenuation of the β-adrenoceptor-coupled adenylyl cyclase activity must result.[5] In the study of Böhm et al,[4] only $G_{i\alpha}$, but neither Gβ subunits of the G proteins nor adenylyl cyclase activity have been determined. Therefore, drawing functional consequences from these findings must be taken with caution.

There are also two publications reporting an improvement of heart function, as measured by left ventricular stroke work index, by anti-TNF-α antibodies in septic patients (see also chapter 10).[6,7] These findings argue for an involvement of TNF-α in the pathophysiology of septic cardiomyopathy, as could be suggested by the overwhelming evidence of experimental findings (see chapters 4 and 8).

Sparse, but very interesting data are also available concerning the NO/cGMP pathway in septic cardiomyopathy; as mentioned earlier, induction of iNOS and an increased content of cGMP have been found in hearts of patients with septic shock,[8] arguing for a relevant role of this pathway in septic cardiomyopathy. This assumption is further supported by the findings of an increased nitric production[9] as well as an increased cGMP output[10] in sepsis. It is further strengthened by an improvement of left ventricular stroke work index after application of methylene blue—a potent inhibitor of guanylyl cyclase—in patients with septic shock.[11]

There is only one clinical finding left documenting the presence of sufficient amounts of cardiodepressant factor (CDF) in patients with septic shock, with a clear-cut inhibition of calcium inward current. The degree of calcium current inhibition by CDF is sufficient to produce a negative inotropic effect (see also chapters 4 and 8).[12]

What is the state of the art concerning the molecular mechanisms of septic cardiomyopathy in 1995? We know a lot of toxins and mediators which are likely candidates of inducing septic cardiomyopathy. And we also know a lot of mechanisms which might bring about this cardiodepression. The real lack of evidence, however, is on the basis of which toxin(s) and/or mediator(s) to what degree are really involved in Gram-negative, in Gram-positive and in fungal septic cardiomyopathy. Hopefully, an answer to these burning questions, with hopefully therapeutical consequences, can be given in the near future. Understanding better the molecular mechanisms of septic cardiomyopathy will have a further benefit. Regarding the dominant role of cytokines playing in this special area, we will also learn a lot how cytokines affect heart function in health and disease in general. We, the authors, are convinced that the next years will document a much broader influence and importance of cytokines with respect to the heart than it is assumed today.

REFERENCES

1. Silverman HJ, Penaranda R, Orens JB et al. Impaired β-adrenergic receptor stimulation of cyclic adenosine monophosphate in human septic shock: Association with myocardial hyporesponsiveness to catecholamines. Crit Care Med 1993; 21:31-39.

2. Ognibene FP, Cunnion RE. Mechanisms of myocardial depression in sepsis. Crit Care Med 1993; 21:6-8.

3. Reithmann C, Hallström S, Pilz G et al. Desensitization of rat cardiomyocyte adenylyl cyclase stimulation by plasma of noradrenaline-treated patients with septic shock. Circ Shock 1993; 41:48-59.

4. Böhm M, Kirchmayr R, Gierschik P et al. Increase of myocardial inhibitory G-proteins in catecholamine-refractory septic shock or in septic multiorgan failure. Am J Med 1995; 98:183-186.

5. Reithmann C, Gierschik P, Werdan K et al. Tumor necrosis factor α up-regulates G_i and G_β proteins and adenylate cyclase responsiveness in rat cardiomyocytes. Eur J Pharmacol (Mol Pharmacol section) 1991; 206:53-60.

6. Vincent J-L, Bakker J, Marecaux G et al. Administration of anti-TNF antibody improves left ventricular function in septic shock patients. Results of a pilot study. Chest 1992; 101:810-815.

7. Boekstegers P, Weidenhöfer S, Zell R et al. Repeated administration of a $F(ab')_2$ fragment of an anti-tumor necrosis factor α monoclonal antibody in patients with severe sepsis: effects on the cardiovascular system and cytokine levels. Shock 1994; 1:237-245.

8. Thoenes M, Förstermann U, Rüdiger J et al. Expression of inducible nitric oxide synthase in failing and non-failing human heart. Naunyn-Schmiedeberg's Arch Pharmacol 1995; 351:R112.

9. Gomez-Jimenez J, Salgado A, Mourelle M et al. L-arginine: Nitric oxide pathway in endotoxemia and human septic shock. Crit Care Med 1995; 23:253-258.

10. Schneider F, Lutun Ph, Couchot A et al. Plasma cyclic guanosine 3'-5' monophosphate concentrations and low vascular resistance in human septic shock. Intensive Care Med 1993; 19:99-104.

11. Preiser J-C, Lejeune P, Roman A et al. Methylene blue administration in septic shock: A clinical trial. Crit Care Med 1995; 23:259-264.

12. Hallström S, Bernhart E, Müller U et al. A cardiodepressant factor (CDF) isolated from hemofiltrates of patients in septic and/or cardiogenic shock blocks calcium inward current in cardiomyocytes. Shock 1994; Suppl to Vol 2:abstract 1.

INDEX

Italics denote figures (f) or tables (t).

MOLECULAR BIOLOGY INTELLIGENCE UNIT

AVAILABLE AND UPCOMING TITLES

NEUROSCIENCE
INTELLIGENCE UNIT

AVAILABLE AND UPCOMING TITLES

MEDICAL INTELLIGENCE UNIT
AVAILABLE AND UPCOMING TITLES

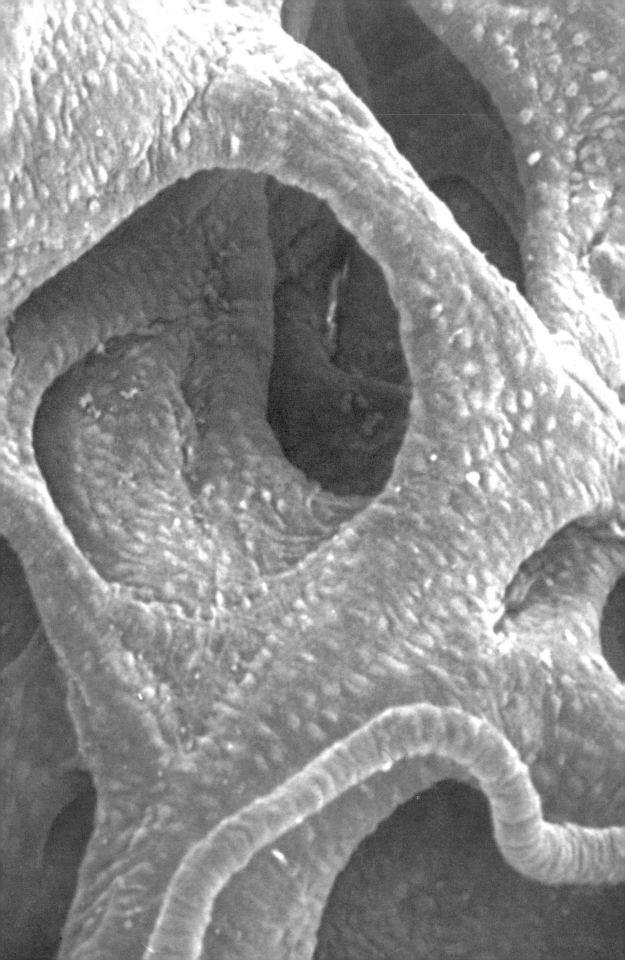